TRACKING MEDICINE

TRACKING
MEDICINE

A RESEARCHER'S QUEST TO
UNDERSTAND HEALTH CARE

JOHN E. WENNBERG

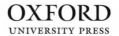

OXFORD

UNIVERSITY PRESS

2010

OXFORD
UNIVERSITY PRESS

Oxford University Press, Inc., publishes works that further
Oxford University's objective of excellence
in research, scholarship, and education.

Oxford   New York
Auckland   Cape Town   Dar es Salaam   Hong Kong   Karachi
Kuala Lumpur   Madrid   Melbourne   Mexico City   Nairobi
New Delhi   Shanghai   Taipei   Toronto

With offices in
Argentina   Austria   Brazil   Chile   Czech Republic   France   Greece
Guatemala   Hungary   Italy   Japan   Poland   Portugal   Singapore
South Korea   Switzerland   Thailand   Turkey   Ukraine   Vietnam

Published by Oxford University Press, Inc.
198 Madison Avenue, New York, New York 10016
www.oup.com

Library of Congress Cataloging-in-Publication Data
CIP data on file
ISBN 978-0-19-973178-7

3 5 7 9 8 6 4 2

Printed in the United States of America
on acid-free paper

For Corky and Emma

Foreword

New forms of knowledge with the power to reshape a major field of human practice emerge once in a generation. This book presents such a body of knowledge. It describes how, as a young physician and epidemiologist, Jack Wennberg first detected and worked to explain striking variations in the delivery of health care services among local areas in the United States. It shows how, over time, Wennberg and his colleagues harnessed these initial discoveries to build a scientific field for the study of practice variation and comparative effectiveness in health care. And it applies findings from this field to set an agenda for action to save our nation's beleaguered health system.

Wennberg's research rises above partisan divisions to provide an objective common ground for critical health policy decisions. It reminds us that health care reform must tackle more than the problem of insurance coverage. Reform efforts must also address performance variation in the delivery strategies that actually bring services to patients. This is the only way to engage the levers that truly drive health care costs and that shape the outcomes patients experience within our health care system. We can be certain that any reform effort that fails to incorporate Wennberg's insights will fall short of success. The good news from Washington is that Wennberg and his colleagues at The Dartmouth Institute for Health Policy and Clinical Practice have become pivotal references for increasing numbers of policy makers across the political spectrum.

The policy solutions Wennberg proposes will not gain easy acceptance. His recommendations imply a profound reconfiguration of health care delivery patterns from which some actors have profited handsomely. The story that Wennberg tells of the "birth and near death" of federal government support for comparative effectiveness research in the 1990s provides an object lesson. It reminds us that some interests will be threatened by resolute action to address unwarranted variation and the overuse of health care. But Wennberg's analyses also make clear how much the health care system, and our country as a whole, stand to gain from the measures he recommends. Equally important, Wennberg documents settings where, in local health care systems from New Hampshire to Minnesota to California, these transformations have already begun to happen, with major gains in efficiency and improved outcomes for patients.

Wennberg argues that health care reform should focus on four goals: (1) promoting organized local systems of care delivery that build on the best examples that currently exist; (2) fighting misuse of medical services by establishing shared decision making between patient and provider as the norm for choices on elective surgeries, tests, and other procedures; (3) strengthening the science of health delivery; and (4) constraining undisciplined growth in health care capacity that fuels the upward spiral in spending.

All four of these aims are critical. Together, they will give us a health care system that uses its resources much more efficiently, that will have a shot at reining in runaway health care costs, and that will improve outcomes for a large number of Americans who are not now receiving the high-quality care they deserve.

In my own view, it is the third of Wennberg's goals—strengthening the science of health care delivery—that has been the least clearly understood by policy makers and the general public, while it is in some respects the most fundamental. The task of improving health care delivery and putting effective delivery on a solid scientific foundation holds the key to all the other objectives. If we fail to attain this goal, we will miss the others, too. For too long, we have assumed that, to improve health care, it was enough to ensure the rapid development of new drugs and technologies. The scientific study of how these technologies are actually delivered to patients by providers, and how those delivery processes can be optimized, was given little or no importance. Witness the fact that students at our major medical schools, while they are rigorously drilled in molecular biology, receive no formal training in delivery science or management skills, or processes that would permit meaningful, informed patient participation in decision making.

Today's spiraling health care costs, for care that too often fails to yield value for patients, are the consequence of this neglect of the field of delivery. Recalling the initial promise of the national Agency for Health Care Policy and Research, briefly supported by the federal government in the late 1980s and early 1990s, Jack Wennberg makes the case for ensuring that a focus on delivery science is front and center in the rebuilding of our health care system that we know is unavoidable.

Recent health care reform debates have again highlighted the need to lay solid foundations for the young science of health care delivery in the United States. We need a national institute of health care delivery science that can support and sustain cutting-edge research on delivery problems. The creation of such an institution would be an opportunity to reestablish American leadership in a critical area of knowledge production. A national institute dedicated to health care delivery would provide the objective evidence needed to guide the ongoing reform and improvement of our health system that must and will unfold in the decades ahead.

The evidence Jack Wennberg distills from his own four decades at the forefront of practice variation research shows the direction we must follow. The future of our health care system and the well-being of our people will depend to a substantial degree on the energy and commitment with which Wennberg's recommendations are taken up by those in a position to shape public policy.

Jim Yong Kim, M.D., Ph.D.
President
Dartmouth College

Acknowledgments

My book is a record of a long intellectual journey to deal with fundamental contradictions in the patterns of medical practice. I have had the incredible good fortune to share this journey with many colleagues, friends, and family who have joined together in an effort to understand and seek remedy for unwarranted variation. Needless to say, but important to emphasize, this has been and remains a team effort.

Let me begin with the project that started it all—the uncovering of small area variations in Vermont. First and foremost, I want to acknowledge the contribution of Alan Gittelsohn, then professor of biostatistics at the Johns Hopkins School of Hygiene. Our collaboration set the stage for most of the research reported in this book. The project would not have been possible without the dedication and innovative work of John Senning, Pat Hickcox, Roger Gillam, David Herr, and Karen Provost; they formed the technical staff that made it possible to solve the numerous, first-of-a-kind tasks encountered in building and analyzing large databases using the primitive computers available at that time. I also want to recognize the contribution of Kerr White, who taught me the importance of using the tools of epidemiology to study the health care system, and of John Mazuzan, who, as assistant dean for regional affairs at the University of Vermont, supported my decision to use RMP funds to build the database and helped interpret its findings to the physicians of Vermont.

Our work in Maine was made possible by the firm commitment of professional leaders to address the unsettling implications of practice variation. I want to acknowledge the pivotal importance of two Maine physicians: Dan Hanley, who challenged Maine physicians to address the inconsistency in their practice patterns and undertake the research required to address scientific uncertainty; and Robert Keller, who kept the commitment alive when he succeeded Dan as director of the Maine Medical Assessment Foundation. Other practicing physicians in Maine who contributed time and energy to the feedback process are Buell Miller, Robert Timothy, Terrance Sheehan, John Adams, and Dennis Shubert. The Maine project also depended on the work of David Soule and John Putnam, who, working for Blue Cross of Maine, built the first Maine database, and Alice Chapin, David Smith, and Suanne Singer of the Maine Health Information Center, and Ellen Schneiter of the Maine Medical Assessment Foundation, who kept the database current and the feedback channels open.

Further development of the small area analysis methodology took place at Dartmouth when I moved there in 1979. For work in the 1980s and early 1990s, Loredo Sola, for his skill and wisdom in managing an ever expanding database in an environment of rapid change in computer technology and a tight budget, and Tom Bubolz for his special knowledge of hospital discharge databases and how to analyze them, need special recognition. The Dartmouth Atlas Project, which began in 1992, greatly expanded the size and complexity of the database. Jim Dykes undertook the required upgrade of our computer software and hardware systems. Megan Cooper came on board as the Atlas editor. In 1990, I had the good fortune to hire Sally Sharp, who had years of experience with claims data. Soon after, Kristy Bronner, a recent Dartmouth graduate, and Stephanie Raymond joined the staff, followed by Zhao Peng, Jia Lan, Dongmei Wang, Phyllis Wright-Slaughter, and Dean Stanley. These folks, the core of the Atlas Project production team, are still on the job today. Special thanks also go to Vin Fusca for providing project management for the Dartmouth Atlas. Without the team's problem-solving skills, corporate memories, and commitment to the goals of the Atlas Project, I am sure we would have lost the war to make sense out of the national Medicare database. Faculty members who have contributed as coauthors of the Dartmouth Atlas series include Elliott Fisher, Alan Gittelsohn, David Goodman, Jonathan Skinner, and Therese Stukel. Special editions of the Dartmouth Atlas were authored by John Birkmeyer, Jack Cronenwett, and David Wennberg.

I need to acknowledge and thank several individuals for their efforts to establish the Foundation of Informed Medical Decision Making: Al Mulley, the cofounder of the foundation; Lyn Hutton, treasurer of Dartmouth College, and Adam Keller, chief financial officer for the medical school, who persuaded the college to make a critical investment that saved the foundation during its start-up phase; Bob Derzon, the first chairman of the board; my colleagues who have served as president of the Foundation: John Billings, Joe Kasper, David Jensen, Jack Fowler, and Mike Barry; and Joe Henderson and Gary Schwitzer, who made major contributions to the design and production of the interactive patient decision aids in the early days of the foundation. Since 1997, because of the success of its commercial partner, Health Dialog, in developing a business model to support shared decision making, the foundation has been on firm financial ground. For this, my thanks go to Health Dialog's founders, George Bennett and Chris McKown; its CEO, Pat Flynn; and my son, David Wennberg, president of Health Dialog Analytics. I am particularly pleased that the Dartmouth-Hitchcock Medical Center can claim to be the first medical center in the United States to implement shared decision making in the routine management of patient care. Among others, thanks for this go to Jim Weinstein, Dale Collins, Kate Clay, Ann Flood, Hilary Llewellyn-Thomas, Annette O'Connor, Blair Brooks, and Nan Cochran.

I am completely in the debt of my colleagues and fellow faculty members who have played major roles in sustaining the intellectual effort to come to terms with practice variation. Several came from outside the walls of Dartmouth, beginning with Alan Gittelsohn. Jack Fowler, whom I first met in 1970, is part of many research stories reported in this book, as is Klim McPherson, whom I met in 1977. I first met Al Mulley in 1983 when he attended a seminar at Dartmouth on practice variations; not long after, Jack, Al, and Mike Barry joined the Maine project to form the nucleus of the research team that would eventually become the Patient Outcomes Research Team (PORT) for prostate disease, which I discuss in Chapters 6 and 7. We have continued to collaborate ever since.

While the history of practice variation research at Dartmouth may have officially begun in 1979 with my recruitment to the faculty by Jim Strickler, dean of the Medical School and Mike Zubkoff, chairman of the Department of Community Medicine, the story really began when Elliott Fisher joined us in 1986, followed in 1990 by Gil Welch, David Goodman (1991), Therese Stukel (1994), and Julie Bynum (2003). In 1995, our research team gained strength when Jonathan Skinner joined the Department of Economics and became an active member of the research team; subsequently, Jon recruited Doug Staiger (1998), Katherine Baicker (1998), and Amitabh Chandra (2000), to the Department of Economics, all of whom have made important contributions to Dartmouth research into practice variation and continue to do so, although some have been recruited elsewhere.

I want to thank and acknowledge those who played an important role in establishing "TDI"—The Dartmouth Institute for Health Policy and Clinical Practice. As leaders of Harvard's Center for the Analysis of Health Practices, Howard Hiatt, Howard Frazier, John Bunker, Benjamin Barnes, and Fred Mosteller were instrumental in showing how the evaluative sciences can be organized to study health care. Dartmouth Medical School's Dean Robert McCollum, Associate Dean Bill Culp, and Mike Zubkoff receive my thanks for their support in establishing in 1988 the Center for the Evaluative Clinical Sciences (now called TDI) as "home base" for research on the science of health care delivery. In addition to faculty members whose work has focused primarily on practice variations and shared decision making, it is important to acknowledge the contributions to the intellectual environment and research productivity of TDI by Paul Batalden, Bill Black, David Malenka, Gerry O'Connor, Rosemary Orgren, Lisa Schwartz, John Wasson, and Steve Woloshin. My thanks and appreciation go to Jim Weinstein for assuming the directorship of TDI when I stepped down in July 2007.

I also want to thank John Iglehart, founding editor of *Health Affairs*, and Uwe Reinhardt, James Madison Professor of Political Economy and Professor of Economics and Public Affairs at Princeton University's Woodrow Wilson School of Public & International Affairs, for their friendship and encouragement that has helped me to sustain a focus on practice variation over the years.

The research and efforts to reform medical practice reported in this book would not have happened were it not for the support of a number of charitable foundations. The early stage of the Maine project was funded by the Commonwealth Foundation. For more than ten years, thanks to the personal attention of John Billings and Richard Sharpe, the Hartford Foundation provided the support that sustained the prostate research discussed in Chapter 6, including the development of the decision aid. Beginning in 1992, the Robert Wood Johnson Foundation, thanks to the interest of Steve Schroeder and Jim Knickman, has sustained the Dartmouth Atlas Project, and more recently, the United Health Foundation, WellPoint Foundation, California HealthCare Foundation, and Aetna, Inc. have joined RWJF in providing support for the Atlas research. Our work has also received funding from the Foundation for Informed Medical Decision Making, the National Institutes of Health, and the Agency for Health Care Policy and Research. Over the years, our research programs have also received generous support from a number of donors who support the TDI mission, including George Bennett,

Bob Derzon, Ross and Eve Jaffe, Dick and Sue Levy, Gordon Russell, and the Thomson Family, whose generous gift established the Peggy Y. Thomson Chair in the Evaluative Sciences, of which I was privileged to be the first occupant.

A number of colleagues and friends generously took time to read parts or all of earlier versions this book. I want to thank Mike Barry, Don Berwick, Catherine Coles, David Durenberger, Jack Fowler, Ben Moulton, Fitzhugh Mullan, Jonathan Skinner, Lisa Schwartz, and Steve Woloshin for their extremely helpful suggestions. Special thanks go to Jim Kim, president of Dartmouth College, for contributing the foreword. I would also like to thank Martha Smith for her splendid administrative support in putting this manuscript together (many times), and Jonathan Sa'adah and Beth Adams for preparing the figures and tables. My thanks go also to Oxford University Press: to my editor Regan Hofmann, production editor Rachel Mayer, Soniya Ashok and the Newgen team, and to Geronna Lyte and Mark LaRiviere for the cover design.

I want to express my special appreciation to Shannon Brownlee, who has been a constant mentor in the writing of this book. Shannon interviewed me while writing *Overtreated*, which the New York Times named the number one economics book of the year in 2007. The book does a terrific job of explaining the practice variation to the general public. It was my lucky day when she agreed to help me make the complicated and interconnected body of research discussed in this book accessible to a broad audience. We worked as a team to bring this book to closure and the book would not have been completed without her. For her skill, commitment, perseverance, good humor, and support I am grateful, almost beyond words.

Finally, my wife, family, and our dear friend Sally Smith supported, encouraged, and just plain put up with me over the years it took to write this book.

Contents

A study of the history of opinion is a necessary preliminary to the emancipation of the mind.

John Maynard Keynes

It is difficult to get a man to understand something when his salary depends on him not understanding it.

Upton Sinclair

PART I

*An Introduction to the Problem of
Unwarranted Variation*

I

In Health Care, Geography Is Destiny

Early in my career, I was hired as director of a federally sponsored program whose goal was to ensure that all Vermonters had access to recent advances in the treatment of heart disease, cancers, and stroke. As part of the program, my colleagues and I developed a data system that we thought would help us identify which Vermont communities were underserved, and thus in need of the program's help. As the results came in, however, rather than evidence for underuse (i.e., patients not getting care they needed), we found extensive and seemingly inexplicable variation in the way health care was delivered from one Vermont community to another. In Stowe, for example, the rate of tonsillectomy was such that by age 15, about 60% of children were without tonsils, while in the bordering town of Waterbury, only 20% had undergone the surgery by that age. Among communities, the chances that a woman would have her uterus surgically removed varied by more than fourfold, and the rate of gallbladder surgery varied by more than threefold. Rates of hospitalizations for a host of different medical conditions also varied in ways that made little sense; on a per capita basis, patients were hospitalized in Randolph two times more often for digestive disease than in Middlebury and three times more often for respiratory disease.

These are just a few examples of the chaotic patterns of utilization and practice our data uncovered—variations that challenged the very premise of the program I had been hired to direct. The rates of hospitalization and surgery appeared to be unrelated to illness or other patient-based factors, and thus the variation was at odds with the conventional wisdom that medicine was driven by science and by an understanding of patient desires and preferences. The data also challenged the assumption that the supply of medical resources and the capacity of the health care system were regulated either by a central professional consensus on the need for medical care, and its effectiveness, or by the invisible hand of the market. It became clear that the amount of care Vermonters received depended on where they lived and on the physicians and hospitals they used.

Over the years since that time, my colleagues and I have pursued the study of practice variation in many places, using a variety of methods, and the Vermont findings have been widely confirmed. Unwarranted variation in health care delivery—variation that cannot be explained on the basis of illness, medical evidence, or patient preference—is ubiquitous. Moreover, as I argue in this book, an understanding of the causes of unwarranted variation has important and sometimes surprising implications for today's debate over health care reform. Most analysts of health care reform expect huge increases in spending once the uninsured gain coverage and begin to consume more health care services. But the understanding I have gained from the study of the practice variation phenomenon provides a counterintuitive, maybe even shocking, prediction: given the important role that the supply of resources plays in determining utilization of medical care, increasing the insured population will have a much smaller impact on the trend in overall health care costs than estimated, provided that the capacity of the health care system is not increased.

Another prediction that emerges from an understanding of practice variation is that controlling costs will not necessarily require rationing—if by "rationing" we mean the withholding of care that patients want, and that is effective in improving outcomes. The studies reviewed in this book show that much of health care is of questionable value and that informed patients often prefer a form of treatment other than the one their physicians actually prescribe. Indeed, when offered a clear explanation of the treatment options, informed patients often choose the less invasive treatment, resulting in a decline in the use of elective surgery and certain cancer screening tests. Moreover, more care is not necessarily better, at least when it comes to managing chronic illness. Care coordination and intelligent management of patients over the course of their illness, which typically lasts until death, count far more than simply providing more medical services. Some of our most respected health care providers—for example, the Mayo Clinic, the Geisinger Clinic, and the Cleveland Clinic—provide high-quality care at a much lower per capita cost than most other providers. If the rest of the nation were equally efficient, we could shave 30% to 40% off the cost of caring for Medicare's chronically ill patients.

If, as I recommend in this book, health care reform concentrates on four goals, the quality and value of care will increase and growth in health care costs will likely decrease. Those goals are as follows:

1. Promoting organized systems of health care delivery
2. Establishing informed patient choice as the ethical and legal standard for decisions surrounding elective surgeries, drugs, tests, and procedures, and care at the end of life
3. Improving the science of health care delivery
4. Constraining undisciplined growth in health care capacity and spending

These are strong conclusions, ones that policy makers should not ignore given today's economic realities. They are supported by a growing body of evidence drawn from practice variation studies and from interventions to improve the scientific basis of clinical decision making and promote informed patient choice. An important goal of this book is to make this complicated and interconnected body of research accessible to a broad audience, including policy makers, health care providers, students, patient advocates, and, I hope, patients and families.

Epidemiology of Medical Care

My understanding of practice variation is based primarily on evidence from "medical care epidemiology," studies that use routinely collected data (primarily from insurance claims) to conduct what we have dubbed "small area analysis of health care delivery." An important feature of the small area methodology is that it is *population-based:* it studies the use of health care services among populations living within the geographic boundaries of "natural" health care markets. Our Vermont studies were extended to Maine and eventually replicated throughout New England and in Iowa. In the early 1990s, anticipating that the Clinton health plan and its provision for regulating health care at the regional level would become law, the Robert Wood Johnson Foundation provided us with the funds to use claims data from the Medicare program to develop a body of data that would provide feedback to both Medicare administrators and providers, and a means of bringing practice variations to the attention of those who would implement reform. By the time it became clear that the Clinton plan had failed, we had completed much of the research but had lost our primary customers.

The failure of the Clinton plan led to the establishment of the Dartmouth Atlas Project. Rather than use the remaining funds solely for research, Dr. Steven Schroeder, then president of the Robert Wood Johnson Foundation, and James Knickman, its vice president, encouraged us to stick to the plan to provide feedback but to target a wider audience, in the hope that information on local and regional practice variation would focus attention on the need to reduce it. With support from several foundations, we have continued to analyze the care delivered to Medicare enrollees and have made the results available on the Dartmouth Atlas website (www.dartmouthatlas.org). Most of our published reports (and much of the data I use in this book) compare the geographic practice patterns among the Medicare enrollees living in 1 of 306 hospital referral regions (Box 1.1).

Box 1.1. *The Geography of Health Care in the United States*

The use of health care resources in the United States is highly localized. Most Americans use the services of physicians whose practices are nearby. Physicians, in turn, are usually affiliated with hospitals that are near their practices. As a result, when patients are admitted to hospitals, the admission generally takes place within a relatively short distance of where the patient lives. This is true across the United States. Although the distances from homes to hospitals vary with geography—people who live in rural areas travel farther than those who live in cities—in general, most patients are admitted to a hospital close to where they live to obtain an appropriate level of care.

The Medicare program maintains exhaustive records of hospitalizations, which makes it possible to trace the patterns of use of hospital care. (Research shows that the pattern of use by patients in the Medicare program is more or less similar to that of younger patients.) In the Dartmouth Atlas Project, 3,436 geographically distinct hospital service areas in the United States were defined. In each hospital service area, most of the care received by Medicare patients is provided in hospitals within the area. Based on the patterns of care for major cardiovascular surgery and neurosurgery (which are generally provided at tertiary care hospitals), hospital service areas were aggregated into 306 hospital referral regions. (Details on how hospital service areas and referral regions are defined are given in the Appendix, and maps showing their location are available in the Methods section of the 1999 Dartmouth Atlas.[1])

It is important for the reader to keep in mind that the comparisons are *population-based*. We look at what happens to groups of patients, not individuals, and we compare what happens to those groups living in different parts of the United States. In calculating the numerator for a population-based rate, all medical services are counted, *regardless of where in the United States care was obtained*. For example, if a resident of the Fort Meyers region goes to a hospital located in the Miami region to get surgery, the procedure is counted as a service delivered to the population living in Fort Meyers. Looking at populations in this way allows us to document large differences in the way care is delivered by different health care providers, but it also offers individuals a way to understand what might happen to them, depending on where they live and where they go to get their care. In making population-based comparisons—whether among regions or populations loyal to a given hospital—the rates are adjusted for differences in important characteristics of the population that influence the use of health care, such as age, gender, race/ethnicity, and, when possible or appropriate, type and severity of illness. For details on the methods used in this book, please consult the Appendix.

One of the more powerful and inescapable conclusions that has emerged from our research is that physician behavior is behind much of the variation. I do not mean that all, or even most, physicians are cynically rubbing their hands together every time a patient walks in the door, thinking of ways to deliver more care, and thus make more money. On the contrary, most physicians are simply trying to do the best job they can to care for patients. Nonetheless, physicians practice in a particular context—in a local market with its own complement of health resources, including the supply of hospital beds and physicians. It is physicians who exert the greatest influence over demand—or really, utilization—because patients traditionally delegate

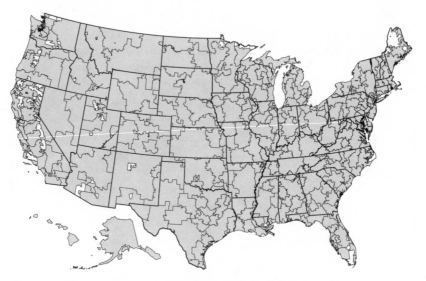

Figure 1.1. The 306 Dartmouth Atlas Hospital Referral Regions.

decision making to them under the assumption that doctors know what is best. Physicians thus control the majority of decisions made in medicine, most of which do not necessarily put money in the physician's pocket. The most costly decisions are those governing the use of acute care hospitals.

Categories of Care

My understanding of the role that physicians play in influencing demand has been greatly facilitated by the realization that the causes and the remedies for unwarranted variation differ according to three categories of care: effective or necessary care, preference-sensitive care, and supply-sensitive care. Until very recently, policy makers have concentrated almost exclusively on what I call the "*effective care*" or "*necessary care*" category—services that, on the basis of reasonably sound medical evidence, are known to work better than any alternative, and for which the benefits of treatment far exceed the side effects or unintended consequences. In other words, effective care includes any treatment that all eligible patients should receive. Demand for effective care is defined and limited by medical science—by objective information, "high-quality" information about the outcomes of treatment and evidence-based clinical guidelines that identify which patients stand to benefit.

For effective care, the problem is underuse—the failure to provide care for patients who should, but did not, get the required treatment. Examples of underuse include failure to provide immunizations to young children or lifesaving drugs to patients with heart attacks. Efforts by policy makers to increase the use of such effective care include monitoring of performance, publication of quality reports on the Internet (such as Medicare's Hospital Compare! Website), and Medicare's Pay for Performance program, which rewards providers who achieve high rates of use of effective care and penalizes those who achieve low quality scores.

Although it is important to reduce underuse, it does not account for much of the overall variation in Medicare spending. Even when one includes the inpatient costs for conditions and treatments for which there is no alternative to hospitalization (e.g., hip fractures and surgery for colon cancer), spending for effective care seems to account for no more than about 15% of total Medicare spending. Ironically, our research shows that greater supply of physicians and greater total Medicare per capita spending are not associated with less underuse of effective care.

A second category of care that varies is elective, or "preference-sensitive" care, interventions for which there is more than one option and where the outcomes will differ according to the option used. This category, which accounts for about 25% of Medicare spending, includes elective surgery, for example, and such cancer screening tests as mammography and the prostate specific antigen test. The treatment of early-stage breast cancer provides a good example of preference-sensitive surgery. For most patients, the options include lumpectomy, or local excision of the cancer, and mastectomy, the complete removal of the breast. The two are equivalent in terms of impact on reducing mortality but have very different impacts on the quality of life; thus, the decision as to which treatment is right for the individual patient should depend on the patient's preference. But for reasons described in this book, because patients delegate decision making to doctors, *physician opinion* rather than *patient preference* often determines which treatment patients receive. I argue that this can result in a serious but commonly overlooked medical error: operating on the wrong patients—on those who, were they fully informed, would not have wanted the operation they received. Figure 1.2 is a graphic representation of the various forces I will discuss in this book that come into play for preference-sensitive care when patients delegate decision making to their physicians.

Finding a remedy for unwarranted variation in preference-sensitive care requires a concentrated, ongoing effort to reduce scientific uncertainty about the outcomes of various treatments. But evidence-based medicine is only

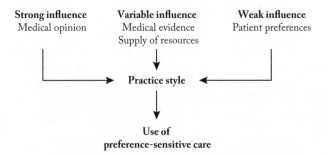

Figure 1.2.   A model of preference-sensitive care under delegated decision making.

part of the answer. The more fundamental reform must involve a shift in the culture of medicine—a change in the doctor-patient relationship that reduces the influence of medical opinion and enhances the role of patient preferences in determining the utilization of preference-sensitive care. This democratization of the doctor-patient relationship requires replacing delegated decision making, and the doctrine of informed consent, with shared decision making and informed patient choice. My book will argue that establishing evidence-based medicine and informed patient choice are feasible as well as necessary goals for health reform.

The third category of care is what we have come to call "supply-sensitive care." It differs in fundamental ways from both effective care and preference-sensitive care. Supply-sensitive care is not about a specific treatment per se; rather, it is about the frequency with which everyday medical care is used in treating patients with acute and chronic illnesses. Here I am talking about physician visits; referrals for a consultation, home health care, and imaging exams; and admissions to hospitals, intensive care units (ICUs), and skilled nursing homes. The physicians whose decisions determine the frequency of such care are not usually surgeons—they are mostly primary care physicians and medical specialists.

This category, which accounts for roughly 60% of Medicare spending, may be difficult to grasp because it runs counter to the widespread belief that medical interventions are driven by explicit medical theories and scientific evidence. Most of us, including most doctors, believe that a physician makes decisions such as when to schedule a patient with diabetes for a follow-up visit, for example, or when to hospitalize a patient with chronic heart failure, or when to call in an infectious disease specialist for a patient with a fever, on the basis of medical science, augmented by some combination of experience and wisdom. As it turns out, medical science is virtually silent on such matters.

There is another factor that influences such decisions. As Figure 1.3 illustrates and the book will demonstrate, physician decisions regarding supply-sensitive care are strongly influenced by the capacity of the local medical market—the per capita numbers of primary care physicians, medical specialists, and hospital or ICU beds, for example. (In the jargon of economics, the market is in disequilibrium—supply pushes demand or utilization.) This may seem deeply counterintuitive, and the effect of supply on professional behavior by and large goes unrecognized by physicians, who are unaware of the effect that capacity has on their decisions. But in the absence of a constraining professional consensus on best practices, and under the cultural assumption that more care is better care, available resources are used up to the point of their exhaustion. Moreover, patients who live in regions of the country where per capita supply of resources is high have no way of knowing that they are destined to spend more days in the ICU, for example, days that they probably would not have spent had they lived in a region of the country where the per capita supply of ICU beds was less.

Remedying variation in supply-sensitive care requires coming to terms with the "more care is better" assumption. Are physician services and hospitals in high-cost, high-use regions overused? Or is valuable care being rationed in regions with low rates of use, even though physicians and their patients are unaware of it? Beginning with the early studies in Vermont, extended to comparisons between Boston and New Haven, and now accomplished on a national scale as part of the Dartmouth Atlas Project, our studies consistently show that more care is not necessarily better.

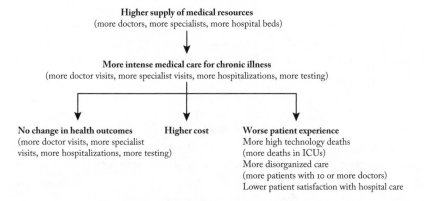

Figure 1.3.   A model of supply-sensitive medical care.

Finding a remedy for unwarranted variations in supply-sensitive care requires improving the science of health care delivery—converting the "black box" of supply-sensitive care into evidence-based care that is effective or preference-sensitive, thus reducing the power that capacity exerts on use. As this book will argue, this is particularly important for patients with severe chronic illness, whose care today is primarily driven by local capacity of the delivery system, not by the wishes of patients and their families, particularly during the last two years of life. Reducing the overuse of supply-sensitive care will also require organized systems of delivery, capable of managing the care of a population of chronically ill patients over time and across locations of care, and adjusting capacity to reflect medical evidence and patient preferences. The good news for the health care economy is that, compared with most providers, organized systems of delivery are relatively efficient. They use fewer resources (and spend less) in serving their chronically ill patients and, by available measures, achieve high-quality care and satisfied patients. The bad news is that the United States does not have enough of them. My book will argue that conducting the necessary research and promoting the growth of organized systems are necessary goals for health reform.

I have organized this book to highlight the importance of, first, preference-sensitive care and, then, supply-sensitive care, which together make up about 85% of Medicare spending. The following chapter tells the story of my first encounter with practice variation in Vermont and how the extent and magnitude of the variations we uncovered challenged me to reconsider some basic assumptions about how health care markets worked. Chapters 3 through 7 are devoted to unwarranted surgical variation, to understanding the patterns of variation, the role of medical opinion as a cause of variation, the role that supply of resources sometimes plays in decisions about preference-sensitive treatments, the importance of reforming the doctor-patient relationship to ensure that patient preferences play a part in determining when surgery is necessary, and to a report on the research project we undertook to learn how well surgical treatments work and to help patients make decisions on the treatment they want. I argue that this project, undertaken over more than ten years, provides a cogent model for how the science of health care delivery can reduce uncertainty, clarify the importance of patient preferences and address significant flaws in the market for health care services.

Chapters 8 through 12 are dedicated to understanding supply-sensitive care. I review the effect that supply exerts on care intensity—the frequency of hospitalization, for example—for those with chronic illness and the evidence that greater care intensity is not driven by differences in illness and that greater intensity is not producing better outcomes, and I make estimates of the waste from the overuse of supply-sensitive services. Even academic medical centers, "America's Best Hospitals," are shown to vary widely in their treatment patterns, much like other hospitals. However, organized systems of care—multispecialty group practices and integrated hospital systems—are generally more efficient: compared with most providers in the United States, they use fewer resources to deliver equal, often higher-quality care. When we use the per capita resources of organized care systems as benchmarks for the rest of the country, I see a glimmer of hope with regard to controlling health care spending. The efficiency achieved by these organized practices suggests that the nation already has more than enough resources and spends more than enough to care for all Americans, provided we can "reengineer," or transform, the rest of the system so that it looks more like those of organized group practices and less like the disorganized, fragmented, inefficient delivery nonsystem that currently exists.

Chapters 13 through 15 focus on the four goals of health care reform that I have set. I suggest strategies for improving the science of health care delivery, promoting the growth of organized systems of care, and establishing informed patient choice as a standard of care. But I want to be clear. While we urgently need to reform the health care delivery system, the nation cannot depend on the reengineering of clinical practice as the primary strategy for achieving the fourth goal: constraining undisciplined growth in capacity and out-of-control expansion in health care spending. Reducing unwarranted variations requires a painful transition from today's chaotic, disorganized care to systems of organized care and a cultural change from patient dependency on the authority of the physician to the democratization of the doctor-patient relationship. How long this will take simply cannot be predicted, but it will likely take years before these reforms can be expected to play a significant role in controlling the growth of costs. In the meantime, unless specific steps are taken to counter the dynamics of growth, the health care spending bubble will continue to expand, further threatening the national economy and limiting our options for designing our future. It is up to policy makers to take the necessary steps. In Chapter 15, I outline five steps that can be taken to place limits on capacity and spending, and buy time for reform to take hold.

* * *

The final chapter is a summing up of the challenges we face. An Epilogue looks at the prospects that federal legislation will advance my goals for health care reform.

2

The Vermont Experience

In 1967, fresh out of my medical training, I took a job as director of Vermont's Regional Medical Program (RMP). Sponsored by the National Institutes of Health as part of President Johnson's vision of the "Great Society," the RMPs were intended to ensure that the miracles of modern medicine were available to all Americans. Advances in biomedical theory and technology had improved the outcomes of such major diseases as cancer, stroke, and heart disease, and health policy makers in Washington, D.C., worried that only those fortunate enough to live near an academic medical center had access to these advances. In the wake of Medicare's passage in 1965, the RMPs were supposed to provide the roadmap to reform U.S. health care and ensure the timely diffusion of innovative and high-quality care based on the latest medical science.

As a young physician at Johns Hopkins Medical Center, in Baltimore, Maryland, I had witnessed the power of some of the most spectacular technologic developments of the postwar decades, including chemotherapy for cancer, open-heart surgery, kidney dialysis, and coronary intensive care. I thus came to my new job in Vermont with a good deal of enthusiasm for the goal of the RMP—to improve the diffusion of new breakthroughs in health care technology. But during my time at Johns Hopkins, I had taken two sidesteps in my education that were to prove critical to the discoveries that would soon emerge in Vermont. I had earned a degree in epidemiology, learning the methods of evaluating medical evidence and measuring events in populations. Epidemiologists are interested in what happens to *groups* of people, as opposed to individual patients. For example, an epidemiologist would look at how many people get heart attacks (*incidence*) and what happens to patients (*outcomes*), according to the natural history of the disease or the treatment they receive. It therefore seemed quite natural, once I arrived in Vermont, to make the health care system itself the object of study, to develop a "medical care epidemiology" capable of measuring the distribution of health care resources and the utilization of services in the state. My motive came out of my belief that improving the health of the state's citizens required measuring current resources and use of care in different communities to guarantee that underserved areas got the necessary medical resources. But, as I was to learn, medical care epidemiology also proved to be a useful tool to facilitate understanding the nature of the health care economy itself.

I also came to Vermont as a student of social systems. While at Johns Hopkins, I was also enrolled in a doctoral program in sociology, which gave me a broad introduction to social theory through readings of the works of Max Weber and Talcott Parsons, for example, and through course work with Professor Arthur Stinchcombe. This exposure helped me view health care as a complex social system, one serving the purposes and needs of many players, not just patients, and to consider a wider set of behavioral explanations for the striking variations in health care utilization my colleagues and I would uncover in Vermont. My days as a doctoral student in sociology also gave me the opportunity to learn from James S. Coleman, a master in the application of quantitative methodologies, whose influential book, *Introduction to Mathematical Sociology*, was required reading for students of the field.[1] Coleman's example inspired me to seek opportunities to test empirically not only the many assumptions concerning how our health care system works but also the proposals for reforming it.

Two lucky breaks made it possible to undertake the studies that would turn out to define the direction of my life's work. First, I had the resources to conduct the studies. As a young investigator without a track record, there was not the slightest chance that I could have obtained grant funds to undertake a research project of the magnitude required to evaluate the performance of a state's health care system. As director of the RMP, however, I could allocate the money needed to build the information system out of my regional planning budget.

The second stroke of luck was that I landed in Vermont, a state tailor-made for uncovering geographic variations. For one thing, the state's population was remarkably homogeneous in terms of race and socioeconomics, two important demographic factors related to a population's health, and therefore the population's need for care. For another, the citizens of individual towns in the state generally received the majority of their care from one hospital and one set of physicians, making it easier to see differences in the care that was being delivered than it might have been in urban areas with multiple hospitals. Finally, the hospital data that would serve as an important component of my research were already in place in most Vermont hospitals. A population-based health information database requires collecting and pooling information from all of the usual sources of care for the target population—the hospital, nursing home, and physicians' offices. And pooling data demands uniform definitions of care and uniformity in coding and collection. No such database existed in the United States until 1955, when the Commission on Professional and Hospital Activities called for the infrastructure to collect and analyze hospital discharge data. Kerr White, widely acknowledged as the father of health services research, had worked at the University of Vermont in the years preceding his appointment as the first professor of health services research at Johns Hopkins. He had persuaded most hospitals in Vermont to subscribe to the commission's database service. During my student days at Johns Hopkins, I had the good fortune of learning many things from him, including his vision of routinely collecting population-based data to understand the health care system. Without his foresight, we could not have developed the Vermont health information database.

The database was designed to include all of the care Vermonters received at their usual places of care. It recorded care for patients no matter where they received it—whether at their local hospital or at a hospital outside of their own community, it all was counted. Data sets from hospitals that did not subscribe to the commission's database were gathered by sending our staff into the hospitals to comb through their records. The database was also designed to obtain information on the full spectrum of care received by Vermonters. Protocols were developed for abstracting home health agency and nursing home utilization, and the needed data were obtained from all locations routinely used by Vermonters to get medical care. The Vermont State Medical Society and the Vermont Hospital Association provided information on physician supply and hospital capacity across the state. We were also fortunate to have information on physician utilization for Vermonters over 65 years of age when the Vermont-New Hampshire Blue Cross program gave us access to Medicare's Part B Claims, the insurance claims submitted by physicians to obtain payment for the care they provided.

I worked with Alan Gittelsohn, a biostatistician from Johns Hopkins, who had also been my teacher. Together, we designed a method to compare population-based rates of care among neighboring hospital service areas. Our strategy of "small area analysis" was intended to examine the distribution of resources, the utilization of care, and, to the extent possible, the outcomes of care delivered in the various hospital service areas of the state.

To compare the utilization patterns among the populations of different regions of the state, we needed to be able to match patients to the providers of their care. To do this, we undertook a "patient origin" study, analyzing the frequency of use of hospitals by patients living in each of Vermont's 251 towns (which served as minor civil divisions in the United States Census). These towns were then aggregated into hospital service areas according to the hospital their residents most often used. Our small area analysis thus defined the geographic boundaries of local health care markets empirically, based on where patients most often went for their care. Altogether, thirteen geographically distinct hospital service areas were defined. In each service area, a large majority of care was delivered by providers whose practices were located within the area.

Our next step was to estimate area measures of per capita expenditures, hospital and nursing home beds, and health care workers, including physicians, according to their specialty.[2] Finally, we measured the rates of utilization, including hospitalization, surgical procedures, and diagnostic procedures.

Chaos in the Patterns of Practice

The results surprised us, to say the least. My training (and the assumptions behind the RMP) had led me to expect that Vermont's largely rural health care system was underserving its population. We found instead a typology of care characterized by wide variations in the deployment of resources and the utilization of services, without any apparent rhyme or reason. Here are some examples of what we found and would eventually publish in *Science* in December 1973.[3]

> *Resource Inputs and Spending:* There were 73% more beds in the region with the most beds per 1,000 compared to the region with the least. The number of physicians serving the population in the area with the most physicians per 1,000 was 57% greater than in the area with the least. When it came to the population-based rate of any particular medical specialty, there was even greater variation. Medicare spending for physician services in the highest cost areas was two-fold to three-fold greater than in the lowest cost area. Nursing home beds per 1,000 population varied more than six-fold among Vermont's 13 hospital service areas.

Use of Care: Tonsillectomy rates per 1,000 population varied eleven-fold; hemorrhoidectomy five-fold; and removal of the uterus (hysterectomy) and surgery for an enlarged prostate (transurethral resection of the prostate, or TURP) varied three-fold from the highest to the lowest area. Hospital discharges per 1,000 in the highest area were 61% greater than in the lowest. Rates of hospitalization for broad classes of disease showed much more variation. Hospitalization rates for respiratory diseases, for example, varied 3.6-fold, while vascular diseases varied more than 2.1-fold.

Implications for the Health Care Economy

It was not just one procedure that varied—virtually everything did, and the extent of variation challenged basic assumptions about how health care markets work. The prevailing assumption was that patient needs and wants drive utilization—that is, unless the supply of medical resources is constrained, in which case patients do not get all the care they need. But on the face of it, we had difficulty believing that variation in patient need could possibly be driving the strange patterns we were seeing. In one region, tonsillectomies would be high, hysterectomies low, nursing home admissions low, and hospitalizations for pneumonia right in the middle. The next region would show a completely different pattern. It was always possible that patients varied that much from place to place, and thus their need for medical care also varied, but that seemed difficult to accept, given the population in Vermont in the early 1970s. The state had fewer than 500,000 inhabitants, mostly of New England stock—a very homogeneous population scattered among its 251 small towns and villages.

To give a personal example of how strange Vermont's health care utilization patterns seemed, our family lived on a farm in Waterbury Center, just south of Stowe, and the children attended the Waterbury elementary school. Proximity and custom dictated that the children in Stowe receive their care from physicians practicing in the Morrisville hospital service area, while the children in Waterbury lived in a different hospital service area and were usually treated by a different group of physicians, despite the close proximity of the two communities. Among the children living in Waterbury Center, less than 20% received a tonsillectomy by age 15. Had our home been located l,000 yards farther north, we would have been in the Stowe school district, where by age 15, more than 60% of children had lost their tonsils.

Other features of conventional wisdom seemed to fall prey to our data. Much of public policy toward nursing homes had been based on the assumption that nursing home beds substituted for acute care beds—that having more nursing home beds would take the pressure off acute care hospitals, leading to the need for fewer hospital beds (and lower hospitalization rates). We found no evidence to support this theory. Indeed, we found that having more nursing home beds was slightly correlated with *more* acute care beds per 1,000.

What per capita utilization rates for some services correlated very nicely with was the local per capita supply of medical resources. Having more hospital beds meant more hospitalizations. The supply and specialty composition of the physician workforce also emerged as strong predictors of utilization, such that the number of procedures performed and their level of complexity were related to the characteristics of the local workforce. Populations living in areas with more surgeons per capita had more surgery at all levels of complexity; areas with more general practitioners who performed surgery had higher rates of less complicated surgery; populations living in hospital service areas with more internists underwent more diagnostic tests, including laboratory tests, x-rays, and electrocardiograms. Vermont populations living in areas with more medical specialists had a greater frequency of follow-up visits with their physicians.

One possible conclusion we could have drawn from our data was that the places that had a lower per capita supply of medical resources, and therefore lower utilization, were suffering from lack of access to care. But when we looked at whether there was an advantage to more spending and higher utilization in terms of outcomes, we could find no supporting evidence. Mortality rates were not lower in regions with more supply or higher utilization, even after adjusting for available demographic factors. Other important outcomes that greater utilization might have produced, such as improvement in the quality of life, were not available in our data. Nonetheless, it was difficult to escape the conclusion that a great deal of the care being delivered in Vermont offered little or no benefit to the population, and might in fact be causing harm. As Alan and I would write in our paper summarizing our Vermont findings in *Science*[3]:

> Given the magnitude of these variations, the possibility of too much medical care and the attendant likelihood of iatrogenic [physician-caused] illness is presumably as strong as the possibility of not enough service and unattended mortality and morbidity.

Naturally, this conclusion did not sit well with our fellow physicians. We published in *Science* only after being turned down by medical journals with wide clinical readerships, such as the *New England Journal of Medicine* and the *Journal of the American Medical Association*. Editors rejected our paper on the assumption that patient demand simply *had* to be the explanation for our observations, and thus the findings would be of no interest to their readers. But the sheer magnitude of the variation in incidence of hospitalization and surgery among these neighboring medical communities suggested that patient demand could not be the sole cause. And that suggested the importance of physician behavior as a major source of variation. The children of Stowe and Waterbury Center did not seem different enough to account for a three-fold variation in tonsillectomy. Neither did the women who were candidates for hysterectomy; nor did it seem plausible that differences in incidence of pneumonia could account for the wide variations in hospitalization for this condition. But support for the hypothesis that patient demand did not explain the variations was at that point indirect—based on census information and local knowledge. Given the implications, we believed that we needed direct evidence as to whether illness or other factors such as health insurance or educational levels could explain the differences in resource allocation and utilization.

Illness Does Not Explain Variation

By the early 1970s, the role of the patient in determining the utilization of health care was under active investigation. Two sociologists at the University of Chicago, Ronald Andersen and John F. Newman, had developed empirical tests of the relative importance of illness, as well as economic and sociological factors, in determining the propensity of an individual to use health care.[4] Their studies had yielded the not surprising result that illness level was by far the most important factor behind the decision patients make to contact a doctor. Socioeconomic factors such as income and educational level, and having health insurance, also mattered. We applied the Chicago findings to evaluate the patterns we uncovered in Vermont. Jack Fowler, a social psychologist at the Center for Survey Research at the University of Massachusetts, was interested in health care issues and was familiar with the work in Chicago. He designed a study to determine whether six contiguous Vermont hospital service areas, which exhibited striking variations in resources allocation, medical spending, and utilization, also exhibited differences in factors that predict patient demand. The six areas included in the study were Burlington and Hanover, New Hampshire, the hospital service areas that contain the two university hospitals serving the region; the Rutland and Montpelier hospital service areas, which contain the state's two largest community hospitals; and the Middlebury and Randolph hospital service areas, which represent areas with smaller hospitals. In each area, we interviewed about 250 households to obtain information on each family member.

We set out to answer the following questions: Are there differences among hospital service areas in illness rates? Are there differences in factors that enable or otherwise influence patients to seek care, such as insurance coverage, educational level, economic circumstances, or ethnic background? Do differences in these factors relate to the observed variations in health care delivery? And, finally, are there any differences in observed access to care—in the propensity of patients to contact their physicians—that could explain the differences in population-based rates of consumption of health care services?

The results confirmed the remarkable homogeneity and stability of the Vermont population. We found nothing on the demand side of the utilization equation to explain the differences in utilization. The vast majority, 99% of Vermonters, were white; most were born in either Vermont or New Hampshire, and almost half of the adults had lived in their hospital service area for longer than 20 years. Educational attainment showed some differences: the hospital areas with large colleges—Burlington, Middlebury, and Hanover, New Hampshire—had slightly more adults who reported having one or more years of college, but neither this difference nor the slight differences among areas in the percentage born in Vermont or New Hampshire showed a meaningful correlation with spending or utilization.

Our study found no significant differences among regions in household economic characteristics known to influence patient demand for care. About 20% of households were at or below poverty and most had health insurance. Of those household members not covered by Medicare or Medicaid, 83% had private insurance, and about half of the policies were from Blue Cross, which at that time provided the same benefits throughout the state. A remarkable 98% of Vermonters had a regular place where they went for physician care.

We observed no net differences in the proportion of household members with illness that explained the regional differences in use of care. Two measures of illness—the percentage of persons whose activity has been restricted by illness within the past two weeks and the percentage confined to bed longer than two weeks in the last year—showed no significant difference among the areas. An estimate for chronic illness was obtained by asking household members if during the last year they had "any health problem or illness" for a period of three months or longer. While there were some differences among areas, the differences were small and bore no relationship to the utilization patterns.

As predicted by the Chicago model, the *individual* Vermonter contacted the health care system on the basis of his or her own perception of need. Having an episode of illness was a powerful predictor of propensity to seek care. However, the similar distribution across the six hospital areas in illness and other factors that relate at the individual *patient level* to the use of health care also predicted that at the *population level*, the six Vermont areas would not differ in their population's ability, need, or interest in consuming medical care.

This expectation was borne out by the remarkably similar rates at which Vermonters contacted their physicians, regardless of where they lived. Take as an example the populations living in the Randolph and the Middlebury hospital service areas (Table 2.1). The two communities were virtually identical with regard to socioeconomic factors and chronic illness level. Access was virtually identical: on an annualized basis, 73.4% of Randolph residents and 72.6% of Middlebury residents contacted their physician one or more times. But there the similarity stopped. In 1973, hospitalization and surgery rates were 66% and 63% greater for residents of the Randolph hospital service area;

Table 2.1. A Test of Consumer Contribution to Small Area Variations in Health Care Delivery: Randolph and Middlebury, Vermont

	Middlebury, Vermont	Randolph, New Hampshire
Socioeconomic characteristics		
White	98%	97%
Born in Vermont or New Hampshire	59	61
Lived in area 20 or more years	47	47
Income level below poverty	20	23
Have health insurance	84	84
Regular place of physician care	97	99
Chronic illness level		
Prevalence	23%	23%
Restricted activity last 2 weeks	5	4
More than 2 weeks in bed last year	4	5
Access to physician		
Contact with physician within year	73%	73%
"Post-access" utilization of health care		
Hospital discharges per 1,000	132	220
Surgery discharges per 1,000	49	80
Medicare Part B spending per Enrollee ($)	92	142

Source: Adapted from Wennberg, J and Fowler, FJ. 1977. A Test of Consumer Contributions to Small Area Variations in Health Care Delivery. *Journal of the Maine Medical Association.* 68(8):275–279. [Used with permission from the Maine Medical Association.]

Medicare spending for physician services was 53% greater on a per person basis. The bottom line was that there was equal demand and equal access but strikingly unequal rates of "postaccess" rates of consumption of health care by demographically similar populations. In other words, what was varying was *what happened after patients met with their physicians, not the rate at which they got sick and went to the doctor.*

The interviews for the test of consumer contribution to practice variation were completed in March of 1973, but it took more than four years before the results were finally published in the *Journal of the Maine Medical Association.*[5] In trying to get our study published, Jack and I encountered pretty much the same resistance that Alan and I had found earlier. I was a bit surprised and not a little disappointed by this, because I had assumed that now that we had "nailed" the evidence that variations were not explained by illness, poverty, or ethnicity, the Vermont findings and their implications would receive serious attention from high-profile academic medical journals. However, we had no such luck.

The Health Care World Turned Upside Down

The uncovering of widespread variations in resource allocation and utilization for elective surgery, hospitals, nursing homes, home health care, and physician services; the strong associations between supply and utilization; and the lack of association with the needs of patients convinced me that the problems facing the Vermont health care system were more profound than the barriers to the diffusion of new technology that the RMP was designed to overcome. The health care system was performing differently than predicted by the mainstream social science I had studied at Johns Hopkins. Social scientists had long recognized that the "exchange relationship" between the physician and the patient was radically different from the exchange relationship that determines the demand for other goods and services in most markets. The doctor-patient relationship is different because of the asymmetry of information. The patient, as a layman, does not know what he or she truly needs; it is the physician who knows the nature of the patient's illness and can select the right treatment. For these reasons, many social scientists thought it was rational for patients to do something they would not dream of doing in most markets—that is, to delegate decision making to the seller of services, the physician, who by virtue of his special knowledge and skill, could act as their "rational agent" in health care purchasing decisions.

From the patient's point of view, the agency model was believed to be rational on the basis of several assumptions. First, it was assumed that clinical decision making is grounded in medical science; physicians have evidence-based knowledge to diagnose illness accurately and estimate the risks and benefits for the treatments they prescribe. Second, physicians make accurate judgments concerning the treatments patients want: they choose the treatment the individual patient would prefer, if only they were themselves physicians, and therefore knew the facts and better understood their own "true" wants and needs. This assumption is implicit when a patient says to his or her physician, "What would you do if you were me?" Third, the ethics of professionalism protects the trust that is the basis for the patient's willingness to delegate decision making to the physician. Despite the fact that the physician benefits financially from higher utilization of his services, professional ethics ensure that he or she will choose what is best for the patient. Finally, egregious behavior by the few unethical physicians who induce patient demand for self-serving motives is detected and controlled through utilization review and other methods the profession adopts to discipline "outlier" behavior.

The delegation of decision making to physicians was also assumed to be rational from society's point of view. A doctor-patient relationship that works in the way I have just described ensures that the supply of medical resources, including physicians, will not influence demand in a way that is wasteful. Professional ethics, bolstered by utilization review and other strategies for patrolling the market for unethical behavior, ensures that the services recommended by the physician agent are both effective and valued. Thus, the physician serves as guarantor of the efficient allocation of society's resources: if capacity exceeds that required to produce effective and valued services, capacity in excess will go unused. Through the physician acting as agent for both patient and society, the market is thus "cleared" of excess capacity. On the other hand, when the resources of the health care system are stressed, when providers express concern about too little capacity, when hospital beds are occupied to the point of overflow, and when physicians' waiting rooms are full, then, under the agency hypothesis, the demand for care exceeds supply. To avoid health care rationing under such circumstances, the proper role of an enlightened public policy is to provide more resources.

Ensuring adequate resources was precisely what public policy for health care sought to accomplish at the time of our Vermont studies—it was the stated goal of both the RMP and of the Hill-Burton Program, the federal subsidies designed to ensure sufficient hospital beds. It also became the goal of physician workforce policy. At that time, the United States had already begun a program that would eventually result in a doubling of the supply of physicians.

Our Vermont studies stood as a direct challenge to the fundamental assumptions of rational agency theory.[6] We were suggesting that supplier-induced demand for medical care seemed to be a central tendency of Vermont's health care market, not an aberration caused by a few unethical, "outlier" physicians. The incidence of disease, and the probability that the patient would show up at the physician's office seeking care for an episode of illness, appeared to be essentially the same from one Vermont community to another. What varied was "post-access" care—the amount and type of care patients received after they entered the health care system. What also varied was the supply of medical resources: the numbers of physicians, hospital beds, and nursing homes, for example. The theories that drove individual physicians' decisions also varied. As we would eventually discover, individual practice styles appeared to be determined in part by specific ideological factors, enthusiasms for a particular diagnostic tool or treatment such as tonsillectomy, and in part by the sheer supply or availability of medical resources. In other words, physicians who practiced in a region of the state where hospital beds were in abundant supply tended to hospitalize their patients more often than their colleagues in regions where beds were less available. And patients were instructed to return for a follow-up office visit more frequently in regions where there were more physicians, particularly medical specialists.

But it was far from clear that more was better—that more beds, more physicians, more hospitalizations, and more surgeries were improving the welfare of Vermonters who were receiving more care. The Vermont studies, by raising questions about which rate was right, thus also challenged the view that the basic problem facing the health care system was a lack of resources that resulted in underservice.

* * *

While the life of the RMP turned out to be a short one, the work we conducted in Vermont defined the research problems and set the research agenda that has consumed my energies over the subsequent years. That research, it turns out, was presaged by earlier studies, which we only discovered after the fact. Had Alan Gittelsohn and I read about the work of J. Alison Glover[7] and Paul Lembcke,[8] researchers who had documented variation in utilization in Great Britain in the 1930s and in New York State in the 1950s, we would have been better prepared for the existence of variations in the rates of surgical procedures we discovered in Vermont, if not for the sheer magnitude and the extent of variations in all types of health care delivery.

PART II

Surgical Variation: Understanding Preference-Sensitive Care

Patients traditionally delegate decision making about treatments to their physicians, under the assumption that physicians prescribe treatments based not only on medical science but also on an understanding of what is best for the individual patient. Embedded in the idea that the physician knows what is best for the patient is the notion that the physician also knows what the patient wants. Yet as early as the 1930s, it was evident that local medical opinion was behind the marked variation in tonsillectomy rates, rather than clinical science or patient (parental) preference. By the mid-1970s, it became clear that the rates of utilization of most common surgical procedures varied extensively among regions, some more than others. Physicians everywhere seemed to differ among themselves on the value of many operations, on who would benefit and who would not, and these differences of opinion directly influenced the incidence of any given surgery. What the patient wanted often appeared not to matter much.

The importance of scientific uncertainty and the misdiagnosis of patient preferences as a cause of practice variation became most clear over the course of a decade-long research effort we undertook to understand why surgery rates for an enlarged prostate showed such great variation among regions in the state of Maine. It turned out that while many urologists undertook surgery under the assumption that it prolonged life, our research showed this was not the case. However, surgery did have a potentially positive effect on the quality of life by reducing symptoms. But this benefit had to be weighed against the harmful effect of surgery on sexual function. It became evident through our research that rational choice required the active engagement of the patient in the choice of treatment. Similar research sponsored by a new federal agency, to investigate practice variations for back surgery and cardiac surgery, came to similar conclusions regarding the importance of patients understanding the benefits and harms of alternative treatments and making informed choices.

Establishing a market where the utilization of preference-sensitive treatments is determined by patient demand will require a profound cultural change in the doctor-patient relationship: replacing delegated decision making, and the doctrine of informed consent, with shared decision making and informed patient choice as the standard for determining the medical necessity of preference-sensitive treatments.

Remedying variation in preference-sensitive care will also require a change in the research culture, a topic that is relevant to today's debate over evidence-based medicine. Under the Agency for Health Care Policy and Research (forerunner to the Agency for Healthcare Research and Quality), a collaborative research model was established that was highly successful in reducing scientific uncertainty and promoting informed patient choice. However, it also challenged the conventional wisdom; it was abruptly interrupted by the U.S. Congress in the mid-1990s, in large part because of strong negative reaction from surgeons over the conclusions of the back surgery research team.

Studies discussed in this section suggest that the implementation of shared decision making will reduce the utilization of surgery and save money. But addressing unwarranted variation in preference-sensitive care is essential not just for economic reasons. By failing to take into account patient preferences, and enabling patients to make informed choices, surgery will be misused. It should be considered a serious form of medical error when surgeons operate on patients who would not have wanted the procedure had they been fully informed and empowered to participate in a meaningful way in the choice of treatment.

3

Tonsillectomy and Medical Opinion

A major surgical intervention is a dramatic event in the life of the patient. It involves a stay in the hospital or clinic, for hours or days. The patient faces the possibility of pain, infection, or an unexpected reaction to anesthesia or a drug. Then there is the risk of error or an adverse event, the unforeseen possibility that something can go horribly wrong. To subject their patients to these rigors and risks, surgeons are by necessity true believers in the efficacy of the operations they perform; they cannot afford psychologically to doubt their clinical necessity. Most surgical patients are also convinced that the benefits of surgery exceed the risks by a wide margin. Yet in the face of such certainty and conviction, it is remarkable how much the rate of surgery can vary from area to area.[1]

No surgical procedure has been studied more, or illustrates better, the role of medical opinion in determining the rate of surgery than tonsillectomy, a procedure that has fallen out of favor in recent years but was practically a rite of passage for children only a few decades ago. (The *rate* of surgery simply means the number of surgeries per 1,000 people. *Incidence* of surgery is another way to express the same idea.) The relevant literature goes back 35 years before our Vermont study, to pre–World War II Britain, when J. Alison Glover, then a medical officer in the Ministry of Health, discovered that a child's chances of undergoing tonsillectomy depended on which school he attended. Calling the phenomenon he observed "the strange bare fact of incidence,"[2] Glover built a convincing case that the major source of variation was differences in the medical opinion of the school health officer responsible for referral for surgery.

Glover built his case on school health records, which revealed a four-fold variation in the per capita utilization of tonsillectomy among British school districts. Just as Alan Gittelsohn and I would do in Vermont some thirty years later, Glover systematically examined and dismissed alternative explanations for this variation. He took pains to rule out the possibility that the differences in tonsillectomy rates were explained by factors on the demand side of the equation. For instance, because the child health services were provided free as part of attending school, economic factors and access to care were not issues in Britain. He looked for but could find no evidence of an association between surgery rates and "any impersonal factor" predictive of illness, such as overcrowding, poverty, bad housing, or climate. He wrote:

> In each of these categories there are extreme variations in the operation rate, the extremes often in adjacent areas.... Possible factors such as the efficiency of school dental service, rainfall, climate, [overcrowding, unemployment] and nutrition returns have been considered, but with one extremely doubtful exception—urbanization—not the slightest suggestion of correlation has been obtained.... But if urbanization be a factor there are inexplicable anomalies ... the highest rates of all are in certain agricultural counties and the [urban areas] with the higher rates include residential towns and health resorts famed for their beauty, climate and spaciousness.[3]

In the end, Glover concluded that differences among children in different school districts could not account for the variation in utilization. That left only one possibility: physician judgment. The school physicians responsible for referring their students for tonsillectomy diverged in their opinion as to which children needed a tonsillectomy.

Glover gave a plausible account for the lack of importance of illness, but his approach was based on an argument of exclusion, and he did not show directly that medical opinion was the source of the variation. Unbeknownst to him, an experiment that demonstrated directly that patient characteristics and illness rates did not drive the tonsillectomy rates had already been reported.[4] In the 1930s, the American Child Health Association, like many volunteer health associations of the day, viewed tonsillectomy as a public health good. The association wanted to make certain that no New York City school child who needed a tonsillectomy had been overlooked. To find out how much unmet need there was, they performed a sophisticated study that, ironically, not only provided direct evidence for the extraordinary variability in physicians' professional judgment but also led to considerable doubt about the notion of unmet need itself.

The American Child Health Association's research design used a random sampling of 1,000 New York City school children. On examination by a school physician, 60% were found to have already had a tonsillectomy, and of the remaining 40%, nearly half were deemed in need of the operation. To make sure that no one in need of a tonsillectomy was left out, the association arranged for the children not selected for tonsillectomy to be reexamined by another group of physicians. The second wave of physicians recommended that 40% of *these* children have the operation. Still not content that unmet need had been adequately detected, the association arranged for a third examination of the twice-rejected children by another group of physicians. On the third try, the physicians produced recommendations that another 44% should have the operation. By the end of the three-examination process, only 65 children of the original 1,000 emerged from the screening examination without a recommendation for tonsillectomy. If the association had put those 65 children through additional rounds of examination, it seems likely that virtually every last one would have been recommended for surgery, a thought that gives new meaning to the phrase "no child left behind."

The most direct clinical evidence supporting Glover's hypothesis that medical opinion was driving rates of tonsillectomy came some forty years after his original report. Compelled by Glover's logic, Michael Bloor, who later became professor of sociology at Aberdeen University, and his colleagues, George A. Venters and Michael L. Samphier, set out to document the role of medical opinion by directly observing physicians as they interacted with their patients in the process of reaching a treatment decision.[5,6] The researchers used as their laboratory two health districts in Scotland with substantially different tonsillectomy rates. The high-rate district, they showed, had higher overall rates of referral from general practitioners to surgeons, as well as higher rates for performing surgery on referred patients, but with considerable differences among individual physicians within each area. With the permission of the surgeons, Bloor and his colleagues sat in on clinical encounters to observe and document variation in the decision rules and practice patterns of the physicians, in an effort to correlate these differences with the physician's propensity to operate. They then met individually with each surgeon to make certain that their observations accurately reflected the surgeon's beliefs and practice.

Differences were found in the specific clinical features that the surgeons thought important in making their decision. In their paper, Bloor and his colleagues[5,6] illustrated these differences with direct quotes from three surgeons who had opposite attitudes concerning the importance of clinical findings suggesting chronic infection, as measured by inflammation in the area near the tonsil (the anterior pillars) or in the cervical lymph nodes (glands in the neck):

Surgeon One
... the anterior pillars being injected (infected) is a fairly constant [i.e., reliable] sign: in the healthy they don't seem to be, whereas in the unhealthy there seems to be a sort of injected ... [appearance].

Surgeon Two
All the anterior pillars will tell you if there's been a recent infection— they'll be a bit reddened. It's not of very great importance. The glands are important—persistent glands are a sign of persistent infection.

Surgeon Three
I don't worry about large cervical glands ... some people say if they're visible it's significant: if a child comes with visible cervical glands I get their blood examined—one child had leukemia ... if they're not visible but palpable it doesn't worry me in the slightest.

The physicians' practice styles also differed regarding the relative importance they gave to the patient's medical history versus the physical examination. Surgeons with a high proclivity to operate tended to stress the importance of the physical examination. For example, one surgeon thought that three physical signs—infected material in the tonsil, reddened anterior pillars, and palpable cervical lymph nodes—were decisive and his rule of thumb was to operate on any child with two or more of these signs. As one more conservative surgeon put it, "Somebody is supposed to have said once that the only point in looking at the child's throat is to make sure the tonsils are still there, that no one else was there before you! That is an exaggeration I'm sure but it puts the point over." Among surgeons who were less quick to operate, the reverse was the case—much more stress was put on the history. A child who had suffered only the occasional bout of tonsillitis probably would not be a candidate for surgery, no matter how inflamed the tonsils might be on physical examination.

Differences among practice styles were also found in the details elicited from the history and the interpretation of the meaning of the referral. One surgeon who was quick to operate thought that the mere fact of referral implied an extensive history of morbidity, and in most cases his decision-making strategy combined an examination of the child with a simple check on his assumption of morbidity by asking the parent if the child suffered "a lot of trouble."[7] In direct contrast, a more conservative physician acted as an independent assessor, seeking to reconstruct the child's clinical history in detail.[8]

Bloor et al. found that such differences among specialists in the depth of their history taking linked directly to differences in the decision rules they used in recommending operations. The conservative physician's decision rules could be characterized as a list of checked boxes: "if a child is of A age, and if the child suffers sore throats of recurrence B, and if attacks are of C severity, and if the examination findings are of D nature, then the child will receive E disposal."[9] Bloor and his colleagues found that the more specific and extensive the decision rules, the more symptomatically differentiated were the patients receiving surgery and the more restrictive were the criteria for surgical admission. Moreover, surgeons who followed well-defined decision algorithms were more conservative in their estimates of the benefits of the tonsillectomy.

Another difference in practice style that was documented by Bloor and colleagues is the physician's belief in "watchful waiting"—observing the natural history of the disease process before making a final decision on the surgery. Conservative surgeons were characterized as having a higher than average tendency to "wait and see" after deciding that an operation was not an immediate necessity and believing that an intermediate approach (such as antibiotic treatment) could be tried. As Bloor et al. quoted one surgeon, "What we're really doing is playing for time. I don't know whether the sulphonamide really helps or not—it certainly helps in the sense that the parents are pleased that she's getting some treatment—but the important thing is that we gain time to allow the trouble to resolve itself."[10] And if children then were like children now, often the symptoms would disappear with time.

Bloor et al.'s detailed observations of the actual behavior of clinicians in reaching their tonsillectomy decisions convinced him that Glover was right. To use their words, the differences in rates between the regions "can be attributed to differences between specialists in their assessment practices: local differences in the nature of specialist practice 'create' local differences in surgical incidence … [The findings] amount to a detailed vindication of Glover's conviction that variations in the incidence of surgery are largely the product of medical opinion rather than the product of the differential distribution of morbidity."[11]

Glover[12] had followed yet another line of reasoning in making his case for the central role of medical opinion in practice variation. He documented the professional controversies concerning the value of tonsillectomy—the disputes over medical theory and fact that made it impossible for the profession to reach consensus on the "best practice" for dealing with chronic tonsillitis. Tonsillectomy was not a lifesaving, emergency operation. Some physicians, Glover among them, were skeptical of its value as a preventive measure, believing the operation to be effective only in properly selected cases with demonstrated morbidity, such as those with "frequently repeated attacks of acute tonsillitis which cannot be explained by extraneous infections."[13] In Glover's opinion, this restricted view of the procedure's value provided no justification for the use of tonsillectomy as a public health intervention where the substantial majority of children were subjected to tonsillectomy, as was the case in some school districts (and as was still the case in the 1960s in Morrisville, Vermont, when Alan Gittelsohn and I came along). In addition to the dubious notion that school children had a high risk of developing serious illness in the future merely because they had a pair of tonsils, it was Glover's judgment that such widespread use of tonsillectomy as a public health strategy denied the "probability that the tonsil serves some useful purpose, its tendency for spontaneous involution, and the success of non-operative methods of treatment that are often likely overlooked.…" Moreover, it ignored the fact that tonsillectomy was a risky procedure; he reported that 424 British school children had died following the surgery between 1931 and 1935.

The final plank in Glover's argument that medical opinion was determining utilization rates came in the form of a natural experiment. He monitored the changes in tonsillectomy rates that followed a change in the school health officer—the physician responsible for the diagnosis and referral of children for tonsillectomy. His most famous case involved Dr. R. P. Garrow, the physician who replaced an unnamed predecessor as school health officer in the Hornsey Borough school district, in the Middlesex region of England. Following Garrow's recruitment, the rates of tonsillectomy fell dramatically and remained below 10% of what it had been before Garrow came on the scene (Figure 3.1).

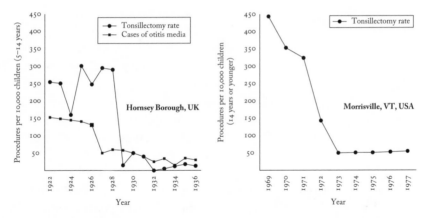

Figure 3.1.   The tonsillectomy rate per 10,000 children in the Hornsey Borough School District (1922 through 1936) and in the Morrisville, Vermont hospital service area (1969 through 1977). *Left,* Tonsillectomy rates and incidence of otitis media or middle ear infections in the years before and after Dr. Garrow's appointment as school physician in 1929. (Adapted from Glover, J. Alison. 1938. The incidence of tonsillectomy in school children. *Proceedings of the Royal Society of Medicine* 31: 1219–1236. Reprinted in the *International Journal of Epidemiology*, 2008;37:9–19. Reproduced by permission of the Royal Society of Medicine Press, London, and Oxford University Press, Oxford, UK.) *Right,* Change following the feedback of information on the rates of tonsillectomy in Morrisville, Vermont. (Adapted with permission from *Pediatrics,* Vol. 59, Pages 821–826, Copyright 1977 by the American Academy of Pediatrics.)

Shifting Practice Patterns

Three decades later, Alan Gittelsohn and I witnessed a similar rapid shift in surgery rates in Vermont, but this time it occurred because of a deliberate change in treatment policy among local physicians. After documenting the variations in local tonsillectomy rates across the state, I provided a report to the Vermont State Medical Society detailing the rates for each area. Dr. Roy Buttles, the society's president, circulated the information among Vermont physicians. Prior to the release of the report, the chances of undergoing tonsillectomy during childhood in the Morrisville area were 60%. On learning of the high rate in their area, two Morrisville physicians, Dr. Lewis Blowers, a general surgeon, and Dr. Robert Parker, a pediatrician, undertook a second opinion process, which led to the rapid decline of their use of the procedure.

In a report published in *Pediatrics*[14] they described what made them change their practice:

> Awareness of the differences among the areas led us to review the literature on indications for tonsillectomy and … to review each candidate for tonsillectomy, whether seen on referral or in our own practices. By the end of 1972, we reviewed most of the tonsillectomies performed at our local hospital. We believe this process of obtaining a second opinion helped us standardize the decision process.

Within two years, the per capita rate of tonsillectomy in Morrisville had dropped to less than 10%, because of changes in local practice styles (see Figure 3.1).

Glover's studies also foreshadowed the use of quasi-experimental designs to evaluate the outcomes of care, designs that we would begin using in Maine in the 1970s. He followed the outcomes of patients for up to eight years after the rapid decline in tonsillectomies following the change in the school physician in the Hornsey Borough. The abrupt change in practice pattern was not associated with an increase in ear infections, the assumed outcome if children were not given the benefit of widespread use of tonsillectomy: "Judging by the [incidence of] otitis media … nothing harmful but rather the reverse has happened from the substitution, in all but the most carefully selected fraction of cases, of conservative methods for operation."[15] In the case of tonsillectomy, more was not better for health.

Although Glover's studies preceded the work we would conduct thirty-five years later, and medical science and technology had galloped forward over that period of time, some things remained the same. Glover began his report on the incidence of tonsillectomy with a brief history of medical opinion that began with his own boyhood, in the 1890s. He wrote that he could not recall a single classmate who had undergone tonsillectomy. By the mid-1930s, more than 50% of students attending his childhood school had received tonsillectomies. The tonsillectomy epidemic also fell on my own family according to generation. My father, born in Norway just after the turn of the century, escaped the procedure entirely, as did most of his generation. I was not so lucky. In the late 1930s my family lived in Bellows Falls, Vermont, and at the age of 5, I underwent my first tonsillectomy in the local hospital. I was one of the lucky ones to have my operation in the hospital. Many of my friends in those Depression-era years were not so fortunate. Their parents could not afford the hospital, so they had their operations in the school gymnasium during "tonsillectectomy day"—a mass surgery event held periodically to ensure that everyone in Bellows Falls who needed an operation received an operation. Although precise statistics are not available, this apparently meant practically every child in town.

My tonsillectomy career wasn't finished with the Bellows Falls operation. At age 12, after my family had moved to the state of Washington, I was sent once again to the operating room for a "redo" tonsillectomy. Apparently, the first surgeon had left a bit of my original tonsils for the next physician to remove.

By the mid-1960s, the epidemic was receding, and as the Vermont data came online, we could monitor the incidence in various communities. Certain "hot spots" such as Morrisville remained, but opinion there changed rapidly once the physicians became aware of the rate at which children were undergoing tonsillectomy. In Bellows Falls, the incidence of tonsillectomy was also quite high until, suddenly, it fell to practically zero. As I looked closer at what was happening in my old hometown, I discovered that the last tonsillectomy performed at the local hospital was recorded as "dead on discharge"—The child had died during or shortly after the operation. It seemed like a painful way to conclude an epidemic of surgery.

* * *

The rise and fall of medical opinion on the value of tonsillectomy serve as a reminder of the importance of paying critical attention to the assumptions behind everyday surgical practice. The treatment theories behind tonsillectomy justified a decades-long pattern of practice that at its height imposed on a large majority of children an operation that proved to be, for the most part, unnecessary. My own children's, and now my grandchildren's, generations have pretty much escaped the procedure, but every age has its tonsillectomy equivalent. Indeed, many routinely performed procedures and surgeries vary as extensively among regions and are backed up with little scientific evidence concerning the outcomes of care and the preferences of patients. Chapter 4 looks closely at several of these situations.

4

Interpreting the Pattern of Surgical Variation

Throughout the 1970s, I sought opportunities to extend our Vermont studies into new territories, in Maine and Rhode Island, and as results became available, we noted an intriguing consistency in the pattern of variation of utilization. A given surgical procedure seemed to obey its own rule in terms of how much its use varied from place to place. For example, the incidence of surgical repair of a hernia, which had shown little variation among Vermont regions, also exhibited little variation in Maine and Rhode Island. Surgery to remove gallstones or the appendix was more variable than hernia repair but, compared with other procedures, exhibited only moderate variation within all three states. By contrast, prostatectomy for noncancerous enlargement of the prostate and hysterectomy were quite variable from area to area and also showed similar patterns between the states. The rate for tonsillectomy was all over the map, the most wildly varying of all (Figure 4.1). As we looked at these patterns, it became apparent that an individual procedure *seemed to have its own characteristic tendency to vary.*

Building on the insights of Glover, I suspected that the more surgeons disagreed among themselves about the efficacy of a procedure, and the indications for which it should be used, the more variation we would see in the surgical rate. I worked with Dr. Benjamin Barnes, a Tufts University transplant surgeon, and Dr. John Bunker, an anesthesiologist who at that time served as director of Harvard University's Center for the Evaluation of

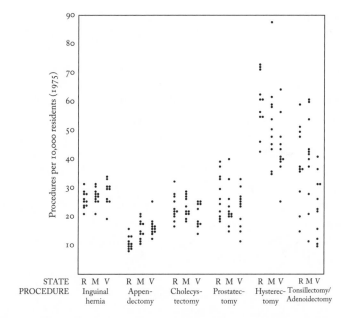

Figure 4.1.   The surgery rates for six common procedures among the eleven most populated hospital service areas in Rhode Island, Maine, and Vermont (1975). The procedures show increasing variation from left to right. Each dot represents a hospital service area: R = Rhode Island; M = Maine; V = Vermont. (Reprinted with permission. Copyright © *Scientific American*. All rights reserved.)

Health Practice, to document the controversies surrounding several different surgeries. We wanted to see if we could find a link between the degree of geographic variation in the rate at which a particular procedure was performed and the degree of disagreement over the use of that procedure in the medical literature.

Just as we predicted, the surgeries that showed the greatest variation from place to place were the subject of the greatest debate within medical science and visa versa.[1] Inguinal hernia repair, the procedure with the least geographic variation, was uniformly recommended as the treatment of choice, at least in the American literature. The medical textbooks and the journal articles we studied did not view the operation as optional or controversial. The relative uniformity in rates, we inferred, reflected the absence of acceptable treatment alternatives, as well as consistency in the way the diagnosis was made by different physicians. An inguinal hernia is usually easy to detect; indeed, the diagnosis is often made by the patient or a family member. At that time in the United States, the prescription for a hernia operation, like hospitalization for hip fracture, was not a "discretionary" decision that could be left to the judgment of the individual physician. Surgery was always deemed necessary, once the diagnosis had been made, to prevent the incarceration or "strangulation" of the bowel, which required emergency surgery. (As I will discuss in a moment, outcomes research in the past few years shows that this consensus was based on an erroneous assumption about how frequently strangulation happens.) However, this uniformity in clinical opinion on the "right" treatment did not extend to the United Kingdom. There, physicians often prescribed a truss as an alternative to surgery, and the availability of this option was consistent with the higher degree of variation seen in rates for inguinal hernia repair in the United Kingdom.[2] (See page 49.)

Our review of the scientific evidence supporting an appendectomy for appendicitis revealed a lack of controversies concerning the theoretical reasons for that surgery. All physicians viewed this operation for patients as nondiscretionary. Yet the procedure rates varied, and they varied sufficiently to suggest that physician opinion might be working to contribute to the variation. As it turned out, the controversy we encountered concerned not the treatment of the condition but rather its diagnosis. Other causes of abdominal pain, nausea, and vomiting are commonly confused with appendicitis, so some patients who do not have appendicitis have an appendectomy. Clinicians whose concerns centered on avoiding delay in operating are more prone to make a false-positive error, that is, to operate on someone who does not have appendicitis. On the other hand, those who delay operating until the cause is clear may miss the opportunity for early intervention and thus have a higher complication rate. In our study of the literature, we could find no empirical evidence concerning the consequences for patient outcomes of these differences in practice styles.

The disagreement over the value of gallbladder surgery centered on its use to remove asymptomatic, or "silent," gallstones.[3] Many Americans—some estimates are as high as 20% for middle-aged adults—harbor these silent gallstones, which are usually discovered by accident through an x-ray or other imaging examination undertaken for some other purpose. At the time of our study, some physicians advocated (as some still do today) the preventive removal of such stones, while others believed the risks of surgery were not worth the potential benefits. The situation for gallstones is thus quite similar to that for tonsillectomy, except that in this case the argument in favor of surgery was based on a hypothesized gain in the length of life that would follow early removal. This "preventive" surgery was justified on the belief that life expectancy is improved because the surgery removes the possibility of serious gallbladder disease sometime in the future, when the patient is older and sicker and therefore more at risk of dying from surgery following a symptomatic attack. Others believed that the risks of developing a complication after surgery and the associated probability of death were sufficiently high, even for a younger patient, that it was not worth doing the surgery before it was really necessary. Some silent gallstones remain silent for the rest of the patient's life, so why perform an operation that might never be needed? Physicians in this camp of opinion advocated what we eventually dubbed "watchful waiting": to observe and operate only if and when the condition and its symptoms becomes severe enough that intervention is warranted.

Prostatectomy and hysterectomy showed considerable variation in different geographic locations, and the controversies surrounding prostatectomy, as I discuss at length in Chapter 6, involved yet another example of surgery as prevention. The theory that lay behind hysterectomy, on the other hand, centered primarily on its value in improving the quality of life. The most common reason for recommending hysterectomy was and still is the treatment of pain and bleeding associated with menopause. Hormonal treatment was an alternative to hysterectomy, as was watchful waiting, because menopause is completed eventually and the bleeding and other symptoms resolve. The recommendation for surgery thus involved judgments about the impact of surgery on the quality of life and whether, given its costs and risks, surgery could be justified when the problem usually goes away on its own in a few months or years. (We found a clear consensus in the literature that surgery was the only appropriate treatment for cancer of the uterus, assuming the cancer had not spread to the point at which an operation was futile. But less than 10% of hysterectomies in the United States were performed for treating cancer.) The controversies in the literature centered in part on questions concerning the possible negative impact of hysterectomy on emotional health and other aspects of the quality of life. As was the case for the other operations that Benjamin, John, and I reviewed, we could find no clinical trials that offered objective evidence to resolve the differences in professional opinion. In other words, physicians were routinely performing many different kinds of surgeries based largely on theories, beliefs, and tradition—but remarkably little valid evidence.

Prognosis, Patient Preference, and Medical Opinion

The lack of evidence for the efficacy of various surgical treatments was remarkable in itself, but there was another aspect of the medical literature that seemed even more astonishing. Although there was considerable debate concerning the prognosis, or outcomes, of surgical treatments, very little of the discussion focused on what patients wanted. What was the patient's preference when faced with surgery? The topic rarely came up and, when it did, the intent was often to dismiss the importance of the patient's role in decision making and to accept unquestioningly the notion that physicians are competent to diagnose what patients desire.

Yet, when physicians themselves are patients, the question of what patients want suddenly becomes a topic of interest. We had been alerted to this idea after we participated in a seminar at Harvard University in the mid-1970s on surgical practice. Our colleague Duncan Neuhauser presented a paper at the seminar arguing for the importance of patient preference, even in the case of an inguinal hernia repair, which in this country was virtually always treated with surgery.[4] In making his case, he cited the experience of two physicians as evidence for interpersonal differences. One noted Boston surgeon who once used a truss said they were "dirty, tight, uncomfortable, hot, and smelly," and he would not wish the elderly, who suffer as it is, to be compelled to use them. Another physician Neuhauser quoted said he had "a painless hernia and preferred to avoid an operation."

In our review of the literature, we found only one example of concern about patient preferences with regard to surgery. It, too, came from a physician, who, in a letter to the editor of the *New England Journal of Medicine*, described his strategy for avoiding surgery for benign prostatic hyperplasia, a diagnosis that often led to a prostatectomy:

> Benign prostatic hyperplasia has awakened me several times a night for years. This past winter … I began to wake up every hour or two with visions of an impending (operation). There was always more urine that could be voided… . I began to spend a minute or more voiding, but carefully not straining, until no more … could be obtained. The results were immediate and dramatic. I now sleep three or four hours at a time and occasionally get up only once in eight hours… . If I am lazy and fail to take plenty of time to void, there is a prompt return of the frequency. It may be that this technic will preclude unnecessary surgery, even without a second opinion.[5]

The notion that a patient's preferences ought to be part of the decision to pursue surgery would turn out to be critical to our analysis of variation in surgical practice patterns. Beginning with our early review of the literature, Benjamin, John, and I, and soon other colleagues, began to think of discretionary surgeries as being "preference-sensitive." In other words, the rate at which they are performed ought to reflect not just medical evidence that the treatment effectively accomplishes its treatment goals and that patients are "appropriate" candidates for the surgery but also the patient's preferences. What a patient wants would depend on his or her perception of symptoms and the tradeoffs that always exist whenever one undergoes an optional medical procedure. And these surgeries were not called "elective" for nothing. They were not absolutely necessary, and the surgeon did not perform them unless the patient elected to go ahead. The patient, we would come to believe, ought to be the final arbiter of necessity, even for a surgery such as the repair of inguinal hernia, a condition whose diagnosis and treatment generated virtually no debate among American physicians.

Perhaps no clinical example better illustrates the importance of knowing what works (outcomes) and what patients want (preference) than the history of treatment for early-stage breast cancer. Beginning in the early 1900s, the predominant treatment for breast cancer was the radical mastectomy, which was first performed in 1882 by the preeminent surgeon William Halsted, whose name would be inextricably attached to the procedure. Chief of surgery at Johns Hopkins Hospital, Halsted believed (and persuaded most of his peers to accept as gospel) that cancer was a local disease that grows outward from the original site, much as a piece of fruit grows from a tiny nub. Halsted argued that removing not just the breast but also the chest muscles beneath it and the lymph nodes in the armpit of the affected side would block the tumor's avenues into the rest of the body and prevent it from spreading. The ascendance of Halsted's treatment was soon followed by the founding of the American Cancer Society, which set out to persuade Americans that early detection would lead to cancer cures. The society campaigned tirelessly, urging women to check their breasts and to go in for surgery as early as possible, and when they did they were likely to be treated with Halsted's draconian procedure. Radical mastectomy came to be used on virtually all breast tumors, no matter how small, despite the fact that the surgery itself posed grave risks to patients.[6]

Halsted's theory that cancer could only be cured by surgically slamming the door in its face held sway until well into the 1950s, when surgeons began adopting a modified version of the treatment. It was not until the 1970s that researchers actually tested the efficacy of mastectomy against lumpectomy with radiation in a randomized controlled trial (RCT), which found that survival was the same for the two techniques.[7]

This trial opened lumpectomy as a viable treatment option for early-stage breast cancer,[8] yet the choice between the two surgeries remained with surgeons, rather than their patients. Twenty years after the RCT showed lumpectomy and mastectomy to be equivalent in terms of survival rate, we would see this in the "strange bare fact of incidence" provided by the Dartmouth Atlas

Project. At that time, the frequency with which lumpectomy was performed remained one of the most varying of surgical procedures, as the first edition of the *Dartmouth Atlas of Health Care*[9] published in 1996, showed. We looked at the variation in surgery among Medicare patients diagnosed with breast cancer and living in the 306 Dartmouth Atlas Project hospital referral regions. In some regions, lumpectomy accounted for less than 2% of breast cancer surgery, whereas in others it made up nearly half.

Now, it is possible that this wide variation reflected differences in the choices that older women were making in different parts of the country. Perhaps nearly all the patients with breast cancer in Rapid City, South Dakota, chose mastectomy, not wanting to bother with radiation that would come after lumpectomy, whereas only half of patients with breast cancer in Elyria, Ohio, were willing to lose an entire breast. But that does not appear to be what was driving the variations in the rates of the two procedures.

One clue to the fact that the rates of the two procedures were heavily influenced by surgeons' preferences, rather than patients' choices, came in the form of a story published in 1996 in *Mirabella* by Laura Green, a New York writer specializing in health issues.[10] Using the Dartmouth Atlas Project data as her starting point, Green set her sights on Rapid City, SouthDakota, where virtually no breast cancer patients underwent a lumpectomy. In a manner reminiscent of Bloor's tonsillectomy study, Green interviewed surgeons in the Rapid City region to learn their attitudes toward cancer surgery. One surgeon was openly biased against lumpectomy. "As far as I'm concerned, the gold standard is still mastectomy. Everything has to be compared to that," he told her. "It is my personal bias that mastectomy does better." Another surgeon seemed to believe that local women wanted mastectomy; he suggested that Western women are less concerned about body image than are women elsewhere in the country. Still another surgeon, who, according to one of his patients, "was very good at presenting options to me," nevertheless held a bias against lumpectomy, as was evident in the way he framed the choice for women. When patients asked him what he would want his wife to do, wrote Green, "He answers that she is a nurse, that they have discussed it, and that she would have a mastectomy, which doesn't require radiation." He also tells his patients that "radiation requires time-consuming, tiring daily trips to the hospital for six weeks, and that 'scatter' from it may touch the lungs and ribs," increasing risk of secondary cancer. Green concludes: "Whatever (he) may intend to convey, the message seems to be: Radiation is not worth the trouble."

Obviously, the degree to which getting radiation treatments is a bother is not a biomedical question, but a deeply personal one. For the patient, the outcome of the two treatments in terms of survival is the same, and the choice between the two involves values and decisions that matter far more to her than to her surgeon. The tradeoffs center on morbidity and the side effects of each treatment. A woman who receives a lumpectomy avoids the loss of her breast, but will probably need to undergo additional therapy, including radiation. Because she also faces a risk that the tumor will recur locally and require further treatment, she should undergo periodic surveillance usually mammographyto detect a recurrence as early as possible. A woman who undergoes a mastectomy avoids the need for radiation and, for the most part, the risk of local recurrence but must deal with the loss of her breast and the additional decision on breast reconstruction, which is in itself an involved and potentially risky procedure.

From a normative perspective, it seems obvious that the choice among these treatments should depend on the preferences of the individual woman. It is well known that women differ in how they evaluate the impact of these two options on their lives and therefore in the treatment they want. Yet, traditionally, women have relied on the physician to make the choice for them, presumably under the assumption that physicians can choose the operation they (the patients) should have. But modern medical training and the tools available to the physician do not equip them to make such judgments. Biomedicine, per se, provides no guidelines on what the preferences of the individual patient might be, what she values, and how she views her own body, and many, if not most, physicians lack the training or skills to elicit those preferences. There is nothing in the clinical history, physical examination, or laboratory test that can be used to accurately "diagnose" the patient's preferences.

As I discuss in Chapter 14, creating a clinical environment where patient preferences play a significant role in determining the utilization rates for discretionary surgery should be a central goal of public policy. Information on the risks and benefits of alternative treatments is key to creating freedom of informed choice. With the completion of clinical trials establishing that radical mastectomy did not improve life expectancy over simple mastectomy, women no longer were required by "medical science" to undergo the mutilating radical procedure—it was not more effective than the less invasive simple mastectomy. With the completion of clinical trials showing that lumpectomy and simple mastectomy were similar in survival benefit, women became free (or should have become free) to choose the treatment that works best for them, to interpret their own health care needs with full knowledge of the risks and benefits.

Information gained recently from another clinical trial is creating a new option for choice for men with inguinal hernias. For decades, what for some men was a preference to avoid the inconvenience, risks, and added costs of surgery had been effectively blocked by physicians who based their advice on the specter of bowel strangulation, emergency surgery, and higher risk of death if surgery was refused. But because nearly everyone who had been diagnosed to have a hernia had been operated upon, the natural history of untreated inguinal hernia was poorly understood: physicians simply did not know the actual risk for strangulation; they just assumed it was bad enough to justify performing an operation on everyone who was fit enough to undergo surgery, at least until recently. In 2006, the *Journal of the American Medical Association* published the results of a multicenter clinical trial that tested the outcomes of watchful waiting versus surgical repair among men with "minimal" symptoms. The researchers found that bowel strangulation was a rare event, even for patients followed for as long as four and one-half years. The conclusion the researchers reached upset the conventional wisdom: "A strategy of watchful waiting is a safe and acceptable option for men with asymptomatic or minimally symptomatic inguinal hernias."[11]

In an accompanying editorial that bore the title, "The Asymptomatic Hernia: 'If It's Not Broken, Don't Fix It,'" David R. Flum, a professor of surgery at the University of Washington, summed up the situation as follows:

> The edict *primum non nocere* (first, do no harm) has deep roots in medicine.... Now, physicians can counsel these patients with regard to both operative and nonoperative strategies, with a better sense of which will do the least harm.... Avoiding harm in this case is easy—it can best be accomplished by counseling and educating patients and only repairing hernias that cause symptoms.[12]

The results of this clinical trial shift the basis for clinical decision making from one dominated by a preventive theory of avoidance of future harm to a quality-of-life tradeoff between the risks of surgery versus the discomfort of symptoms.

The treatment of chronic chest pain due to coronary artery disease with stents appears to be in the throes of a similar change brought about by new information. Stenting—the placement of a hollow tube into the coronary arteries to reduce blockage due to atherosclerosis or "plaque"—has grown enormously in popularity over the past fifteen years. For patients who have a sudden occlusion of their artery—in other words, those who are suffering a heart attack—clinical trials have shown that stenting can save lives and prevent subsequent morbidity. If done in time, it reestablishes blood flow before damage to the heart muscle has become irreversible.

Most stents, however, are used in patients who are not having a heart attack but who have a narrowing in their coronary artery that is caused by plaque, which has been detected by angiography or, increasingly, by computed tomography (CT) scan. The theory has been that these narrowings need to be treated because, if left alone, they may rupture and cause a heart attack. This idea of preventive surgery—attacking the narrowing due to plaque before it causes a heart attack—is under revision today. Several leading cardiologists have long maintained that the underlying problem leading to heart attack is not the rupture of plaque that can be treated with stents. Patients susceptible to heart attacks typically have numerous sites with vulnerable plaques, most of which go undetected by angiography or CT scan. The way to reduce the risk of heart attack is not to use stents but rather to address the underlying cause of the proliferation of vulnerable plaque in the patient, by reducing blood pressure, controlling cholesterol and blood sugar, and encouraging the patient to stop smoking.

A recent clinical trial, which compared drug treatment alone to stenting plus drug treatment, provides substantial support to the multiple plaque theory.[13] Coming as a shock to many cardiologists, it showed that stents provide no added benefit over drugs alone in preventing heart attacks and other cardiovascular events. In other words, attacking plaque with stents does not increase life expectancy compared to more conservative treatment. It can improve symptoms of chest pain, but so can drugs alone, in many cases. As in the breast cancer and hernia examples, reliable information on the outcomes of care opens up options for patients: they need no longer be driven to surgery on the basis of fear of sudden death or a debilitating heart attack; they are free to weigh the risks and benefits and to select the treatment strategy that corresponds best to their preferences for managing their chest pain.

For still other conditions, the clinical trials required to clarify the main outcome are inconclusive or have yet to be completed; in these examples, patient preferences are as important as they are in situations where the outcomes are reasonably well studied. The value of the prostate specific antigen (PSA) test in detecting early-stage prostate cancer is an important contemporary example. The PSA test is highly sensitive, picking up potential prostate cancers as much as two years earlier than a digital rectal examination. Yet it is not clear if the treatment of early prostate cancer discovered by the PSA screening test offers benefit over no treatment.[14] What is clear is that the choice of treatment, once a cancer is discovered, involves different risks. Men who undergo surgery experience a high rate of impotence and incontinence. Men who undergo radiation also experience some risk for incontinence and impotence, although less so, but may experience radiation damage to the bowel and rectum. Neither treatment can guarantee that the patient will not die of metastatic disease. Men who choose watchful waiting avoid the immediate risks of intervention but may suffer incontinence, impotence, and death from prostate cancer if their tumor progresses.

The decision to undergo a PSA test is thus best characterized as a wager: men with early-stage prostate cancer discovered through PSA who undergo active treatment are betting that the risks and significant side effects of treatment (which are well known) are worth taking, even though they cannot be certain that there is a benefit in terms of survival from cancer, much less how great the benefit might be. As I will argue in other sections of this book, the various choices, including whether to have a PSA test in the first place, ought to be made not by the physician on the basis of his or her beliefs about both the value of the test and resulting treatments but rather by the patient. Indeed, the decision about tests and treatments for many conditions ought to be shared by doctor and patient.

The Ubiquitous Nature of Practice Variation

Over the years, my colleagues and I replicated the studies of variation in surgery in as many states as we could. The same patterns of variation for the highly disputed procedures were seen in studies in Massachusetts, Iowa, and California. We also reasoned that the patterns should generally be similar from one nation to another, at least among Western countries. Clinicians in different parts of the world generally have similar clinical options and they share a common world medical literature. Difficulties in interpreting physical signs and symptoms, evaluating disease severity, and diagnosing patient preferences respect neither state nor international boundaries.

Two colleagues from Europe, Klim McPherson and Oli Hovind, and I tested this hypothesis by studying the patterns of variation among New England hospital referral areas, Norwegian counties, and British health districts, which correspond roughly to our hospital service areas.[15] Altogether, we studied nine surgeries: hernia operations, appendectomy, gallbladder surgery, hysterectomy, prostate surgery for an enlarged prostate, tonsillectomy, lens extraction for cataracts, hemorrhoidectomy, and varicose vein stripping. Despite the differences in the organization of medical practices, payment systems, the numbers of surgeons, and the ethnic and social characteristics of Norwegians, Americans, and the British, the degree of variation for a given procedure was essentially the same in each country. The exceptions were for inguinal hernia repair, which was more variable among British health districts than between New England and Norwegian areas, and for hysterectomy, which was less variable in Norway. The clinical reasons for increased variability for inguinal hernia repair in the United Kingdom were discussed earlier—British physicians sometimes recommended a truss. The reasons for the lower hysterectomy rates in Norway remain unclear. Despite these minor differences, our finding of the consistency of variation was astonishing in many ways. Differences in the methods of organizing and financing health care have less to do with the decisions surgeons make than with the lack of solid evidence available for diagnosing and treating different conditions.

In recent years, the Dartmouth Atlas Project has been reporting on a regular basis the variation in surgical uptake across the United States for Medicare recipients enrolled in the traditional fee-for-service Medicare program. Discretionary surgery varies about as much today as in the time of Glover and in our early studies in New England.

Consider first the use of surgery for three common cancers. The incidence of colectomy for cancer of the colon shows relatively little variation among the 306 Dartmouth Atlas Project regions (Figure 4.2). The reason? Surgery is not really optional; it is required. For patients whose cancers have not spread, surgery can cure; for those whose cancer has already spread, it prevents obstruction of the bowel, a painful and fatal complication if not prevented (or treated) with surgery. Thus, virtually all patients with cancer of the bowel will receive a colectomy, such that the incidence of surgery closely follows the incidence of the cancer itself.

This is not so, however, for surgery for cancer of the breast and cancer of the prostate. Mastectomy is much more variable than colectomy for cancer of the colon. As discussed earlier, for most patients with early-stage breast cancer, the options include lumpectomy and mastectomy; the frequency of use of each option varies from region to region, creating variation in the treatment patterns well beyond that which might be expected based on the natural incidence of disease or distribution of patient preferences. For example, the incidence of mastectomy in the highest region is nearly eight times greater than in the lowest region. Prostatectomy for early-stage cancer of the prostate is even more variable. As discussed earlier, the increased variation here reflects underlying differences in the use of the PSA test for cancer screening, "creating" a higher incidence of prostate cancer in regions with higher screening rates. It is also reflected in the frequency of use of surgery, radiation, and watchful waiting among those who are diagnosed with prostate cancer. The range of variation in the use of surgery is extraordinary: rates of prostatectomy in the highest region are nearly nineteen times greater than in the lowest.

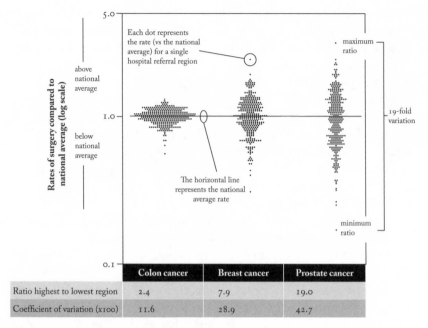

Figure 4.2.   The rates of surgery for colon cancer, breast cancer, and prostate cancer among hospital referral regions (2003 through 2005). (Source: Dartmouth Atlas Project database.)

Consider now the incidence of surgical interventions for narrowing of the arteries due to atherosclerosis. Figure 4.3 shows the pattern of variation among the 306 regions for coronary artery bypass graft surgery (CABG) and for percutaneous coronary intervention (PCI) (stents and angioplasty), which are undertaken to treat blockage in the arteries that feed the heart, carotid artery endarterectomy to treat the arteries in the neck that feed the brain, and lower extremity bypass surgery to treat blockage of arteries delivering blood to the legs.

It's my theory that each procedure varies much more than can reasonably be expected on the basis of illness rates or patient preferences. CABG, the least variable of the four procedures, is more variable than colectomy for colon cancer (one of the few procedures where incidence of illness appears to account for most of the variation). Carotid artery surgery, stenting of coronary arteries, and lower extremity bypass are substantially more variable. The rate in the highest region for CABG is nearly five times greater than in the lowest; for the other procedures, the ratio of highest to lowest is tenfold or

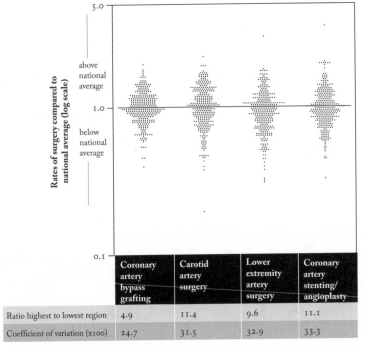

	Coronary artery bypass grafting	Carotid artery surgery	Lower extremity artery surgery	Coronary artery stenting/ angioplasty
Ratio highest to lowest region	4.9	11.4	9.6	11.1
Coefficient of variation (x100)	24.7	31.5	32.9	33.3

Figure 4.3.   The rates of surgery for atherosclerosis of selected arteries among hospital referral regions (2003 through 2005). (Source: Dartmouth Atlas Project database.)

greater. Interestingly, we find no evidence that stenting is being substituted for CABG: regions with higher rates of CABG also tend to have higher rates for stenting. Some of the treatment controversies associated with these procedures were discussed earlier.

Finally, consider the pattern of variation among four orthopedic procedures: hip fracture repair, knee and hip replacement undertaken to treat disability due to advanced arthritis of knee and hip joints, and back surgery, undertaken to treat back pain due to herniated disc or arthritis of the spine (Figure 4.4).

Why does hip fracture repair vary so little? Clinicians treating patients with hip fractures have little or no choice. The patient faces a life-threatening situation. He or she must be hospitalized and most undergo some form of procedure. The incidence of surgical repair of the hip thus corresponds closely to the incidence of hip fracture and the profile for hip fracture is "low variation," consistent with our theory that degree of variation signals degree of discretion. While the range in rates from high regions to

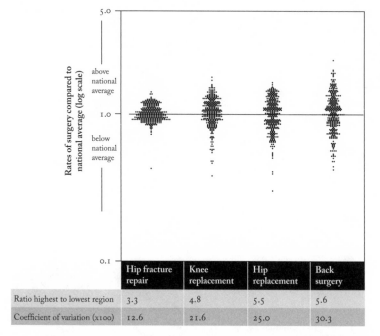

	Hip fracture repair	Knee replacement	Hip replacement	Back surgery
Ratio highest to lowest region	3.3	4.8	5.5	5.6
Coefficient of variation (x100)	12.6	21.6	25.0	30.3

Figure 4.4. The rates of surgery for selected orthopedic procedures among hospital referral regions (2003 through 2005). (Source: Dartmouth Atlas Project database.)

low regions is quite high, this is explained by very low rates in one region, namely Hawaii, which consistently registers as an extreme outlier in the Atlas database. This should not be interpreted to mean that hip fracture patients in Hawaii are not being treated in the hospital; the database shows that they are. Rather, for some reason, the incidence of hip fracture is incredibly low in the Hawaii region. Hip fracture hospitalizations are one of the few examples of health care utilization where variation reliably tracks variation in disease incidence. For example, the pattern of utilization, documented over many years in the Dartmouth Atlas Project, draws attention to an elevation in the incidence of hip fracture repair throughout the inland south, raising intriguing questions about what factor(s) might be causing this difference in illness rates.

The profile for the other orthopedic procedures displayed in Figure 4.4 shows considerably greater variation, primarily because the conditions for which these procedures are performed can be treated in more than one way. Osteoarthritis of the knee and hip can be treated surgically or medically, including lifestyle modification and weight loss. Disc disease and arthritis of the spine (spondylosis) can be treated surgically (using several procedures and devices), as well as medically, including with watchful waiting.

* * *

Variations in discretionary surgery of the magnitude displayed in this chapter pose an important challenge to the assumption that the demand for medical care is controlled by clinical science and patient preference. The remarkable variation in common procedures seen among Dartmouth Atlas Project regions is a consequence of the way decisions about preference-sensitive treatments are routinely made, and the rates of utilization of such treatments could shift, simply by changing physician opinion. Establishing a true market for preference-sensitive care, where utilization is determined by patient demand, will require a cultural change in the doctor-patient relationship. These are topics for Chapter 5.

5

Understanding the Market for Preference-Sensitive Surgery

Looking at the variations in rates of surgical procedures among geographic regions provides a highly aggregated snapshot of comparative performance, but these variations have their origins in the microcosm of the doctor-patient relationship, in the one-on-one exchange between an individual physician and a patient that results in the choice of treatment. When patients delegate decision making, as most now do, physicians are for the most part free to choose their own favorite treatments, so long as the treatment selected falls within the domain of a "clinically appropriate" option, that is, an option that conforms to prevailing theory and clinical science (whatever the quality and quantity of the evidence in support of that "science" may be). The medical opinions of referring physicians and surgeons who specialize in a specific procedure thus combine to determine the rate for any particular procedure in a given market.

As this chapter will show, the variation in the incidence of any particular surgery between regions tends to remain quite constant, even when measured over a decade or more. Thus regions have characteristic "surgical signatures" and regions with high rates of a surgery in the early 1990s still tend to have high rates today, and the cumulative effect is to expose large numbers of patients to surgical interventions that they may or may not have wanted. Rates can be reduced by setting quotas and otherwise imposing limits, but this will not guarantee that the right patients—those who are fully informed and choose surgery—will receive it.

The Surgical Signature Phenomenon

In our early studies in Maine, we noted that each community seemed to have its own characteristic pattern of surgical variation, which we came to call the "surgical signature."[1] You can actually identify a hospital service area by looking at its profile of rates for a handful of surgeries, as shown in Figure 5.1. In each hospital service area, a different procedure was performed most often. In Portland, prostatectomy for an enlarged prostate was the most commonly performed operation, exceeding the state average by 40% and the lowest region (Bangor) by more than 100%. In Lewiston, hysterectomy exceeded the state average by more than 60% and the lowest area for hysterectomy (neighboring Augusta) by more than 125%. Augusta led in surgery for varicose veins, with a rate almost 90% higher than the state average and

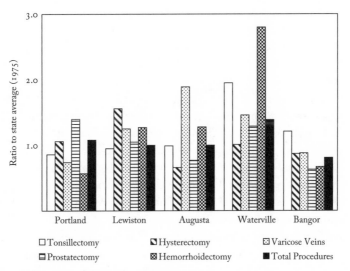

Figure 5.1.   The surgical signatures of the five most populous hospital service areas in Maine (1975). For each area, the rate relative to the state average for five surgical procedures is displayed. (Adapted from Wennberg, J. and A. Gittelsohn. 1975. Health Care Delivery in Maine I: Patterns of Use of Common Surgical Procedures. *Journal of the Maine Medical Association* 66:123–130, 149. Used with the permission of the Maine Medical Association.)

more than 2.5 times that of Portland. Surgeons practicing in the Waterville area were particularly prone to operate on hemorrhoids, achieving a rate 2.8 times greater than the state average and 4.6 times greater than the surgeons serving Portland. In Bangor, surgery rates overall were lower than in the other regions.

When confronted with the surgical signatures in their own community, physicians want to believe their practice profiles are the result of patient need. Time and time again, when my colleagues and I have presented our data to physicians, many in the audience argue vigorously against the notion that it is their opinions that play a major role in determining what kind of care their patients receive. Yet simply changing the opinions of local practitioners can have a remarkable effect on the rate of surgery in a region. In the case of tonsillectomy, as discussed in Chapter 3, Glover documented what happened when Dr. R. P. Garrow replaced a retiring school health officer who had great enthusiasm for the surgery, and in Morrisville, Vermont, local physicians dramatically and swiftly reduced the rate of tonsillectomy after deciding to seek a second opinion before recommending it.

Our monitoring of the rates of surgery in Maine—and the publication of the results in the *Journal of the Maine Medical Association*—provides yet a third example of abrupt change, this one explained when the management of a hospital in Lewiston, Maine, embarrassed by knowledge of its high-surgery rate for hysterectomy, imposed a quota on the number of procedures that should be performed. Over one four-year period in the 1970s, hysterectomy rates in Lewiston were such that over 800 more women were operated on than would have experienced surgery had the average rate for the state applied.[2] Most of the surgeries were undertaken by two very enthusiastic surgeons in Lewiston, who kept themselves so busy that about 60% of women in the region were estimated to be uterus-free by age 70.

The intervention in Lewiston was organized by Dr. Daniel Hanley, the editor of the *Journal of the Maine Medical Association* and secretary of the Maine Medical Association. Like Dr. Buttles in Vermont, who used our data to inform physicians in Morrisville about their high rate of tonsillectomy, Dan went from town to town in Maine, showing physicians our data on the patterns of variation in surgery in the state. Hanley met with Dr. Buell Miller and several of his colleagues from the state chapter of the American College of Gynecology to devise a plan to challenge the practice patterns of the gynecologists in Lewiston. After several meetings, the medical leadership in the hospital serving the Lewiston area decided to govern the quantity of surgery by imposing a quota on the number of hysterectomies the surgeons could perform over the course of a year. The quota was set to bring the rate of hysterectomies performed down to the state average. The efficacy of this policy of limits and its stability over time were quite remarkable. By 1981, the rate of hysterectomy had declined 45%, where it remained until at least 1994 (Figure 5.2).

The data in Figure 5.2 attest to the precision with which providers can control the rate of elective surgery. They met their production goal, year in and year out. Yet despite the success of the quota in bringing down the rate of hysterectomy, the physicians were not necessarily operating on the right women. There was no way to ensure that physicians were not doing unnecessary surgeries in some cases and failing to perform needed (or wanted) operations in others, because the quota did not guarantee that the surgeons were taking into account their patients' own preferences. Perhaps there were women in Lewiston whose symptoms were so bothersome that they wanted hysterectomies but were not offered surgery. It was also possible that women whose uterus was removed would have chosen watchful waiting or hormone therapy, had they been given an opportunity to truly understand the tradeoffs of the surgery, its very real risks as well as its potential benefits.

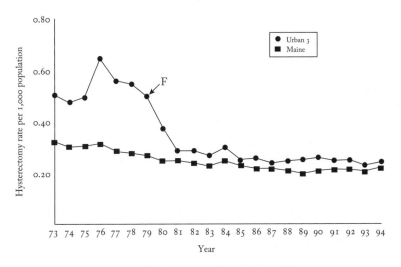

Figure 5.2.   Hysterectomy rates for Maine and for residents of hospital service area III from 1973 through 1994. The figure gives the age-adjusted hysterectomy rate over a twenty-four-year period for residents of Lewiston, Maine (Urban 3). Data feedback (F) first took place in 1979. (Source: Keller, R.B., D. E. Wennberg, and D. N. Soule. 1997. Changing physician behavior: The Maine Medical Assessment Foundation. *Quality Management in Health Care* Summer;5(4):1–11. Reproduced with permission from *Quality Management in Health Care*, Lippincott Williams & Wilkins, publishers.)

This is the essential fallacy of quotas, or indeed any other attempt to control demand for discretionary surgery on the basis of rules of thumb, or "practice guidelines" that fail to take the individual patient's own preference into account. The state's average for hysterectomy was, after all, merely the weighted average of the variation in medical opinion among the physicians and surgeons practicing in the Maine's hospital service areas. To put this another way, the Maine average would have been different had a different group of surgeons decided to practice there. Making medical decisions for preference-sensitive care on the basis of statistical averages provides no assurance that procedures are being performed on patients who need or want the operations they get.

Ubiquitous and Persistent

The surgical signature phenomenon has turned out to be commonplace, a characteristic of health care in every region of the country, including care delivered by the most prestigious of providers. One of my favorite small area comparisons focused on Boston and New Haven, two communities whose residents receive most of their care from faculty members of some of the nation's most renowned medical schools. One would assume that because of the credentials of these hospitals and physicians, the care received by the populations in these two cities would be of the highest quality, based on the most credible medical evidence. Yet how that "high quality" care differed! For some operations, the chances of surgery were much higher in New Haven than in Boston, while for others, Bostonians were much more likely to undergo surgery. During the 1980s, for example, a resident of New Haven was twice as likely to undergo a hysterectomy or coronary artery bypass graft (CABG) as a Bostonian. For carotid endarterectomy (surgery to unblock the major arteries feeding the brain) and hip replacement surgery, the risk was, respectively, 2.4 and 1.6 times greater for residents of Boston.[3]

The common cause for these differences between these two areas served by academic medical centers could be traced, once again, to Glover's theory of medical opinions strongly held by small groups of physicians concerning medical efficacy or value to patients. Through interviews with physicians in both Boston and New Haven, I learned that the low rate of carotid endarterectomy rates in New Haven compared to Boston could be attributed to a group of skeptical neurologists who simply did not believe in the procedure, preferring aspirin to surgery for any patient who came to them for advice. By contrast, the physicians in Boston had, on average, greater "faith" in carotid artery surgery (although relative to many other parts of the country, the Boston rates were rather low). The conservative medical management of coronary artery disease and symptoms of menopause was more popular in Boston, whereas clinicians in New Haven more often preferred surgical management, which meant that more CABG and hysterectomies were performed. On the other hand, New Haven physicians were more enthusiastic about the conservative management of arthritis of the hip.

Beginning in the 1990s, our work on the Dartmouth Atlas Project has made it possible to monitor the surgical signature phenomenon throughout the United States, and the pattern is the same writ large. Take the rates for surgery for degenerative diseases of the hip and knee, conditions that are often treated by orthopedic surgeons. In Chapter 4, I illustrated the striking variation among the 306 Dartmouth Atlas Project regions in the use of knee or hip replacement for these conditions. The chance of having a knee or hip replacement *varied about five times* from the lowest to the highest region in the country.

Yet within a given region, there is a remarkable constancy in the pattern of practice over time: regions that rank high in a procedure rate at one period in time tend to do so in subsequent periods. This is evident through the correlations in Figure 5.3, which shows the relationship between rates for hip replacement and knee replacement in 1996 and 2005. The coefficient

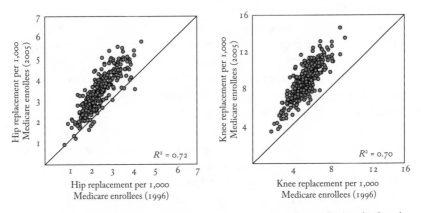

Figure 5.3. The association between surgery rates in 1996 and 2005 for hip (*left*) and knee replacement (*right*) among hospital referral regions. (Source: Dartmouth Atlas Project database.)

of determination (the R^2 statistic) indicates a strong association: a large majority—about 70%—of the variation in surgery rates for knee and hip replacement in 2005 was "explained" by the variation in surgery rates in 1996, a decade earlier. (See page 274 in the Appendix for an explanation of the R^2 statistic and regression lines.) This constancy was maintained, even though there was a substantial trend upward in overall rate; the U.S. average rate of surgery increased 61% for knee replacement and 37% for total hip replacement. Most regions experienced substantial increases and there was little evidence of regression to the mean.

Consistency in the rates of specific procedures over time is seen for other procedures, although to a lesser degree. The correlation between inpatient surgery in 1996 and 2005 for back surgery was $R^2 = 0.48$; for carotid artery surgery, $R^2 = 0.43$; for radical prostatectomy, $R^2 = 0.38$; for mastectomy, $R^2 = 0.33$; for coronary artery surgery, $R^2 = 0.32$; and for PCI, $R^2 = 0.32$.

The Paradoxical Role of Surgeon Supply in Rates of Surgery

What about the relationship between the supply of resources and the use of preference-sensitive surgery? For years, health service researchers have documented that more surgeons per capita means more surgery per capita, but these studies have been primarily concerned with the association between the overall supply of surgeons and the overall rate of surgery.[4] More recently, we have been looking at the association between the rate for an *individual* procedure and the supply of the surgical specialists who perform the surgery. Given the evidence that more surgeons means more surgery, it came as a surprise to find out that among the 306 hospital referral regions, *there is little or no relationship between the rate of a given procedure and the supply of the surgeons trained in the specialty that performs that procedure.*

Take the case of the per capita number of orthopedic surgeons and the rates of hip replacement and knee replacement (Figure 5.4). What can account for this puzzling lack of correlation? In a "rational" health care market, an incremental increase in professional capacity would presumably be spread on the basis of clinical need. In the case of capacity to treat patients with orthopedic conditions, it would be spread among surgical management of all the conditions that can be treated by orthopedists: arthritis of the hip, knee, and back; carpal tunnel disease; shoulder conditions; impairments of the foot and ankle; sports medicine and trauma; etc. One would thus expect to see a positive association between individual procedures and overall surgical capacity. In other words, if the health care market functioned in the way

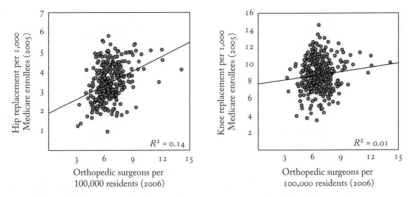

Figure 5.4. The association between supply of orthopedic surgeons (2006) and rates for hip (*left*) and knee replacement (*right*) (2005) among hospital referral regions. (Source: Dartmouth Atlas Project database.)

predicted by rational agency theory, surgical utilization in regions that gain orthopedists would be allocated in a way that ensured that all bases were covered, and patients with different conditions would get the surgeries they need. Moreover, regions with low rates for a given procedure, and thus presumably greater unmet need, would be expected to increase the number of orthopedists capable of providing those procedures. Capacity in high-rate regions for that procedure ought to decline. In other words, you would expect to see regression toward the mean. But this is not what we see.

I think an important explanation for this phenomenon is subspecialization. In their initial training programs, orthopedic surgeons are exposed to a cross-section of conditions that members of their specialty treat, such as arthritis of the knee and hip, which can be treated surgically with joint replacements. Other conditions orthopedists encounter include carpel tunnel syndrome (surgical repair), trauma (various procedures), and a number of conditions affecting the shoulder, ankle, and foot (surgical repairs). However, later in their training or early in their practice years, they tend to specialize in one or two of these conditions, achieving greater competence in a narrow range of surgical procedures, with some specializing in backs, others in hip and knee replacement, and still others in shoulder surgery. When it all gets added up at the local market level, or the regional level, there is little correlation between *overall* supply of orthopedic surgeons and the number who devote their workload to a particular subset of procedures. Some regions may have a lot of orthopedists who primarily perform back surgery, while others may have a handful who perform back surgery, some who perform hip surgery, and others who perform shoulders and hand surgery.

We have seen a similar lack of correlation between the supply of vascular surgeons and carotid artery surgery and lower extremity arterial bypass procedures, between general surgeons and mastectomy and gallbladder surgery, and between urologists and prostatectomy.[5]

The exception—and one that seems to prove the rule—is the association between the supply of interventional cardiologists and cardiac catheterization laboratories and the rate of angiography, the invasive diagnostic test used to pinpoint the location of blockages to the arteries of the heart. Unlike orthopedic surgeons who perform many different procedures, invasive cardiologists are trained to focus on two interconnected procedures—angiography and percutaneous coronary interventions (PCIs) (see discussion in Chapter 4). Angiography and PCIs must take place in a specially equipped clinic, the "cath lab." Angiography and PCI thus require both a specialized workforce specifically trained in the procedures and a specialized workplace where the procedures can be performed. Not surprisingly, the supply of invasive cardiologists and cardiac catheterization laboratories is correlated with the incidence of angiography and PCI (Figure 5.5). Together, the supply of invasive cardiologists and catheterization laboratories account for about 40% of the variation in rates of angiography and PCIs.

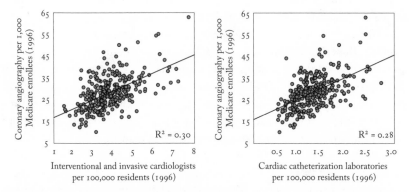

Figure 5.5.   The association between supply of interventional cardiologists (*left*) and cardiac catheterization laboratories (*right*) and rates of angiography among hospital referral regions (1996). (Source: Wennberg, D. E., and J. D. Birkmeyer, eds. 1999. *The Dartmouth Atlas of Cardiovascular Health Care.* The Center for the Evaluative Clinical Sciences, Dartmouth Medical School; and the Center for Outcomes Research and Evaluation, Maine Medical Center. Chicago: AHA Press.)

Does this mean that the PCI procedure should be classified as a supply-sensitive service (a concept that I will discuss at greater length later in this book)? Not at all. When done as a means for treating a heart attack, clinical trials show that the procedure is highly effective in reducing mortality and cardiac damage. When undertaken for this purpose, the procedure is an example of effective care. However, in most examples of its use, the primary purpose is to treat chest pain or stable angina, and for this indication, as discussed in Chapter 4, the procedure is elective and thus preference-sensitive—there is more than one effective treatment and the choice should depend on patient preference, not on local medical opinion.

High Rates Do Not Necessarily Mean Unnecessary Care from the Physician's Point of View

A study done in 2000 by Gillian Hawker and her colleagues in Ontario, Canada,[6] provides the missing link to gaining an understanding of the market for preference-sensitive care: it helps us understand why the variations in knee and hip replacement are so stable over time; why surgery rates show little regression to the mean; why there are no apparent barriers to the market entry of orthopedic surgeons who specialize in knee and hip replacements into regions where the rates of surgery are already high; and why all of this can occur without transgressing professional standards and norms—at least under the prevalent rational agency model that delegates clinical decisions to physicians. Hawker and her colleagues sought to understand the need for joint replacement in two Canadian regions, one with a high-surgery rate and the other with a low rate. Initially they focused on defining medical need in the traditional way. Using the latest evidence-based guidelines for identifying candidates who were clinically appropriate for surgery, they interviewed a representative sample of the general population over 40 years of age. A standardized questionnaire was used to identify those with limitation of motion and symptoms of arthritis of the hip and knee sufficiently poor to warrant further assessment of need for surgery. The "patients" who passed this initial screen were then given an imaging examination to define the patient population who, according to practice guidelines, needed surgery.

The first surprise came when the researchers found that the population-based *need* defined in this way was much higher than the observed rates of joint replacement surgery, even in the region where rates of surgery were higher. This suggested substantial *underuse* of surgery, not exactly good news for the Canadian health care system, which already operates under the cloud of suspicion that it withholds valuable care for economic reasons. Indeed, it was not good news for the American health care system, either. The per capita number of patients whom the study identified as clinically appropriate for joint replacement exceeded the surgery rates found in the Dartmouth Atlas Project region in the United States where joint replacement rates are the highest, suggesting underuse in this country as well.

But the final step in the Hawker group's assessment process produced an even greater surprise. The patients who met the evidence-based clinical guidelines for undergoing joint replacement were then asked a series of questions designed to ascertain their desire and willingness to undergo surgery. Much of the interview focused on the patient's preferences—given their clinical situation, would they prefer surgery, or would they prefer more conservative means of managing their disability? Only *14.9% of the patients in the high-rate region and only 8.5% in the low-rate region who were eligible for surgery, according to evidence-based clinical guidelines, actually wanted surgery.* That means that given the current stage in the evolution of their clinical problem, between 86% and 91% preferred medical management. A revised estimate of need that included patient preferences thus suggested that the surgery rates in Canada were close to meeting need, *if only those who wanted surgery were the ones who actually got it.*

The Hawker study provides an important insight into the limitations of the prevalent method for determining surgical need based on "objective" clinical information, as obtained from clinical history (progression of morbidity), the clinical interview (current symptom level), the physical examination (limitation of mobility), and biomedical tests (presence of joint disease documented by imaging examinations). Even when evidence-based, the method can lead to unnecessary surgery—that is, surgery on patients who do not want the operation.

The Hawker study also points to the weakness of delegated decision making in constraining demand. At least in the case of knee and hip replacement, the number of patients who meet "best practices" appropriateness criteria for medical need established in this fashion exceeds the amount of surgery now provided, even in regions where the rate of the surgery is the highest. However, the Hawker benchmark indicates a much lower level of demand when clinical decision making is based on choices made by fully informed patients, rather than a decision that has been delegated to the physician (or made by a less than fully informed patient). In other words, when the market for surgery operates under the assumption that it is rational to delegate decision making to the physicians, orthopedic surgeons have a nearly bottomless well of potential patients to work on, at least according to their clinical criteria for appropriateness—even when their criteria are evidence-based. This means that if a new surgeon comes to town specializing in knee replacement, more patients will get new knees. And if that town happens to become the home for yet another orthopedist who performs knee replacements, even more patients will undergo knee replacement. But having more surgeons does not mean the right patients (i.e., those who not only "need" new knees according to professional judgment but also want them) are undergoing surgery.

* * *

For a few surgical procedures, notably hip fractures repair and colectomy for colon cancer, the incidence of illness imposes a natural limit on the demand for surgery. In other words, the rate of surgery tracks the incidence of the condition. For most procedures, however, the rate of surgery varies substantially from one market area to another, unrelated to variation in illness—or patient preferences. Because patient preferences are not now routinely and systematically elicited, and the clinical decision process does not recognize the central importance of an accurate diagnosis of what patients want (as opposed to what physicians think they need), many patients are likely undergoing surgery that they would not want if they were fully informed and empowered to participate in a meaningful way in the choice of treatment.

Establishing a market where the utilization of preference-sensitive treatment is determined by patient demand will require a cultural change in the doctor-patient relationship. It will require replacing delegated decision making with shared decision making, and establishing informed patient choice as the standard of care for determining medical necessity.

Chapter 6 describes a decade-long research project targeted at understanding the clinical reasons for practice variation in the surgical treatment of benign prostate hyperplasia, or BPH, a condition that affects many men as they age. This research led to an experiment to replace delegated decision making with shared decision making, to empower meaningful patient participation in treatment choice.

6

Learning What Works and What Patients Want

In the late 1970s, our research team was able to move beyond the statistical description of surgical variation to undertake a series of detailed studies in the state of Maine that led to a diagnosis of the clinical causes of variation and a strategy for reducing unwarranted variation in preference-sensitive treatments. The opportunity evolved from the publication in 1975 in the *Journal of the Maine Medical Association* of our data on geographic variation (including the surgical signature for the five largest Maine communities discussed in Chapter 5).[1] In our paper, we made the then rather novel argument that variations that cannot be attributed to illness or access to care should be interpreted as an indication of variation in professional opinion, and the remedy for that variation ought to be outcomes research.

In an accompanying editorial, Dr. Daniel Hanley, the editor of the journal, challenged his fellow physicians to respond. "All this will require a series of detailed looks by those who know the situation best—the Physicians themselves," he wrote. "This means time and effort, but the rewards are great: a better understanding of the decision-making process in Medicine (Surgery)…and a chance to build a medical education program that is tailored to demonstrated needs."[2]

Dan titled his editorial, in his typical tongue-in-cheek fashion, "A Tool for All Committees," and he acknowledged that our work and recommendations would undoubtedly raise some hackles. But as secretary of the Maine Medical

Association and a well-known and highly respected physician in his state, Dan had a way of smoothing the way for us. He was for many years an active member of the U.S. Olympic Committee, serving as its principal advisor in dealing with the epidemic of drug use among Olympic athletes that broke out in the mid-1970s; he was also the beloved campus physician for Bowdoin College. Moreover, he was extremely proud of his profession but insistent on its need to take responsibility for the quality of health care. Primarily because of Dan's advocacy, the Commonwealth Fund agreed to invest some capital into what became the Maine Medical Assessment Foundation, a nonprofit group that served as a focal point for promoting professional accountability for practice variations and treatment outcomes (Box 6.1).

Box 6.1.   *A Short History of the Maine Medical Assessment Foundation*

The Foundation had its beginning in 1980 as the Maine Medical Assessment Program, organized by Dr. Daniel Hanley under the Commonwealth Fund's grant to facilitate the feedback of information on practice variation to Maine physicians. Over its first ten years, the project organized study groups in internal medicine, pediatrics, urology, gynecology, and orthopedics to examine practice variations related to their specialties. Each of these groups undertook the "three-step process." Step One was to identify blatant examples of overuse or underuse of care and urge local physicians to change their practices. This approach worked reasonably well in the case of hysterectomies in Lewiston, Maine, as I described in Chapter 5. If the variation was not obviously due to the delivery of unnecessary care, Step Two was to undertake a review of the scientific literature to identify what would nowadays be called "best practices." If disagreement remained after review of the scientific literature, our third step was to undertake "outcomes" research to reduce scientific uncertainty.[3]

The pediatrics, gynecology, and orthopedic study groups carried out "Step One" interventions that led to a rapid reduction of the utilization rates in high-rate regions. Three of the study groups joined with academic researchers to undertake "Step Three" outcomes research for low back pain (spine surgery), abnormal uterine bleeding (hysterectomy), and an enlarged prostate (prostate surgery).

(continued)

In 1989, the program was reorganized as The Maine Medical Assessment Foundation, and Dr. Robert Keller, an orthopedic surgeon from Belfast, Maine, succeeded Dan Hanley as executive director of the foundation. Over the next several years, Bob worked to enlarge the feedback network to include fourteen active study groups, and my son David Wennberg, along with David Soule, a senior data analyst who had been a coauthor on our surgical paper in the *Journal of Maine Medical Association*, created most of the feedback reports to the study groups. The success of the foundation in changing practice patterns and in organizing physicians in everyday practice to study the outcomes of their care, attracted a good deal of attention in Washington, thanks in large part to the friendship between Dan Hanley and Senate majority leader George Mitchell. Through this avenue of influence, the Maine Medical Assessment Foundation came to serve as the model for Section 5008 of the Clintons' Health Security Act calling for the establishment of Regional Professional Foundations to provide infrastructure for physicians to investigate practice variations and participate in studies to reduce unwarranted variation.[4] But this was not to be. Without federal support or consistent support from payers, the financial condition of the foundation grew more and more precarious and ultimately, in 2000, it had to close its doors.

We worked as a team to get Maine physicians on board for a program aimed at understanding practice variation and improving clinical decision making. Our research team prepared reports for "feedback" to Maine physicians, much along the lines of those we used in Vermont. The feedback sessions took place over a two-day retreat at Dartmouth's Minary Center, an idyllic lodge on the shores of Squam Lake, the setting of the 1981 movie "On Golden Pond." The sessions were organized around specialty groups and the targets for feedback were the procedures they performed. Typically, the first hour or so was spent establishing credibility of the data, a task that, by then, I thought I had more or less mastered—at least I thought so until I met Dr. Robert Keller, who led the orthopedic study group. After I went through a series of reports showing variation in knee, hip, and back surgery—and thinking I saw an emerging consensus that the variation was related to surgical opinion—I showed the pattern of variation in hospitalizations for a fractured hip. Bob Keller immediately challenged the validity of the data. Our reports showed that hip fractures varied nearly as extensively as back surgery. But Keller knew that hip fractures left no room for discretion: everyone had to be admitted to hospital; illness is a primary driver of utilization; and the Dartmouth data just did not make sense. David Soule and I quickly regrouped and took another look at the data. We had made a mistake—miscoding hip fracture to include several other fractures that did not belong in the group—thus creating variation that was not real. Within a few hours we were able to rerun the data and establish that hip fracture hospitalizations showed little variation among Maine communities.

Eventually, Bob became a strong advocate for the Maine project and ultimately succeeded Dan as the executive director of the Maine Medical Assessment Foundation. Indeed, one of the most important outcomes of these early forays into improving clinical decision making was the recognition of the importance of involving practicing physicians in the process of assessing evidence. We also formulated a systematic method, involving three separate but interlocking steps, for assessing existing medical evidence and conducting outcomes research (see Box 6.1).

A key—and revolutionary—component of our conception of outcomes research was including the patient's view of the consequences of different treatment options.[5] This research would lead to the development of systematic methods for gathering outcomes data and probing the preferences of patients—methods that would have a brief moment on the national stage until they were sidelined in the mid-1990s, when the U.S. Congress pulled the rug out from under comparative effectiveness research.

Doing the Three-Step for Prostate Disease

The most successful and longest lasting research program to grow out of the Maine experience proved to be the study of the outcomes of treatment for an enlarged prostate, or "BPH" (Box 6.2). The John A. Hartford Foundation, through the advocacy of, first, John Billings and then his successor, Richard Sharpe, provided the generous and long-term funding required to sustain the program. Starting in the early 1980s, it continued for more than a decade: it led to the development of a series of methods and strategies for outcomes research and, as I discuss in Chapter 7, provided the prototype for the Patient Outcomes Research Teams (PORTs) organized by the federal government in 1988.

Box 6.2.   *What Is BPH?*

The reader who is not familiar with BPH will need a little background on the clinical issues involved. First, BPH is the abbreviation for "benign prostatic hyperplasia," a noncancerous growth of the prostate gland that is part of the normal aging process in men. Sometime beyond their 50th birthday, most men become aware of changes in their patterns of urination and many experience annoying urinary tract symptoms. The symptoms include difficulty in urination, the need to get up frequently at night to urinate, and an uncomfortable urgency to urinate. Some men experience an embarrassing dribbling after urination and a few will have acute urinary retention, a very painful episode during which they cannot urinate at all and must seek immediate medical attention to have a catheter put into the bladder to drain the urine. At the time of our initial research, prostatectomy—the surgical removal of the prostate gland, which sits at the base of the penis near the outlet of the bladder—was the only active treatment available for BPH.

In Maine in the late 1970s, the probability of undergoing a prostate operation for BPH by age 75 ranged from less than 20% of men in some parts of the state to more than 60% in other parts. A study group consisting of urologists from around the state was formed to address the reasons for these striking variations in surgery rates, under the leadership of Dr. Robert Timothy, a urologist practicing at the Maine Medical Center in Portland. Reports were made available to each urologist comparing the rates of prostatectomy for BPH in his own and in all other hospital service areas in Maine. Because most hospitals in Maine had only one or two urologists, and most hospital areas had only one hospital, the connection between the surgical decisions made by the physicians receiving the reports and the rates of surgery in their hospital service area was inescapable.

The project began with a two-day Minary Center retreat with our research team and the urologists from Maine that illuminated why rates of treatment varied. Maine urologists held two distinctly different surgical theories, which they used to justify their decisions to operate. Most urologists practiced under the "preventive" theory of surgery, which was rooted in the idea that the operation should be done early to prevent disease progression and bad outcomes from occurring at a later date. The assumption was similar to the silent gallstone assumption discussed in Chapter 4—that early removal solved a problem that would only get worse if nothing was done. By operating early on the prostate, the backup of urine behind the enlarged prostate could be avoided—a backup that could damage the bladder and kidneys and even prove fatal upon occasion. Moreover, by operating early—when the patient was younger and healthier—the surgery carried less risk than it might if performed later. Thus, life expectancy for the population of patients with early BPH would be increased and morbidity would be reduced by early surgery. Or so the adherents to the preventive theory of BPH believed.

A minority of Maine urologists did not hold such a pessimistic view of the natural history of untreated BPH. In their opinion, for most men the disease would not progress to the point where surgery was needed to prevent damage to the bladder or the kidneys or to save the patient's life. Under their theory, surgery was justified by its superior ability to improve the quality of life by reducing troublesome urinary tract *symptoms,* such as difficulty in voiding, frequency of urination, and urgency, as well as its power to reduce the risk of acute urinary retention and urinary tract infections.

In addition to these disagreements concerning the theoretical basis for undertaking surgery (differences sometimes found even among urologists working together in the same hospital), physicians also varied according to the clinical rules of thumb they used to determine medical need. Some physicians relied primarily on a simple biomedical test to determine need, namely urine flow rate—the volume of urine a patient could void into a collection device per minute. If urine flow fell below a critical minimum, in their opinion, surgery was needed. Others measured postvoid residual (the amount of urine that was left in the bladder after urination). Others, like some physicians Bloor encountered in his tonsillectomy study, relied mostly on clinical history, recommending surgery for patients who were getting up two or more times a night.

In the lively conversations and sometimes heated debates over the reasons to operate, it became apparent that opinions differed as much over actual fact as over theory. We asked the physicians to estimate the probability that a patient would have a bad outcome from surgery, such as an operative death, impotence, postoperative leakage of urine (incontinence), and strictures caused by urethral scarring (urethral stricture). Opinions diverged markedly. Estimates of the chances for acute urinary retention were similarly varied. Recurrent growth of prostate tissue and the occasional need for another operation were recognized as problems, but opinions differed substantially on how much of a problem these issues represented. There was uniform agreement among all physicians—the preventive as well as the quality-of-life camps—that surgery improved symptoms and functional status but little agreement as to how much improvement it could provide, and for which patients. Indeed, more fundamentally, there was no agreed-on method for objectively measuring the burden of urinary symptoms.

As a result of these conversations, our research team quickly proceeded to the second step in the three-step process. We reviewed the textbooks and journal articles on BPH to see if the medical literature could be used to come up with recommendations for best practices that would reduce the uncertainty and disagreements over fact and theory. The results of the literature review were disappointing. We found no reports of randomized controlled clinical trials (RCTs) comparing prostatectomy to watchful waiting. Indeed, we could not even find any population-based cohort studies—the "second-best" methodology for evaluating outcomes. Perhaps most astonishing of all, even studies that were designed to look at quality-of-life improvement asked physicians rather than patients to evaluate symptom relief.

It simply was not possible to get a handle on the risks and benefits. The estimates on which the urologists depended came from hospital-based case series of patients. Case history studies can suffer from what is called *publication bias*. Because the decision to publish is voluntary, only institutions with good results are motivated to publish. The literature thus tends to give a more optimistic estimate for benefits and an underestimation of harms than would be the case if all hospitals were routinely reporting their findings.

The inadequacies in the literature left us with puzzling uncertainties about what the results of prostate surgery actually were. Were patients' symptoms eased? Was the risk of acute urinary retention reduced, or the risk of serious injury to the kidneys and bladder? There was no way to know from the available literature. We needed to proceed to the third step—conducting outcome research. This was to give our group the opportunity to test a number of ideas and concepts for applying interdisciplinary research teams to evaluate the effectiveness of medical care, many of which I had first encountered during the five years that I was a member of the Center for the Analysis of Health Practices at the Harvard School of Public Health (Box 6.3).

Large Databases Provide Some Answers

At the time our group was seeking to help the urologists of Maine come to grips with practice variations, we were also conducting research into new ways to study outcomes using data from Medicare claims. Because most BPH operations are done on men over 65 years of age, the Medicare claims data were well suited for studying this condition. Medicare claims data make a certain type of outcomes study—population-based cohort studies—possible

Box 6.3. *The Center for the Analysis of Health Practices at the Harvard School of Public Health*

The Center for the Analysis of Health Practices was the inspiration of Howard Hiatt, then dean of Harvard's School of Public Health. Howard, an accomplished professor of medicine and well-known biomedical researcher, was one of the first to recognize the important role that physicians play in the growth of health care costs, and given his background in clinical medicine, he was acutely aware of its scientific weaknesses. On becoming dean of the School of Public Health, he decided to something about it. He understood, as had Kerr White at Johns Hopkins, that the sciences that prospered in schools of public health, such as epidemiology, biostatistics, decision analysis, and the social sciences, were of vital importance to the orderly development of the scientific basis of clinical medicine. In 1974, he created the Center for the Analysis of Health Practices as the focal point for integrating these disciplines into a "science of health care delivery" and brought on board John Bunker, the chair of the Department of Anesthesiology at Stanford University. While at Stanford, John, together with Fred Mosteller, head of Harvard's statistics department, was instrumental in a groundbreaking investigation into "unexplained" variations in surgical death rates among hospitals—a study euphemistically known as "the institutional differences study."[6] The study raised many issues concerning the quality of surgical practices in the United States and set the agenda for much of our discussion at the center at Harvard.

Under Bunker's and Mosteller's leadership, the focus of intellectual development became a biweekly seminar over dinner held at the Harvard Faculty Club. The price of membership was agreement by each participant to present a paper on some aspect of the evaluation of surgery and to agree that the paper be included in the proceedings of the seminar, which ultimately were published by Oxford University Press.[7] The seminar members included economists, decision analysts, sociologists, biostatisticians, epidemiologists, and clinicians, each with different perspectives and different contributions to make to the group goal of understanding surgical practice. It was during this time that John Bunker, Jack Fowler, and I first conducted open-ended interviews

(continued)

with patients who had undergone hysterectomies, learning firsthand about their surgical experiences. It became clear from their stories that the outcomes that mattered to patients were not necessarily high on the list of those valued by physicians. For patients, depression and decreased interest in sex following hysterectomy were important outcomes, ones that few physicians seemed to recognize as noteworthy. Although this research remained preliminary and did not lead to a publication, the experience anchored in my mind the importance of direct dialog with the patient to establish the list of outcomes that should be the target of outcomes research.

The experience proved to be a formative one, setting the stage for the interdisciplinary approach that would come to characterize our research efforts in Maine and, ultimately, the organization of Dartmouth's Center for the Evaluative Clinical Sciences in 1988.

on a grand scale. Thus, the large majority of American men who are over 65 years of age and have had a prostatectomy can be included in a cohort study of the outcomes of this operation. For this segment of the population, there is no selection bias, because we could look at virtually every man over age 65 who underwent surgery.

The value of the Medicare database rests in part in the completeness of the transaction information it contains. Each time a hospital or a physician provides a medical service (such as a prostatectomy), a bill is submitted to Medicare that identifies the services performed. When another service is performed, another bill is submitted, and these events can be linked for each patient. If a second prostate surgery is performed, this becomes known; if further diagnostic studies are done, this is recorded. If the patient dies, this too is noted. By linking these data together for all patients in Maine, a complete enumeration of important outcomes and the time between events could be obtained for patients 65 years of age and older,[8] making it possible to calculate the risk for reoperation, for subsequent diagnostic interventions, and for mortality.

Our initial (unpublished) study identified all Medicare patients in Maine who had a prostatectomy over a three-year period. The importance of publication bias in the previously published literature quickly became apparent. The actual outcomes for Maine patients who underwent surgery were substantially worse than predicted by the published medical literature. An extensive review of the literature for a 1975 National Institutes of Health conference on BPH estimated postoperative mortality of prostatectomy to be "less than one percent even though poor risk patients are rarely denied the operation."[9] In reality, at least in Maine, 4.7% of Medicare patients 65 years of age and older were dead within three months of their prostatectomy. For some men, the risk was much higher. Mortality reached 35% by six months for men who resided in nursing homes before their operation. How much of this mortality was attributable to the operation and how much was due to other illnesses could not be ascertained without a clinical trial. However, as our research was to show, the principal reason for undertaking the operation for most patients was to improve the quality of life. In the months following the operation, quality of life is low because of the short-term effects of the surgery, so men who die so soon after surgery gain very little, if anything.

The literature-based estimates for long-term morbidity were also quite optimistic: According to the 1975 literature review,[10] "Long-term morbidity is limited. The procedure provides correction of urinary stasis in approximately 90–98 percent of patients operated upon. The need for further operative treatment is uncommon." Again, the Medicare data showed a very different picture for Maine. We used the claims to identify complications from surgery. Over a four-year period after surgery, 13% of surgery patients experienced a scarring (stricture) of the urethra that required treatment—sometimes additional surgery; 20% of men underwent further diagnostic workups, usually involving having a cystoscope inserted into the urethra; and 10% had a second prostatectomy. At the end of four years, only 52% of patients having a prostatectomy were still alive and free from one or more of the postoperative complications just listed. This pessimistic estimate for the long-term cure rate (i.e., those who were alive and free from subsequent urological intervention) was in stark contrast to the conclusion reached in the literature.

The claims data studies had an immediate impact on Maine's Urology Study Group. The information changed the way they treated urinary symptoms in men who were also chronically ill, as most physicians became much more reluctant to recommend a prostatectomy to their elderly, high-risk patients, particularly those residing in nursing homes.

Feedback of information on the outcomes of the patients whom the urologists of Maine were responsible for treating proved decisive in opening the door to the next step in the assessment process: evaluation of the specific theories behind the variation in practice we were documenting. But to do this, I needed to expand the research team beyond medical care epidemiologists. Fortunately, several colleagues with the necessary skills had already become deeply interested in studying practice variation and their recruitment to the Maine project would prove decisive to its ultimate success. Jack Fowler, whose skills as a social psychologist were critical in measuring patient outcomes, continued to stay in touch and we had already conducted some preliminary studies. In 1983, Dr. Albert Mulley, who at a young age had become head of primary care medicine at the Massachusetts General Hospital (MGH), attended a seminar I gave that included early data from Maine and immediately saw the broad importance of practice variation for clinical medicine. His interest in health policy and decision analysis had been piqued by a year at Harvard University's Kennedy School of Government, and he had built his MGH research team around the applications of decision sciences to clinical decision making and had recruited Dr. Michael "Mike" Barry, a promising young decision analyst who was also trained as a primary care clinician. With the recruitment of Jack, Al, and Mike to the Maine project, we were ready to tackle Step Three in rationalizing practice variations for BPH.

Evaluating the Theories

By the mid-1980s, a sense of trust and cooperation between the Maine Urology Study Group and the outcomes researchers was firmly established. The troubling conflicts in their surgical theories had been exposed and the studies we could do with claims data had been done. Everyone agreed that the next step should be to test the preventive theory of prostatectomy. When compared to "watchful waiting," does early prostatectomy prevent BPH from progressing to a point where blockage of urine flow obstructs the bladder and kidneys, leading to higher mortality and morbidity? Nobody knew the answer, in large measure because nobody knew the natural history of untreated BPH—its rate of progression to chronic obstruction if left untreated. To test the preventive theory, two members of the assessment team, Mike and Al, both physicians and experts in decision analysis, constructed a model to compare life expectancy among patients who underwent surgery to those who chose watchful waiting. The model made it clear that the probabilities governing four critical events needed to be understood:

1. The chance of death immediately following surgery (given the age and illness level of the patient)
2. Life expectancy (given the age and illness level of the patient)
3. The risk of a second prostatectomy over time
4. The chance that untreated BPH will progress to the point where a patient who elected watchful waiting needs an operation to prevent death or serious bladder decompensation from upper urinary tract obstruction

The way in which our research team identified and put together the various strands of evidence to estimate these probabilities illustrates the eclectic, opportunistic approach sometimes required for successful outcomes research. Three sources of data were used. The information on the chances for reoperation and for operative mortality came from the Medicare claims data. The information on life expectancy came from the vital records. The information on the natural history of untreated BPH came from the medical literature. Using information from these various sources, Mike and Al were able to show that the preventive theory was very likely incorrect: *no matter what the age or illness level of the patient at the time of surgery, the chances of death from the surgery was not made up for by gains in life expectancy among those who survived the operation.*[11] The older or sicker the patient, the greater the loss of life expectancy was from prostatectomy for patients with BPH who did not have overt bladder or kidney failure. For example, an 80-year-old man in average health appeared to lose about 2.4 months of life, while a 60-year-old, also in average health, lost about two weeks.

Disproving the preventive theory meant that the use of the operation for most patients had to be justified on the basis of its value for reducing symptoms and improving the quality of life. But how good was the evidence that the operation actually worked? The data available from the medical literature and the Medicare claims had not helped. To fill in the gaps in knowledge, we wanted to conduct an RCT to define the symptomatic outcomes of men who had a prostatectomy. By now, our urology colleagues in Maine viewed this information as critical to their ability to advise their patients on treatment options and they volunteered their practices as the source of patients for a follow-up study of the effect of prostate surgery on symptoms, complications, and functional status. They insisted, however, that we use a case-series approach, not the RCT we researchers recommended. While they were not sure exactly what were the probabilities for outcomes, they were united in their belief that prostate surgery offered much better relief from symptoms than watchful waiting. They thought it would not be ethical for them to claim that they were uncertain about this fact; they were not at the equipoise in professional opinion that is traditionally required to justify an experiment.

There was, however, considerable disagreement about what outcomes were actually important to patients and how they should be evaluated. Our urology colleagues, like most physicians trained in the traditions of biomedical science, had spent little time worrying about the subjective side of medical practice, the measurement of "soft" outcomes such as symptoms, incontinence, impotence, and functional status. Nor did they give much thought to their ability to diagnose patient preferences. Most held that the proper metric for evaluating prostate patients and their treatments was urine flow; it served as an indicator both of the need for treatment (when it indicates outlet obstruction) and of the success of treatment (when urine flow improves because the obstruction has been relieved). Urine flow, as a "biomarker" for both diagnosis of need and outcome of care, seemed to fit neatly into their conceptualization of medicine as a science.

What Matters to Patients

We looked at the research problem a little differently. A distinguishing feature of our approach to outcomes was the insistence we placed on obtaining information about *all of the outcomes that matter to patients*. While we respected the urologists' opinions that urine flow might be correlated both with the patient's perception of need and with the improvements he might experience as a result of treatment, we insisted that the proper focus for outcomes research is on the list of problems that actually bother patients—not biomedical surrogates for these problems as viewed through professional eyes. The relationship between improvement in urine flow and the outcomes that mattered to patients had never been established.

We already had a good idea that what matters to patients—what they believe is relevant to their choice of treatments—cannot be intuited by researchers any more than it can by physicians. We had gained this insight in part through a series of interviews conducted in Boston with women following hysterectomy, many of whom were troubled by depression and loss of interest in sex—side effects of the surgery that generally did not concern their surgeons. We knew that patients needed to be asked about these matters in a systematic way.

Jack Fowler conducted interviews with patients with BPH to develop an extensive list of concerns and expectations for the different treatments. The patients interviewed included those with symptoms, some of whom were contemplating surgery and some who had already had surgery. Events that patients considered to be complications or unpleasant outcomes for surgery and watchful waiting were carefully solicited. During the sessions with patients considering surgery, Jack and his team asked a series of open-ended questions designed to elicit how patients felt about their symptoms and their reasons for considering the operation.

The questions they asked illustrated another important, distinguishing feature of our approach to outcomes research. Not only were we interested in obtaining knowledge about the range of problems and concerns that matter to patients, but we also focused on the value patients place on their fears, concerns, and expectations about their condition and the possible treatments. Because patients are not all the same in how they react to their symptoms, we were eager to learn from individuals how bothersome their symptoms seemed. For patients who had had surgery, we concentrated on their reaction to the surgical experience. Not surprisingly, Jack found important differences among patients. He also found that some patients who had already had surgery did not have a proper understanding of the actual purpose of the treatment. For example, some patients (it turned out to be about 15%) underwent surgery under the false expectation that surgery would prevent cancer of the prostate.

The literature review and the results of the interviews were then used to develop a questionnaire for measuring symptoms, complications of treatment, and subjective attitudes toward symptoms and risk. This method, of first interviewing patients with open-ended questions, then using their concerns to develop a questionnaire, would eventually become a standard procedure for developing objective measures of important subjective outcomes.

The alliance between practicing physicians and outcomes researchers was critically important in learning what works. Using the questionnaire, we studied the impact of prostatectomy on symptoms, functional status, and patient-reported complications among patients all over the state of Maine who had undergone BPH surgery. Interviews were conducted prior to surgery and at intervals of three, six, and twelve months after surgery. We found that for most men with symptoms due to BPH, the improvements following surgery were quite spectacular.[12] The urologists were right. An RCT was not needed to test the hypothesis that prostatectomy relieved symptoms better than watchful waiting; for this outcome, the surgery was a slam-dunk.

But it turned out that once men fully understood the potential downside to surgery, the decision to go under the knife was no longer so easy. The gains in symptom relief were purchased at a price. First, they were available only to patients who were willing to take the risks of the operation, including death, urethral stricture, and retrograde ejaculation, a postoperation complication in which ejaculation occurs into the bladder rather than out of the penis—a problem that the great majority of men are left with after surgery. Although urologists tend to think of retrograde ejaculation as a "normal" outcome of surgery, we learned from our interviews that some men were quite upset by it. As a result, retrograde ejaculation led to a net decline in quality of life for some men, regardless of their newfound ease in urination. Moreover, it became clear that not all patients were equally bothered by their urinary tract symptoms, including those who were severely symptomatic. There was virtually no correlation between objective clinical measures like urine flow and how greatly men were bothered by their symptoms. In view of the tradeoffs and the differing subjective responses to a given level of symptoms, it seemed likely that not all men, if offered a choice, would want surgery. Some might well choose watchful waiting. Mike and Al completed our assessment by confirming, with a formal decision analysis, that rational choice of treatment was indeed highly dependent on patients' preferences for outcomes and their attitudes toward the risks.[13]

We were now in a position to diagnose the clinical causes of the small area variations in prostatectomy rate. They were due to incorrect medical opinion favoring the preventive theory of early prostatectomy and to the failure of physicians to take patient preferences adequately into account in recommending prostatectomy.[14]

Addressing the Predicament of Choice

With a diagnosis of the cause of geographic variation in prostatectomy rates in hand, we could now think about a remedy. We began to conceive of a very different model for how physicians and patients should come to decisions about a course of treatment, a model that depends on patient preferences. We came to see that delegated decision making and its ethical foundation in informed consent should be replaced by a process of shared decision making, grounded in a different ethic—the ethic of informed patient choice. Under the model we envisioned, the patient must be invited to participate actively in the decision, learn to look ahead at the possible outcomes he might face following alternative treatments, and to think about how each of those scenarios might affect him. In the case of BPH, this means being aware of the advantages of surgery, but also its harms—the risks for incontinence, acute retention, retrograde ejaculation, and other sexual dysfunctions. It means being aware of the hazards of watchful waiting, including acute urinary retention. It also means understanding the current limits of medical science and what is known and not known about the prognoses for the outcomes that matter to patients.

We found a way to provide decision support for shared decision making to men contemplating surgery for BPH by using a new technology that first became available in the late 1980s, the interactive videodisc player. The videodisc player, a precursor of the Internet and today's DVD technology, married the computer to video. The computer solved the problem of conveying probability information about outcomes, tailored to the individual (or, really, his patient subgroup).[15] The video helped us find a solution to the problem of representing possible outcomes in a way that made them seem real to patients. Our decision aid video included films of patients who had experienced good outcomes as well as those who had complications following both watchful waiting and surgery. We called these videos shared decision-making programs (SDPs). (An excerpt of the original SDP is available for download from YouTube at: www.youtube.com/original SDP)

The patient decision aid was designed to support shared decision making in everyday practice. In our original BPH video,[16] the narrator set the stage:

> There is a decision to be made by you and your doctor. How you decide depends on how you feel about your symptoms and how you feel about the possible harms and benefits of surgery compared to the possible harms and benefits of watchful waiting. We'll tell you how likely it is that these harms and benefits might occur, but then you must decide, based on how you would feel about these harms and benefits if they happened to you. Keep in mind that either choice has possible harms and benefits. How you decide should involve your own evaluation of them.

Following this narration were interviews with two physician-patients, both of whom experienced severe symptoms from their prostate condition but chose different treatments. Our logic for selecting physicians was that if patients see that physicians can choose differently, they will understand that they, too, have a choice. Dr. X, who chose watchful waiting, explained to the patient his approach to risk assessment: "I considered the advantage of the operation against the amount of trouble I am having with the symptoms and the extent to which (the operation) might relieve them. And I felt that I am not bothered enough even by these fairly severe symptoms to undertake the risk of incontinence which the operation involves." Dr. Y, on the other hand, emphasized the amount of trouble he was having with the symptoms and how they interfered with the quality of his life: "(It was) the feeling that I had a full bladder, to know that it took a long time to empty it ... and the fact that I would have to wake up more often at night. And again, the restrictive features, to be able to do less and less things or to worry about more and more things as I began to plan my daily routine."

The two physician patients had typical outcomes following surgery and watchful waiting. Dr. Y was among the 80% of men who have a very satisfactory result from surgery. The narrator asks him how he fared: "Oh, infinitely better. Just a totally different situation. Such a feeling of relief. I remember the day when I walked into my urologist's office, and [began singing]: 'Summertime, and the peeing is easy.' That's the way I felt. I remember another occasion when he asked me about strength of stream and length of stream and all that. I described my ability—my regained ability to put my initials in the snow. That was great to be able to do!!"

Dr. X, who was severely symptomatic, had symptoms that were worse than most BPH patients who watched the video. For such patients, his description of his status as a watchful waiter offered viewers insight into the future they might face if they chose watchful waiting:

> Q.   The symptoms you have mentioned ... to what extent do they interfere with your activities of daily living?
> Dr. X: I suppose we've made a lot of adjustments and it has taken a lot of planning and anticipation. For example, all tickets on the airliner or concerts or theaters had better be on the aisle side so I can get out in a hurry if I need to.
> Dr. X: I don't go through a three-hour movie without having to leave.
> Q.   You've said that the symptoms are getting gradually worse. How close are you to changing your mind?
> Dr. X: It's hard to quantitate, but I think I still see a margin principally because there is such irregularity in this.

We designed our program to inform patients that either choice can have its problems as well as its advantages. Viewers saw interviews with patients who experienced complications, one on the watchful waiting side and one on the surgery side. The two complications we chose to illustrate had about the same chance of occurring. A patient with surgically induced incontinence reported:

> I have leakage. I think the word is *incontinence* or something like that. And I was getting wet all the time and of course I didn't know what to do about all that so my wife and I figured it out. I went out and bought some jockey shorts and sort of Kotex type stuff and put it inside and I would have to change that three or four times a day, which I am still doing. It didn't pour out, but it would on occasion leak out and was much worse when I walked around a lot or stood a lot ... this came out of the blue (following surgery). This was a minus, a big minus.

A watchful waiter who had an episode of acute retention answered questions about his experience:

Q. Were you in a lot of pain?

A. Yes, a lot of pain; pain that I couldn't control or help. So finally, in getting up to the doctor, I got on the table to be interviewed there and I said, "Hold on doctor, before you go any further, the first thing you do is drain that bladder."

Q. How did it feel when they finally did use the catheter?

A. Heavenly! It was like being under water longer than you wanted to be and you had to hold your breath longer than you wanted to and the moment that catheter cleared the passage there, it was a relief like that pain was leaving all the time—right up until it got comfortable—the doctor made two or three trips with the urinal bowl until there was no more.

In keeping with our patient-oriented perspective, the patient decision aid was designed to include the full gamut of information required by the patient, as ascertained by extensive focus groups. Patients were asked to explain their perceptions about their condition, the symptoms that bothered them, and what they wanted to know in choosing a treatment. Those with complications were asked what they would have wanted to know about possible complications before they made their decision. The fears patients have, and their expectations and misunderstandings, were identified and this information was used to plan the presentation to correct significant misperceptions. For example, some men thought having a prostatectomy would eliminate their chances of getting prostate cancer, a completely wrong perception that led to wrong decisions. To deal with this misperception, we added a section to the program:

You should know that an operation can't be considered a cure for cancer because it doesn't remove all prostate tissue; for the same reason, an operation doesn't prevent future prostate cancer. Worries about cancer shouldn't influence your decision to choose surgery or watchful waiting.

We also thought it was important to inform patients about current limits to medical knowledge. The risk of serious urinary tract retention among watchful waiting patients was a good example:

The risk of serious urinary tract infections hasn't been very well studied in men with BPH, but it's safe to assume that it happens even less often than acute retention, that is, less than 2% of men over 5 years.

In designing the BPH patient decision aid, we faced three tasks. The first was to get the science right. We believed that this was reasonably assured by our adherence to scientific methods and peer review, and our insistence on informing patients of our uncertainty, as in the example of probabilities for urinary tract infection. The second was to make clear and comprehensible the essential features of the decision. Our success in communicating information was evaluated by testing viewer reactions and in testing whether viewers understood the objective content of the presentation.[17] The third task was to achieve balance and fairness in the presentation of treatment options. This was in many ways the most difficult task. We found no "gold standard" methods for evaluation and depended primarily on the judgments of focus groups with patients as well as clinicians (of varying specialties). After several revisions, consensus was reached that the program was considered fair. (The emergence of patient preferences as a key to rational decision making opens up a whole new field of medical research dealing with the communication of risk and the balanced description of treatment choices, issues I will discuss briefly in Chapter 7.)

What Do Patients Want?

After the BPH patient decision aid was finalized, it was installed in a number of urological practices in the United States and Canada. The impact on patients' decisions has been tested with hundreds of patients with BPH who were possible candidates for surgery, but whose clinicians believed they could also safely choose watchful waiting without immediate risk of acute urinary retention. Prior to viewing the program, patients were asked to fill out questionnaires regarding their symptoms and information relevant to their treatment preferences. After viewing the program, patients rated the experience. They also agreed to fill out questionnaires periodically about their treatment choices, their symptoms, their preferences, and how they felt things were working out.

The evaluation process allowed us to answer two important questions concerning the feasibility and impact of shared decision making.

1. Do Patients Really Want to Participate in the Choice of Treatment?

Following their session with the SDP, most patients were ready to make up their minds about their treatment. Concerns that patients would not want as much information as we presented or that they would not want to play an important role in decision making were not substantiated. Impressive evidence for the empowerment of patients with SDPs occurred early in the course of our evaluation when fifteen patients already scheduled for surgery at a Veterans Administration (VA) Hospital were inadvertently shown the SDP. Half of the patients decided against surgery, even though they had already accepted their physician's recommendation to have it.

2. When Patients Are Informed about Options, Do They Choose More Rationally from Their Own Point of View?

This is the bottom-line question: Does the use of decision aids and the implementation of a shared decision-making process promote informed patient choice? An answer was provided by an important study spearheaded by Mike Barry and Jack Fowler.[18] First, they found that symptoms mattered in predicting choice. Compared to those with moderate symptoms, patients who were severely symptomatic were about twice as likely to choose surgery, the treatment with the best chance of improving symptoms. But even among the most severely symptomatic, only a minority of patients wanted surgery: 11% of those with moderate symptoms, and 22% of those with severe symptoms chose surgery.

What mattered most in determining choice was not symptoms, but two other factors governing the patient's decision: the patient's own attitudes toward his symptoms—how much he was bothered by them—and the *patient's degree of concern about risks to his sexuality (impotence and problems with ejaculation).*

It is worth following the logic of Mike's and Jack's study to examine the means by which they investigated how these two spheres—the "objective" state of symptom level and the attitude of the patient toward them—interact to predict the choice that patients will make in the shared decision-making environment. The researchers used a standardized questionnaire to evaluate the patient's symptoms and asked the following question to rank their attitudes toward their symptoms: Suppose your urinary symptoms stayed just about the same as they are now for the rest of your life. How would you feel about that? Surprisingly, only a minority of patients was bothered very much by the prospect that their symptoms would remain the same, even among those who were severely symptomatic[19] (Table 6.1).

Patients were also asked questions about their degree of concern about complications: Suppose a treatment cured your urinary symptoms, but you were unable to have sexual erections. How would you feel about your

Table 6.1.   How Patients with an Enlarged Prostate Felt about Their Symptoms
According to Symptom Severity

Symptom Level	Attitude Toward Their Symptoms		
	Mostly Satisfied	Mixed Reaction	Mostly Dissatisfied
Mild	84%	8	8
Moderate	58%	21	21
Severe	39%	18	42

Source: Floyd Jackson Fowler, Jr., "The Role of Patient Preferences in Medical Care" (Paper presented at the Distinguished Lecture Series, Office of Graduate Studies and Research, University of Massachusetts, November 1994). [Used by permission of Floyd Jackson Fowler, Jr.]

situation? The individual patient's attitudes about the possibility for impotence and the degree to which he was bothered by his symptoms proved to be very strong predictors of choice of treatment. Patients who were negative about their symptoms were seven times more likely to choose surgery than those who had a positive or a mixed attitude; those who were negative about the prospect of impotence were five times more likely to choose watchful waiting than those who had mixed feelings or didn't seem to care. Thus, while the "objective" reason for doing surgery was to reduce symptoms, the assessment of the "need" for surgery requires the evaluation of how much the patient is bothered by his symptoms and his concerns about the impact of surgery on sexuality.

Which Rate Is Right?

Our BPH studies also held intriguing hints that the "right rate" for prostatectomy—that happens when demand for discretionary surgery is based on informed patient choice—might be lower than the rate at which men were actually undergoing the procedure. The evidence came from a study our group conducted among BPH patients enrolled in two prepaid group practices: the Kaiser Permanente Medical Group in Denver, Colorado, and Group Health Cooperative in Seattle, Washington. After shared decision making for BPH was implemented in these plans, the rates for surgery dropped an astonishing 40% below baseline and in comparison to a control population.[20] The rates for surgery in these organizations were already below the national average prior to our study. After shared decision making was widely implemented for BPH, their

rates were at the bottom of the national distribution (Figure 6.1). If the preference patterns of men in these two HMOs reflected the average for Americans,
then the amount of surgery prescribed and performed in the United States for
BPH during the study years would have exceeded the amount that informed
patients wanted in virtually every region of the country.

The Value of Outcomes Research

Let me summarize the progress that was made over the fourteen-year period
(1975 through 1989) of the Maine phase of our outcomes research project.
In response to feedback on variation, Dan Hanley was able to organize the
urologists in Maine to come together to debate the reasons for variation. The
conversations soon focused on the differences in theory among the urologists
themselves and this, in turn, led to a series of studies that resulted in showing that the preventive theory of surgical intervention was counterfactual—
that surgery on large numbers of elderly men could not be justified on the

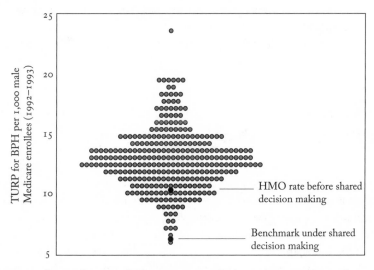

Figure 6.1.   Rates of transurethral prostatectomy for benign prostatic hyperplasia
(TURP) among hospital referral regions (1992 through 1993) compared to rates for
two staff model HMOs before and after introduction of shared decision making. The
data from the two HMOs have been pooled. The rate before shared decision making
is for 1987 through 1989; the benchmark under shared decision making is for 1990 and
1991. (Source: Dartmouth Atlas Project database.)

basis of the procedure's ability to prevent death and disability due to obstruction of the urinary tract. By contrast, the quality of life theory was sustained: the procedure was quite effective in reducing symptoms, but rational choice depended on the patient deciding between the procedure's superior ability to reduce urinary tract symptoms and its negative impact on sexuality and other complications. Studies of the preferences of men, even those with severe symptoms, demonstrated that only a minority would want surgery, given the tradeoffs that surgery imposes.

Rational choice thus depended on sorting out the individual patient's preferences. Patient preferences could not be predicted by any of the traditional tools available to physicians, including patient history, physical examination, or biological tests such as urine flow. Urine flow was found to be uncorrelated with symptom level and therefore unhelpful in evaluating need.[21] In turn, while symptom level was an important predictor of need—and could be measured "objectively" with a standardized questionnaire, it provided no reliable rule of thumb on which to base decisions: only a minority of even the most severely symptomatic men wanted surgery once they were informed of the full scope of tradeoffs. Rather, it was two subjective aspects of patient choice—how much they were bothered by their symptoms and their concern about the impact of surgery on sexuality—that proved to be more important in predicting patient choice than symptom level. The critical nature of these factors only became clear through implementing a shared decision-making process.

* * *

Outcomes research does not take place within the controlled environment of a research laboratory; it requires the active engagement of physicians themselves—those whose very theories and patterns of practice are to become the subject of evaluation. It requires trust and, because the research is long term and often iterative in nature, a stable infrastructure to support the research. Our studies in Maine helped to clarify the rationale for using surgery to treat benign prostatic hyperplasia and provided a strategy for estimating the "true demand" of discretionary surgery through shared decision making. By the end of the 1980s, the value of outcomes research had wider recognition, and the Maine Medical Assessment Program became the prototype for a national research program to address unwarranted practice variation. For a few years, it seemed as if the nation might actually be prepared to invest in the research that is necessary to provide medicine with a firm scientific footing and base the utilization of discretionary surgery both on what works and what patients want. Chapter 7 describes some of the lessons learned.

7

The Birth and Near Death of
Comparative Effectiveness Research

During the 1980s, practice variations and outcomes research attracted a good deal of attention among members of the U.S. Congress, stimulated by a growing world literature documenting the ubiquity of practice variation and its connection to medical spending. In 1987, Senator David Durenberger, a Republican from Minnesota and chair of the Senate Finance Subcommittee on Health, used his influence to establish an outcomes research program, which became known as the Patient Outcomes Research Team, or PORT program. Modeled after our Maine project on benign prostatic hyperplasia (BPH) (discussed in Chapter 6), four teams were funded under the National Center for Health Services Research: each focused on conditions for which surgical treatment rates varied extensively among regions. The conditions included angina or chest pain due to coronary artery disease, low back pain due to herniated intervertebral disc or spinal stenosis, cataracts, and prostate disease. Our research group became the prostate disease PORT, expanding its BPH focus to include early-stage prostate cancer. Two years later, Congress brought into being the Agency for Health Care Policy and Research (AHCPR [name changed in 1999 to the Agency for Healthcare Research and Quality (AHRQ)], with the much more ambitious agenda of organizing a comprehensive national approach to improving the scientific basis for both clinical practice and policy decision making in health care. The PORT project became part of AHCPR's medical effectiveness program.[1]

It was the hope of our research group that the new agency would provide a "home base" of sufficient scale to establish the evaluative clinical sciences as central to the scientific mission of America's academic medical centers. Early success with the PORT program seemed to justify optimism. AHCPR established strict procedures for scientific review patterned after those in place at the National Institutes of Health (NIH), as well as a process for setting priorities to ensure that costly conditions with highly variable treatment patterns were the focus of research. The funding level, while modest (indeed, miniscule by NIH standards), was sufficient to induce academic medicine to commit resources and talent to the PORT agenda. Interdisciplinary teams of investigators—clinicians, epidemiologists, decision analysts, social scientists, and statisticians—were formed to address practice variation for some of the most variable conditions. In keeping with the Maine experience, the PORTs focused on pragmatic, problem-solving approaches to research methods and strategies for evaluating treatment theories, and they also monitored medical innovations in an effort to evaluate promising new technologies as soon as possible. Additional PORT duties included collaboration with clinical leaders to promote both physician allegiance to the ethic of evaluation and broad participation in evaluation networks similar to the one formed by the Maine Medical Assessment Foundation and the practicing urologists in Maine. Finally, they disseminated the results of research findings directly to patients, and promoted informed patient choice as a strategy for improving care and reducing unwarranted practice variations—and health care spending.[2]

The future of medical effectiveness research seemed particularly bright as the ideas of outcomes research and advancing the patient's role in decision making became incorporated into the Clinton health plan. Al Mulley and I met with Hillary Clinton during a visit to Hanover and had the opportunity to show her the results of our BPH research projects and to convey to her the importance of involving patients as active partners in the choice of treatment. When the Clinton health plan neared readiness for delivery to Congress, she invited me to Washington to read the draft legislation and to suggest changes to ensure that shared decision making and outcomes research were well represented in the final bill. I was particularly pleased when the administration agreed to our recommendation to establish regional professional foundations under Section 5008 of the Health Security Act. The proposal was directly modeled after the Maine Medical Assessment Foundation and its link to the research community through the PORT concept. We envisioned that, like the Maine Medical Assessment Foundation, professional foundations would serve as a focus for feedback of information on practice patterns and for organizing active engagement of practicing physicians in resolving unwarranted variation. As Bob Keller and I explained in an article in *Health Affairs,* the professional foundations would focus on "building a professional infrastructure for quality, outcomes research, and lifetime learning in local communities and regions."[3]

But then the political climate in Washington changed abruptly. The Clinton health plan failed to pass in Congress. In 1995, Congress withdrew much of its support for AHCPR, doing away with the illusion that Congress and federal science policy had made a broad commitment to the evaluative sciences.[4] Many lessons were learned, however, and they are of value, not just historically but also for practical reasons. The nation is once again struggling with the problem of medical effectiveness and contemplating a new effort to establish the evaluative sciences. The PORT model should inform any renewed effort to develop a national program to improve the scientific basis of clinical decision making. This chapter discusses key aspects of the mission and accomplishments of the PORTs, which I believe are relevant to today's effort to reestablish comparative effectiveness research as a national priority.

The Nature of the Innovative Process

The design of comparative effectiveness research must capture the complexity of the innovative process. Contrary to popular opinion, medical innovation rarely follows a linear process—a consecutive series of studies that begins with the ideas of the biomedical scientist, proceeds to the laboratory bench, moves from there to an applied technology that is tested in animal and human populations and subjected to proof of efficacy through randomized clinical trials (RCTs), before finally being made available to the medical profession and patients. In the real world, innovation is often chaotic, with the line blurred between what is experimental and what is evidence-based and effective. Physicians often invent new treatments on the fly, and serendipity plays a hand as a treatment used for one purpose is applied to another. This process is much too complex, dynamic, and multidimensional for evaluation policy to be based primarily on regulation, such as the constraints the U.S. Food and Drug Administration (FDA) places on market entry for drugs and devices.

Our experience in evaluating treatments for BPH illustrates this. Although we spent years tracking innovation in treatment theory—attending national clinical meetings, reading medical journals, and networking with clinical leadership in the United States and elsewhere—only one treatment innovation that we encountered corresponded to the linear model of innovation captured by the FDA model of regulation of market entry: Merck's drug Proscar (finasteride), which was specifically designed to treat BPH. The drug blocks a key hormone that is responsible in part for prostate growth. In clinical trials, it works better than a placebo, at least to increase urine flow, although its effects on other symptoms are not dramatic.[5] Based on its effect on urine flow, Proscar won regulatory approval as an effective BPH treatment.

By contrast, we found many examples of medical innovations that had become (or threatened to become) part of everyday practice but were untouched by sound biomedical research or FDA evaluation. Sometimes, new treatments were discovered by serendipity by practicing physicians. In our networking to identify emerging practice theories, we found that urologists were beginning to use alpha-blocker drugs—a class of drugs that had won FDA approval for an entirely different purpose (the treatment of hypertension)—to treat BPH. Some patients who have high blood pressure also have an enlarged prostate. Observant physicians (or patients) noted that the drug appeared to improve urine flow and subsequent studies have shown that it has a beneficial effect on prostate symptoms. Alpha-blockers were soon widely used to treat BPH, a good example of a common phenomenon, the "off-label" use of drugs, in which physicians end up prescribing drugs for purposes other than an approved use. Through networking with practicing physicians, PORTs were specifically designed to detect and bring forward for early evaluation such treatment theories that were following these sorts of nonlinear pathways into everyday practice.

While medical devices are subject to FDA approval, the process often requires only evidence of safety. One example we encountered was balloon dilation, a technique that involved inserting a deflated balloon into the urethra, lodging it against the base of the bladder, and then inflating it to push back the prostate tissue. The idea crept into urology on the basis of reasoning by analogy. Another form of balloon dilation—cardiac angioplasty had been used since the late 1970s to unclog the arteries of the heart. So why wouldn't the same strategy work for prostate disease? An enterprising urologist designed and patented such a balloon and then went off to form his own company to produce and sell the balloons to his fellow urologists. But because the balloons did not come under the strict FDA requirements for proof of efficacy that was required of new drugs, his company and others that pursued this idea were not required to invest the resources needed to evaluate their product, as they would have had to do if their technology had been a drug. The use of the balloons thus slipped into practice with little information on efficacy. Over the course of our PORT work, balloon dilation dipped out of favor, again without proper evaluation of whether it worked.

A new treatment based on microwave diathermy, or "thermotherapy," entered into practice through yet another back door of innovation. The theory was that symptoms would be improved when prostate tissue was destroyed by the heat generated from the microwave. For more than a decade, the NIH had poured money into the development of a device to heat tumors, using a form of microwave that scientists hoped would improve the effectiveness of chemotherapy. The idea that heat might help has its theoretical origins in cellular physiology and its experimental basis in animal experiments, which show that animal tumors shrink when the tumor cells' metabolic rates speed up due to microwaves. This discovery led to a large government investment in bioengineering projects to produce devices that could be used in the treatment of human cancers. Although this strategy ultimately did not pay off for the treatment of human cancers, the availability of machinery that can selectively heat a local organ led some enterprising physicians to look for other uses. One idea was to try it out on the prostate. Local heat, it was found, does indeed destroy prostate tissue, and subsequent clinical trials have shown that the procedure may work better than watchful waiting in reducing symptoms but less well than surgery.[6]

Surgical treatment provides many examples of how medical ideas and innovations evolve, often without much formal evaluation. The surgical treatment of BPH originated from the desperate need to reestablish urine flow in patients with large prostates who could not urinate at all or whose kidneys were so severely obstructed that the patients were in renal failure. As surgery became safer, the preventive theory became more popular among urologists, and an array of new surgical techniques were invented and put to use on patients, all without much formal evaluation. One example is the transurethral resection of the prostate (TURP), which is accomplished without a surgical incision by passing what urologists call a resectoscope through the urethra to chip away parts of the obstructing prostate tissue. Then there is the open operation, or total prostatectomy, which involves an incision through the skin, the surgical exposure of the prostate gland, and its removal with surgical instruments under direct visualization. Over the three decades prior to our studies, TURP had become increasingly more popular until it virtually replaced the older total prostatectomy. This substitution of technique occurred without benefit of prospective clinical trials, reflecting the intuitive belief on the part of urologists that the TURP had to be safer, less invasive, and equally effective in the long term.

During the period in which our research team patrolled the market looking for emerging treatments for BPH, innovators produced a number of new devices to cut, vaporize, or coagulate the prostate and various approaches to gain access to it. Some urologists began to advocate a less invasive surgical approach called a prostatotomy—rather than removing pieces of the prostate, this procedure involved simply making slits in the offending gland to widen the passage.[7] Other surgeons pursued yet another idea: the use of "stents" or little metal braces, which are implanted inside the urethra to "tent up" the obstructing prostate tissue, a strategy that seems analogous to miners using timber beams to shore up the roofs of mineshafts.[8]

Evaluating Treatment Theories

Capturing the complexity of the innovation process was the first step for PORTs. Next came evaluation. The duties included balanced evaluation of all relevant treatment options, those in current use as well as new and promising alternatives—much the same sorts of "head to head" comparisons of treatment options as those being discussed today in the context of a comparative effectiveness program. The PORTs' methods for evaluation were eclectic, designed to make the most of available evidence, while continually focusing on the key issues that mattered most to patients. They included the following:

Structured reviews of the medical literature: PORTs carried out an assessment of the published medical evidence (much like the systematic reviews now done by the Cochrane Collaboration), in which all relevant articles were collected and evaluated as to methodological merit using standard epidemiologic principles. The literature was synthesized to obtain the best possible estimates for the outcomes according to treatment used and patient condition. The synthesis was then made available to researchers in the field and published in medical journals.[9]

Patient focus groups: PORTs conducted focus groups and other forms of patient interviews to obtain as complete an inventory as possible of concerns, outcomes, and other issues that matter to patients. For example, in our work with patients with BPH, focus groups led to the discovery of the importance to some (but not to all) men of the negative effect of surgery on sexual function, and of the variation in the degree to which men with severe symptoms from an enlarged prostate were actually bothered by their symptoms.

Standardized measures of symptoms and subjective states: In keeping with their focus on patients, PORTs developed quantitative measures of patient perception. For example, for BPH, working jointly with the American Urological Association (AUA) (see later discussion), we developed a BPH symptom questionnaire,[10] something we called the prostate "bother" questionnaire,[11] designed to quantify the impact of urinary symptoms on patients' lives, and a questionnaire for measuring sexual function.[12]

Decision models of treatment options and relevant outcomes: PORTs used decision models to test relevant controversies, such as the assumption under the preventive theory that early BPH surgery increased life expectancy. Decision models also served as a guide for understanding the key factors on which the treatment decision should depend. In our work in Maine, for example, the decision model served as the framework for understanding the importance of patient values in the choice of treatment.[13]

Estimating the probabilities for different outcomes: The methods for evaluating treatment theories were eclectic, depending on the outcome in question and the complexity of inferring causal relationships between treatment and outcomes. An important innovation for estimating outcome probabilities that emerged out of the prostate PORT was the systematic follow-up of patient cohorts according to their choice of treatment after the use of decision aids. In the BPH studies conducted in the Kaiser Permanente Medical Group in Denver and Group Cooperative of Puget Sound (described in Chapter 6), patients who chose surgery and those who chose watchful waiting were followed up for a year or more.[14] The data from this follow-up, which included about 1,000 men who chose not to have surgery, answered important questions concerning the natural history of untreated disease. For example, we learned that the incidence of both acute retention and urinary tract infections are low among watchful waiters, no more than 1% per year, even though clinicians have often argued for surgery on the basis of the need to prevent these complications. We then used the information gained from these new outcomes studies to improve the estimates for various outcomes in subsequent editions of the decision aids.

In our research team's conceptualization of its mission, RCTs were also to play an important role in the PORT program. Together with the AUA, we developed a collaborative model for evaluating competing clinical theories, one we believed could serve as a model for how professional societies and independent research teams could work together to improve the science of health care delivery.

Professional Accountability and the Ethic of Evaluation

Professionalism, I argue, must be grounded in a commitment to learn from experience, to evaluate the outcomes of clinical practice for the benefit of today's, as well as tomorrow's, patients. By providing an infrastructure for evaluation, the federal PORT program, like the Maine Medical Assessment Foundation, held out the promise to clinicians and researchers that resources would be made available for the orderly evaluation of everyday practice. By the early 1990s, the program had begun to mobilize the academic community and practicing physicians to take on the duties required for the effective evaluation of treatment theory. The PORT program had also seen its findings adopted into everyday practice, and it was well on its way to securing the commitment of the leaders of American medicine to the ethic of evaluation, using the tried and true methods of peer-reviewed science.

The work of the AUA is a case in point. Prior to 1988, our interactions were primarily with the urology community in Maine. By 1988, we had finished our assessment of watchful waiting and prostatectomy and published our conclusions pointing to the fundamental importance of patient preference in choosing treatment. At about the same time, the initial version of the interactive videodisc patient decision aid was ready for early testing and word about it had crept out into the press. It was featured in an article in *Fortune* magazine and in several press reports.

Our relationship with the leadership of the AUA was triggered by a story by Michael L. Millenson in the *Chicago Tribune*.[15] Millenson, who had visited us in Hanover and seen the interactive videodisc, reported on our efforts to inform patients. He also called Dr. Paul C. Peters, then president of the AUA, to ask his opinion about the approach of informing patients. We were embarrassed to learn that Peters knew nothing about our project. I called Peters and invited senior leadership of the AUA to come to Hanover. Dr. Abraham Cockett, a professor of urology at the University of Rochester and Dr. Logan Holtgrewe, a practicing urologist in Annapolis, Maryland, and the president-elect of the AUA, met with us to discuss our project and see the interactive video program. The result of that visit was a lasting collaboration with the AUA and a commitment from its leadership to conduct a clinical trial into a crucial set of questions about the efficacy and safety of the two main surgical methods for treating BPH.

Which was better—the TURP operation or the older total prostatectomy to remove the prostate? The review of the scientific literature failed to find even a single example of a prospective clinical study that compared the two approaches. We did find several large administrative databases (including Medicare's) that allowed us to compare some of the important outcomes for these two surgical approaches. By the 1980s, in the United States, the TURP had virtually replaced the total prostatectomy, yet buried in the piles of data was evidence that transurethral surgery might be less effective and more dangerous. Patients with an open operation had significantly lower rates for stricture and reoperation, suggesting that the more complete removal of the prostate was less traumatizing to the urethra and resulted in better long-term reduction in symptoms. More puzzling and disturbing was the unexplained elevation in risk of death following TURP. In studies undertaken in Maine and Manitoba, Canada,[16] and Oxford, England, and Denmark,[17] the risk of death was found to be about 50% higher in the five years following surgery, even when the claims data controlled for possible differences in comorbidity. These findings were subsequently confirmed by researchers in the Kaiser Permanente Medical Care Program,[18] and by a small RCT in Denmark.[19] Although no convincing biological explanation or hypothesis as to why TURPs might cause an increase in death rate existed, the available data, limited as they were, pointed in this direction.[20] The consistency of the findings, and our failure to explain them on the basis of data available in medical charts,[21] led us to conclude that differences in comorbidity and other patient risk factors was not an adequate explanation. We concluded that a prospective RCT was needed to evaluate this problem.

But how should such a trial be organized? Who would be responsible for taking the initiative? Well before the results of our study were published, we met with the leadership of the AUA to discuss the idea for a clinical trial. They not only saw the necessity for such a trial—they agreed that it should be the responsibility of the AUA to sponsor it.

The publication of our cohort study showing *increased* mortality after TURP, and the subsequent publicity in the lay press caused a stir in the medical community, motivating one urologist to accuse the journal's editor of "a great disservice to the urological community," for which he "deserves extreme censure."[22] Other urologists were less defensive about our results, and the prestigious British medical journal *The Lancet*, in an editorial about our study whimsically entitled, "TU(RP) or not TU(RP)," wrote, "Urologists are a quiet, unassuming group proud of their role in the development of endoscopic surgery. It takes more than a few stones to ripple their pond, but a boulder just rolled in." The editorial went on to discuss possible mechanisms for the increased mortality and urged members of the profession to take the results seriously. It ended on a note of alarm: "The urologists' boat is being rocked and there is no room for complacency."[23]

But the AUA was well ahead of everyone in providing the leadership to deal with the situation. At the AUA annual meeting in September of 1989, a press conference was held to announce the decision to conduct a trial. A pilot study, funded by the AUA itself, would start immediately. Five academic centers—the University of Rochester, Texas Medical College, the University of Iowa, George Washington University, and Walter Reed Army Medical

Center—quickly volunteered, and more than twenty-five others wanted to join in the full project, which would go forward once a grant was obtained from the federal government.

The AUA's understanding of its role in the evaluation of medical practice and its relationship to the PORT evolved considerably as the pilot study and the grant application proceeded. The potential for harm raised by TURP versus total prostatectomy studies remained the central scientific question of the trial. However, it was also recognized that questions about the efficacy of TURP in terms of reducing symptoms were relevant because of inadequacies in the way TURP and other surgical procedures were evaluated in the first place. The AUA and the PORT saw the opportunity to build a lasting system for evaluating new technologies and medical procedures (as well as the established ones) for many conditions, not just BPH. The pilot study and the grant proposal to extend the project to twenty academic sites around the country was designed in a way that would have brought each of the new urological technologies—balloons, off-label drugs as well as those approved for BPH treatment, stents, incision surgery, and microwave thermotherapy—under evaluation, starting with the most promising.

The AUA-PORT collaboration also facilitated other efforts to rationalize the decision process and outcomes research. While symptom relief is what most men with BPH are looking for, it became clear in preparing for the clinical trial that the various ad hoc ways of measuring prostate symptoms made it almost impossible to compare the outcomes of alternative treatments. There was no standard method for reporting symptom level in patients' clinical records. Researchers, along with drug and device manufacturers, simply invented their own ways to measure symptoms. The AUA appointed a measurement committee to work with our PORT to recommend a set of uniform questionnaires. The report of the committee, published in the AUA's official journal *Urology*, recommended that all studies sponsored by manufacturers of devices and drugs, as well as studies undertaken by independent investigators, use the standardized patient questionnaires developed by the PORT.[24] The committee that was to select new treatments for evaluation by the AUA network would require that the preliminary studies by manufacturers or independent investigators also use the recommended standardized outcome measures. We anticipated that this would guarantee broad compliance, at least by those who hoped that their technology would be eligible to enter the long-awaited AUA trial.

But the AUA clinical trial network was not to be. Despite the nagging questions regarding the safety and effectiveness of the TURP; the obvious rationality of setting up evaluation networks to promote a balanced assessment of all treatments for BPH; the investment of the AUA of over $1 million of its own money; and a federal grant application process that dragged on for more than three years, the AUA-PORT collaboration dissolved. The proximal reason was that the Agency for Health Care Policy and Research, which we were counting on for the development of a national program for the evaluative clinical sciences, lost nearly all of its funding after the release of a 1994 report from the low back pain PORT.[25] The PORT's twenty-three–member panel of experts had found poor evidence for the use of surgery as a first-line treatment for low back pain, a simple enough statement of fact. But the report was seen as a threat by a large contingent of back surgeons, who mounted a lobbying campaign aimed at the Congress. Their arguments found a sympathetic ear in the newly elected Republican majority in the U.S. House of Representatives. The back surgeons' charge that a government agency was trying to regulate the practice of medicine resonated with the Republican enthusiasm for downsizing government, and in 1995, the House voted (twice) to zero out the agency's budget. AHCPR was saved with the help of Republican supporters in the Senate, including Dr. William Frist, a physician from Tennessee. But with a significantly reduced budget and mission, the Agency (which was renamed to be the Agency for Healthcare Research and Quality) no longer supported the "dangerous" medical effectiveness program and the PORTs.[26]

Foundation for Informed Medical Decision Making

The downsizing of AHCPR was a serious blow to those of us who wanted to see medicine put on a firmer scientific footing and the implementation of informed patient choice put into place. Yet there were lasting effects of those PORTs. Under the assumption that PORTs would remain stable instruments of public policy for outcomes research, we anticipated the need for continuously updating the patient decision aids to reflect new information on outcomes. Moreover, the integrity of the decision aids required that the scenarios for presenting treatment options and medical tradeoffs, for communicating benefits and harms, and other issues concerning the predicament of choice, be evaluated and progressively improved upon. But who, we asked ourselves, should be responsible for building and maintaining an expanding library of decision aids?

The first and obvious answer was that it could not be organizations that have a vested interest in a particular treatment option—the AUA or Merck, the maker of Proscar, for example. While the AUA was keenly interested in an objective evaluation of treatment options, the credibility of any prostate decision aid would be compromised if the organization was involved in its creation. It also would be extremely difficult for an insurance company or other payer (such as the Health Care Financing Administration, now called the Centers for Medicare & Medicaid Services [CMS]) to be credible sponsors of decision aids, given their not-so-hidden bias to reduce health care costs. In theory, the federal government might have provided funding for creating more decision aids, but there were no provisions in federal science policy for this task. Our solution was to create the Foundation for Informed Medical Decision Making, a 501(c)(3) medical education and research organization established in 1988 (Box 7.1).

Box 7.1.   *A Brief History of FIMDM*

The Foundation for Informed Medical Decision Making (FIMDM) came into being in 1988 in Santa Monica, California, following a meeting with Dr. Robert Brook, of the RAND Corporation. The meeting was organized by the Hartford Foundation, which funded our research in Maine, as well as studies conducted by RAND. The program director of the Foundation, Richard Sharpe, wanted us to iron out our differences with RAND regarding the best way to remedy the problem of variation in surgical practices. The ideas my colleagues and I were promoting, that medical necessity should depend on informed patient choice, and that patients must therefore be encouraged to participate in making choices about discretionary surgery, stood in contrast to the approach being championed by Brook. He argued that the ultimate authority for determining medical necessity lies with the physician, not the patient. His strategy involved panels of medical experts charged with creating appropriateness guidelines—detailed classification of patients into groups the experts felt would definitely benefit, might benefit, or would not benefit from surgery, based on such clinical criteria as age, diagnosis, and comorbidity. Brook also devised a plan by which physicians would talk over the telephone with a consultant, who would help the physician decide whether an individual patient needed surgery—a sort of second opinion system that had physicians sorting patients according to how well each case fit the appropriateness criteria. If the patient's case was "clinically appropriate," then the insurance company or HMO sponsoring the review would agree to pay for the procedure. After several hours of fruitless discussion, my colleagues Al Mulley, Jack Fowler, Mike Barry, and I were walking along the beach at Santa Monica during a break, when the idea was born for a foundation dedicated to researching how patients make decisions, creating ways to help them understand the tradeoffs, and promoting informed patient choice as the standard of practice.

As originally conceived, FIMDM's role was restricted to incorporating the results of PORT assessments into decision aids and then marketing the decision aids, with the goal of making them available on an unrestricted basis to patients, through their doctors and hospitals. We envisioned FIMDM as an essential part of the infrastructure required to reduce unwarranted variation, by ensuring that the information in the decision aids was up to date and that its representation of treatment options was as fair and balanced as possible. But with the demise of the PORTs, FIMDM found itself on the horns of a dilemma: it would need to bear the costs of the scientific assessments of decision aids. Even if, as indeed happened, FIMDM scaled back the scientific assessment to include only systematic reviews of the literature, the expense of maintaining the library of decision aids would be hard to meet without new sources of revenue. Worse still, with the failure of the Clinton health plan (which included provisions to support shared decision making), any thought that reimbursement reform would pay doctors to implement decision aids went out the window.

By the mid-1990s, the situation had reached a crisis, as the second of two efforts to establish a commercial partner to distribute decision aids failed. At this point, Al approached George Bennett, a Boston entrepreneur, who became intrigued with our project. This led to the founding of Health Dialog as a commercial partner of FIMDM, dedicated to implementing shared decision making and improving the management of chronic illness. The commercial success of Health Dialog has stabilized the FIMDM mission, leading to the development of a large library of decision aids and support for FIMDM's research agenda to implement shared decision making.

The Prostate Cancer Screening Decision

One of the first patient decision aids we developed focused on the decision to undergo the prostate specific antigen (PSA) screening test to detect early stage prostate cancer. During the late 1980s and early 1990s, the nation was experiencing a prostate cancer epidemic. Each year the rate of prostate cancer reported by the NIH rose in spectacular fashion, resulting in a two-fold increase from 1987 to 1992. Naturally, as more cancer was discovered, rates of invasive treatment also rose. An important factor behind the epidemic in incidence and the resulting surgery was the increasingly widespread use of the PSA test to screen for cancer. The PSA was originally approved by the FDA as a test for monitoring prostate cancers that had already been diagnosed. However, in the late 1980s, some prostate cancer specialists began to promote the use of PSA as a screening test to detect prostate cancer before it had spread and before, for many men, it could be detected by the old screening method, a digital rectal exam. The theory that early detection would result in longer life expectancy was soon widely accepted by many clinicians, patients, and the press, and a PSA test became part of routine annual health examinations for middle-aged men in a growing number of communities across the country.

However, official medical opinion on the value of PSA screening was divided, and the public was getting mixed signals about what to do. The National Cancer Institute and the U.S. Preventive Services Task Force[27] recommended against performing the PSA test, on the grounds that the evidence that screening led to improved life expectancy was not strong enough to warrant its use as a public health measure. On the other hand, the American Cancer Society[28] and the AUA urged all men 50 years of age and older to be screened for prostate cancer with PSA. In some parts of the country, county health departments were entering the fray, undertaking mass education programs to persuade men to get screened.

The PORT team reached a different conclusion: that the decision to use the PSA test should be viewed as a preference-sensitive decision, not as something either to be urged on men or prohibited by physicians or the public health sector. Our reasoning went as follows. The advantages of the aggressive treatment of prostate cancer found through the PSA were (and still are) unclear.[29] PSA testing, in the words of one colleague, "is like a license to biopsy." Biopsying men over 50 will uncover a lot of early stage cancers. In this we agreed with the U.S. Preventive Services Task Force. The lack of evidence that treatment works any better when the cancer is caught earlier, and the risk of incontinence, impotence, and rectal damage associated with invasive treatment, meant that the PSA test did not qualify as proven effective care, where benefits clearly exceed the potential harms. Indeed, it was and still is experimental, in the sense that there is no strong evidence for or against its efficacy, and there is clear evidence of significant adverse effects from treatment. Using the power of a public health campaign to persuade patients to undergo PSA screening was clearly inappropriate. However, the PSA test was quite effective in discovering early-stage cancers, and aggressive treatment for prostate cancer might eventually turn out to be effective. It was certainly already part of everyday medical practice. A blanket recommendation not to use the PSA test, particularly if translated into a public health campaign to discourage its use, was perhaps equally inappropriate. Moreover, given the increasing number of vociferous and highly placed "cancer survivors" who were advocating for its use—General Norman Schwarzkopf and former U.S. Senator Robert Dole, for instance—and the broad assumption that it is always better to discover cancer earlier rather than later, a mass effort to dissuade American men from undergoing PSA screening seemed doomed to failure.

This line of reasoning led us to develop a decision aid to help patients with the PSA decision. Designed along the lines of the BPH decision aid, the PSA decision aid presented the screening decision as one that should depend on the patient's own values. The program emphasized that a decision to undergo PSA screening was linked to a second preference-sensitive decision, namely the choice of treatment for prostate cancer, and that the patient should take their treatment preferences into consideration before embarking upon a PSA test. Our video went into considerable detail in describing the potential harms of treatment, and viewers were informed about the controversy as to whether invasive treatment actually improved life expectancy among patients whose cancers were discovered by PSA testing.

The initial clinical test of the video was conducted in the General Medicine division of the Dartmouth-Hitchcock Clinic, where the video was shown to men scheduled for a routine (nonurgent) appointment with their primary care physician.[30] Prior to their appointment, men were sent a video and asked to fill out a questionnaire to test their knowledge about the PSA test and prostate cancer. The questionnaire also probed their preference for screening and, under the hypothetical scenario that cancer was discovered, what treatment they would want. The control group was given the same questionnaire but not the video.

Use of the patient decision aid had a major impact on patient knowledge about prostate cancer. Among the control group, only 41% of men understood that because most prostate cancers are slow growing, most men with prostate cancer will not die from prostate cancer, but rather from some other disease such as heart disease, stroke, or another cancer. Among men who saw the video, a large majority, 93%, got it right. When asked about the efficacy of prostate cancer treatment—whether active treatment extends life—those in the control group had a much more optimistic opinion than warranted by the facts: 76% assumed that treatment prolonged life and only 11% gave the answer that was closest to the truth, that they were not sure. By contrast, among those who saw the video, only 15% said that they thought that treatment extended life expectancy, while 70% said they were unsure.

The decision aid also altered the patients' view of screening. When asked if they intended to have a PSA test in the next two years, almost everyone in the control group, 97%, said yes. This overwhelming vote for screening seemed to reflect the widespread consensus, at least in the United States, that early detection of cancer must be a good thing. However, among informed men (those who saw the video) *only 50% wanted to be screened.* At least in the clinic we studied, the "right rate"—the amount chosen by informed patients—appears to be substantially less than the amount uninformed patients want. The two-to-one difference in stated preference between naïve and informed patients translated into actual behavior: when we checked in the claims data, 23% of men in the control group and 12% in the decision aid intervention group actually got a PSA test in association with their next visit.

Subsequently, other researchers have investigated the effect of the PSA decision aid on patients' decisions to be screened, including three RCTs comparing usual practice to shared decision making with FIMDM's decision aid.[31-33] The studies show a consistent, favorable impact of the decision aid on patient knowledge about the natural history of prostate cancer and the clinical uncertainties associated with invasive treatment. Moreover, the aid also decreased the rate of PSA screening compared to the control group. When the results of these three clinical trials are combined, the average reduction in screening rate among patients participating in shared decision making compared to those in usual practice is an absolute difference in the percentage screened of about 38%.

Our Dartmouth-Hitchcock study uncovered another interesting difference in preferences between informed men and those in the usual practice control group. We asked patients to tell us which treatment they would prefer if cancer were discovered in them. Among the control (uninformed) group, 61% answered that they would want either radiation or surgery. But among those who saw the PSA video, which alerted the viewer about the scientific uncertainty concerning the impact of treatment on PSA-discovered cancer, *only 14% said that, if they had cancer, they would choose invasive treatment;* the majority stated that they would want watchful waiting. Interestingly, we found no association between stated preference for screening and preference for invasive treatment. Patients who said they wanted to be screened were just as likely to prefer watchful waiting as were those who did not want to be screened. This result surprised me and continues to puzzle me. I had assumed that the desire to be screened and the desire to be treated aggressively would be closely linked—that men who would want conservative treatment would rather not be bothered with the knowledge that they have cancer and vice versa. This was not the case. It appears that for some men, knowledge about their cancer status has intrinsic value, independent of whether they would seek active treatment.

We do not, of course, know if patients' stated treatment preferences would change if they were to undergo a PSA test and be diagnosed with cancer. The mere thought of being at risk for cancer may have a very different impact on a patient's decisions compared with actually being diagnosed with it. We would like to know what treatment men with prostate cancer would actually choose if they had access to a patient decision aid and shared decision making. Unfortunately, such studies have not been organized, even though they are essential to a full understanding of the impact shared decision making might have on the demand for prostate cancer treatment. It seems reasonable to assume, however, that patients whose expectations have been shaped at the beginning by knowledge of the natural history of prostate cancer, who are made aware of the limitations of clinical science, and whose physicians are partnered with them in sorting out what is best for the individual patient, might well avoid rash treatment decisions based on an uninformed fear of prostate cancer.

As yet, the PSA decision aid has not been widely used in everyday practice, even though patients who use it are much more knowledgeable about the benefits and harms of screening, report favorably about the shared decision-making experience, and end up being screened much less often than those who do not use the decision aid, thus avoiding the problem of overdiagnosis of early stage cancers. Because it questions the need for cancer screening, the PSA decision aid runs counter to a powerful assumption—the belief that early detection is an unqualified good, one that all patients should have as if it were an example of effective care. My colleague Gil Welch is widely recognized for his research into the problem of overdiagnosis of early cancers. For a summary of his critique of PSA screening, see Box 7.2.

Box 7.2.   *Overdiagnosis: Why Cancer Screening Is a Two-Edged Sword*

Everyone knows the potential benefit of screening: you may avoid death from cancer. Relatively few understand the more certain harm: you may be diagnosed and treated for a cancer that was never going to bother you. This problem is called overdiagnosis.

To understand prostate cancer overdiagnosis you need to understand two things. First, from microscopic examinations of the prostates of men who are autopsied following an accidental death doctors have learned that more than 50% of older men have pathologic evidence of prostate cancer.[34] Second, the lifetime risk of prostate cancer death for the typical American male is only about 3%.[35] So, although the prevalence of the cancer may sound alarming, 97% of men will die from something else.

These two observations have forced doctors to rethink exactly what it means to have this cancer. Some have envisioned the problem to be like an iceberg. In the past, we only saw the part of the iceberg above the waterline—the cancers that caused clinical disease and death. Now, with early detection, we can see below the waterline—and there's a lot more cancer there. Many of these will never cause men problems. They are overdiagnosed.

But physicians cannot tell who is overdiagnosed and who is not. In other words, we cannot reliably distinguish between prostate cancers that will never cause symptoms and those that are deadly. So we tend to treat everyone. That means that overdiagnosed men are treated. And men who are overdiagnosed cannot benefit from treatment—there is nothing to fix. But many of them will be harmed. Treatment causes significant side effects in roughly 30% of those treated: most commonly a decline in sexual function, leaking urine, and/or rectal irritation.

That's why prostate cancer screening is such a challenging issue. Yes, it may save some men's lives, but it will harm many others along the way. Using the most optimistic data from the randomized trials the tradeoff looks like this: screen 1,000 men for 10 years and about 1 man will avoid a prostate cancer death. About 4 men will die from prostate cancer anyway. And about 50 will be overdiagnosed and needlessly treated for prostate cancer.

Thus, most men who view their life as being "saved" by prostate cancer screening (the prostate cancer survivors) are instead being over-diagnosed. Ironically, overdiagnosis creates a powerful cycle of positive feedback for more screening, as an ever increasing proportion of the population knows someone—a friend, a family member, an acquaintance, or a celebrity—who "owes their life" to early cancer detection. Some have labeled this the popularity paradox of screening: the more overdiagnosis screening causes, the more people who feel they owe it their life, and the more popular screening becomes.[36]

Although the problem of overdiagnosis is most dramatic in prostate cancer, it is not confined to prostate cancer. In fact, some degree of overdiagnosis in cancer screening is probably the rule, not the exception.

The Treatment Decision for Stable Angina

Our model for helping patients come to informed decisions about prostate disease was soon broadened to encompass other conditions. The Foundation for Informed Medical Decision Making began collaborating with other PORTs, including the ischemic heart disease (IHD) PORT. This PORT's research agenda encompassed treatments for stable angina, or chest pain due to narrowing of the coronary arteries, a common problem in the United States and throughout the Western world. Sometimes severe pain that begins rapidly may signal that a heart attack is imminent. Pain of this nature requires immediate attention. More often, the chest pain is what cardiologists would call stable angina, which is associated with exercise; sometimes severe, but relieved by rest; and helped by medication such as aspirin, nitroglycerine, and drugs known as beta-blockers. In addition to medications that affect the functioning of the heart, modern medicine offers a number of treatment options for stable angina, including medications to lower cholesterol, lifestyle modification such as exercise and weight reduction, and invasive treatment, including surgery and percutaneous coronary intervention (PCI). The PCI treatment involves snaking a catheter through the groin and up into the arteries of the heart, where blockages can be opened by dilation of a small balloon, or angioplasty, and, more recently, by the insertion of a metal stent.

For cardiologists, the coronary angiogram is a crucial diagnostic test. It provides a map of the arteries of the heart and shows where and by how much they are blocked. Some patients suffering from angina will be found to have a significant (50% or greater) blockage of the "left main" coronary artery. Blockage of this type is associated with markedly increased risk of death, and clinical trials have shown that coronary artery bypass graft (CABG) surgery can reduce that risk. However, the majority of patients who undergo an angiogram have blockages in other arteries, for which invasive treatment probably does not increase life expectancy; rather, its purpose is to improve the quality of life by reducing chest pain and the need for medication.

The collaboration between the IHD PORT and FIMDM resulted in a decision aid that, like the decision aid for BPH, was an interactive video program offering individualized information on treatment options. The video also presented interviews with patients who had experienced various outcomes that the PORT's research indicated were important for patients to know about. The IHD decision aid was tested in an RCT conducted in Toronto, Ontario.[37] The patients in the study all had stable angina and were eligible for invasive treatment, but could also be managed medically without incurring an increased risk of death. Patients with significant blockage of the left main artery were not included. In Canada, the decision to undergo invasive treatment at that time was a two-stage process. For patients being considered by their physicians for CABG surgery, information on the anatomy of the coronary arteries was obtained by angiography and a recommendation for surgery made by the cardiologist who conducted or ordered the cardiac catheterization and interpreted its findings. This information was then discussed with the patient and a decision on treatment ultimately made. In the randomized trial, the decision aid was shown to the patient before the decision was finally made.

Consistent with other trials, patients exposed to the decision aid were more knowledgeable about the decision than the controls; moreover, they chose to pursue invasive treatment less often: 75% of the control group indicated they wanted invasive treatment, while 58% of the group that saw the decision aid did. When the researchers checked six months later to see who had actually gone ahead and received invasive care, the difference held: by that time, 66% of the control group and 52% of the patient decision aid group had undergone invasive treatment.

The fact that this study was conducted in Ontario, Canada, where the patterns of practice for invasive cardiac procedures are much more conservative than in the United States, has important implications for both nations in terms of health care quality and cost. The study showed that even in conservative Ontario, the true demand for invasive cardiac treatment, as determined by informed patients, was less than the amount provided under usual practice. It also documented the interesting divergence between the angiographer's recommendation for invasive treatment (based primarily on their interpretation of biomedical tests) and the patient's preference. In the control group, 16% of patients disagreed with the treatment recommendation of the cardiologist who performed the angiography, and in the patient decision aid group, a full 35% of patients disagreed, preferring medical treatment alone rather than the recommended invasive treatment. Again, we learned that for preference-sensitive care, the treatment that patients prefer can neither be diagnosed by biomedical tests nor inferred from review of the medical history. Even in Ontario, a significant number of those identified as needing treatment did not actually want it, preferring the alternative instead.

The Treatment Decision for Low Back Pain

Back pain is an enormous medical problem in the United States. It is a major source of disability, absenteeism, and costly worker's compensation cases. For patients with severe, chronic back pain, surgery is often recommended. The rates of back surgery, however, show striking variation across the country. During the 1990s, FIMDM worked with the back pain PORT to incorporate their findings on the potential harms and benefits of alternative treatments into a low back pain decision aid. The aid addressed the treatment decision for two quite different causes of back pain.

Herniated disc is a major cause of chronic back pain. The disc is the shock absorber that sits between the vertebrae. It is made of soft, cartilage-like material and, sometimes under mechanical stress, or for no apparent reason at all, it ruptures or "herniates," putting pressure on surrounding nerves. Back and leg pain may result, and sometimes loss of function of the affected nerve may occur as well. Surgery for a herniated disc involves removal of the offending fragment of disc that is impinging on the nerve. While surgery seems to work to relieve pain and restore function, there are risks; moreover, the benefit of surgery over the more conservative management is measured in months. After three years, the problem seems to resolve for most patients, regardless of which treatment they receive. Patients thus face a tradeoff: more immediate relief from surgery, but at the risk of a bad surgical outcome—a risk that can be avoided by choosing conservative management, which generally comes at the cost of a longer interval of pain.

Spinal stenosis is another cause of back pain and disability, but the mechanism of damage is quite different. Patients with spinal stenosis have a form of arthritis of the spine, which narrows the channel through which the nerves pass. Like a herniated disc, the pressure on the nerves can cause pain and loss of function. Surgical treatment involves removal of the arthritic growth of bone that is putting pressure on the nerves. In contrast to a herniated disc, this condition does not tend to improve over time, but it also may not worsen. The surgical decision thus involves an assessment of the degree to which the pain and disability bother the patient versus the risk of surgery.

The clinical trial of the low back pain decision aid took place at Group Health Cooperative of Puget Sound and the University of Iowa Hospital.[38] The design of the trial differed from others in that the control group was not usual practice but rather patients who received a brochure that described the nature of the decision and the importance of patient preferences in the choice of treatment. For the intervention arm of the study, patients received the brochure and viewed the interactive video. The video proved a better decision aid: patients who saw it did better on tests of their knowledge. The effect of the video on their choice of surgery depended on the condition. For patients with herniated discs, those viewing the video decision aid were less likely to choose surgery than the brochure controls: 32% versus 47%, a 32% decline in surgery rate. The result was unlikely to be due to chance. For spinal stenosis patients, the effect seemed to be in the opposite direction: the patients who viewed the decision aid chose more surgery than the brochure control group: 39% versus 29%, a 34% increase, but, given the small sample size, the difference was not large enough to reach statistical significance.

A key aspect of this study was the fact that the control group was not "usual care"; the same physicians who saw the patients receiving the video decision aid also saw the brochure patients, and presumably they endorsed the concept of shared decision making. The focus of the study was thus on two different ways of communicating information to patients. Even though the information on treatment options was available in the brochure, the video format resulted in better knowledge scores and was judged by patients to be easier to use and more informative than the brochure alone.

What about the outcomes? At one year, for herniated disc patients, the functional outcomes for the video group and the brochure group were about the same, leading the PORT researchers to conclude that the rate of surgery was reduced without worse patient outcomes. For spinal stenosis patients, at one year, the outcomes for the video group appeared to be better, but there were not enough patients to pin down the association between surgery and outcomes. For both conditions, the central question of the efficacy of surgery in reducing symptoms remained open, awaiting a definitive RCT.

A Path Forward?

Today, there is renewed interest in federal support for comparative effectiveness research as an essential part of the health reform agenda, and my colleagues and I are once again hopeful that the critical weaknesses in the science of clinical decision making can be successfully addressed. The transition from delegated to shared decision making has important implications for how that research should be conducted.

First and foremost, we need an organized research agenda that is capable of continuously evaluating clinical theories that are used to justify interventions and emerging technologies. Rational decision making requires an accurate, up to date, evidence-based assessment of the outcomes that matter to patients. I believe the PORT model provides the basis for a contemporary research strategy for achieving this goal.

The importance of patient preferences also has implications for the content of clinical research. The shift from delegated decision making to shared decision making—from a decision model based on the assumption that patient preferences can be diagnosed by the physician to an open recognition of the role of the patient—means that the clinical research agenda must be expanded to include medical communication. We need studies that can pin down how best to inform patients. When a decision is well understood, it can be represented in a standardized scenario to be communicated to patients, as demonstrated by the patient decision aid research. The intervention can be evaluated to determine if choices better reflect the concerns that matter most to patients. And through research, the methods for communicating risks and for characterizing the medical tradeoffs can be progressively improved upon.

There are also important implications for the conduct of clinical trials. Patients who accept randomization are very likely different from patients who actively choose their treatment, and it is simply not reasonable to assume that the outcomes of care measured in an RCT will accurately predict what the outcomes would be for those who actively choose their treatment.[39] The inclusion of "preference arms" is a new way of thinking about clinical trials. Such trials seek to include *all* patients who, on the basis of today's evidence-based clinical guidelines, would qualify for surgical treatment if they preferred it. As illustrated by a recent large-scale, multicenter clinical trial of back surgery led by my colleague Dr. James Weinstein, decision aids can play an important role in organizing clinical trials, such that the research can include both randomized cohorts and patients who choose their treatment. By following patients who accept randomization as well as those that do not, the Weinstein study is helping to resolve a number of pressing problems in developing an understanding of the impact of patient choice on outcomes. His research also opens avenues for studying the validity of information from RCTs in predicting what happens when patients choose their treatments.[40] This design may be particularly important for organizing trials of common surgical interventions where informed patients often have strong preferences for either surgery or conservative treatment.

A second important feature of the Weinstein trial was the implied shift in the ethics of conducting clinical trials from a standard based on physician equipoise to one based on *patient* equipoise. Traditional ethics have required that before the surgeon recommends that a patient enter a trial, he must be convinced that the evidence for efficacy is so weak that an experiment in which the flip of the coin determines who gets surgery is required. Since surgeons are rarely uncertain about the value of their surgeries, successful clinical trials involving common surgical interventions are rare. The low back pain trial changed the ethics of trial entry from surgeon equipoise to one that depended on the informed patient's own decision to accept randomization. Patient decision aids provided extensive information to the patient concerning what was known and not known about the outcomes of the treatment options, and then explained the reason for conducting a clinical trial. Patients were invited to participate in the RCT to help improve clinical science; those who had a firm preference were invited to participate in the "preference trial," an outcome study involving the same protocol for data collection and follow-up as those who were randomized. The Weinstein approach resulted in the enrollment of more than 1,000 patients in the randomized arm. Wide adoption of shared decision making as a strategy for enrollment of patients might increase the success rate for surgical clinical trials.

Finally, understanding the implications of the shift from delegated decision making to shared decision making for the health care economy should be a major focus of today's comparative effectiveness research agenda. The first priority should be to understand and predict the demand for discretionary care under informed patient choice. The HMO study of BPH, described in Chapter 6, and the Hawker study of osteoarthritis of the knee, described in Chapter 5, distinguish clearly between clinically appropriate need (defined by medical experts) and preference-defined demand (defined by patients). Studies such as these are needed for predicting utilization and cost once high-quality shared decision-making processes are implemented. The research should directly address the effects of copayment and other forms of patient cost sharing on patient preferences for the more expensive treatment option.

This research is essential if rising patient demand requires policy makers to initiate patient cost sharing to reduce demand for expensive treatments.

* * *

This chapter reviewed a model for conducting comparative effectiveness research for preference-sensitive surgery. Such research depends on a stable scientific infrastructure: an orderly process for setting research priorities and accomplishing peer review, and sustained funding, including support for the practice networks, which are the vital "research laboratories" of the evaluative sciences. It also depends on the translation of research findings into effective interventions to reduce unwarranted variations, which, for preference-sensitive conditions, involves the conversion of research findings into patient decision aids that promote informed patient choice.

With the withdrawal of federal support for AHCPR's medical effectiveness program and its flagship PORT projects, the nation lost an effective program for conducting such research. With the failure of the Clinton health plan, we lost the opportunity to institutionalize the Maine Medical Assessment Foundation as an essential component of the feedback loop on practice variation, and the infrastructure needed to engage practicing physicians in the evaluation of clinical practices. The resulting gap in federal policy has yet to be filled, and the evidence needed by both physicians and patients has been set back fifteen years. In the meantime, treatment theories continue to evolve without sufficient evaluation, and medical opinion, rather than evidence-based medicine and patient preferences, continues to dominate utilization for conditions where treatment decisions should be made by informed patients in concert with their doctors. Action on the part of Congress and the administration to restore the lost opportunity to evaluate the everyday practice of medicine is urgently required if the problem of unwarranted variation is to be addressed.

PART III

Medical Variation: Understanding Supply-Sensitive Care

Supply-sensitive care differs in several fundamental ways from preference-sensitive surgical procedures. First, the physicians whose decisions determine the frequency of the use of supply-sensitive care are mostly primary care physicians and medical specialists, not surgeons. Second, supply-sensitive care is not about deciding on a specific treatment but rather about how frequently numerous, everyday medical services are provided in the process of managing acute and chronic illnesses. Supply-sensitive care covers a range of services, including physician visits, referrals to specialists, diagnostic tests, imaging exams, hospitalizations, and stays in intensive care units. Third, such decisions are not governed by strong medical theory, much less medical evidence. Indeed, practice guidelines governing clinical decisions involving supply-sensitive care are virtually nonexistent.

In the absence of evidence concerning effectiveness but under the prevailing cultural belief held by both patients and physicians that more health care is better, physicians use available capacity up to the point of its exhaustion. They schedule revisits up to the point where they have no time for more, they hospitalize patients until hospital beds become scarce, and they order more imaging exams whenever imaging equipment is available. In other words, as illustrated in Chapter 8, clinical decision making on the part of physicians determining the use of such care is sensitive to the level of supply of the resources available in a region.

This accommodation to supply seems to occur without awareness on the part of physicians that per capita supply varies from place to place or that it influences their behavior. As I will show, physicians practicing in Boston and New Haven (and affiliated with some of the nation's most prestigious academic medical centers) were largely unaware that bed capacity (and hospitalization rates for supply-sensitive conditions) in Boston was 60% greater than that in New Haven on a per capita basis. Moreover, decisions that led to an expansion in capacity in Boston were made without information on baseline supply or what the expected benefits of an increase in supply might be.

Not surprisingly, the idea that the supply of resources exerts such a strong effect on utilization has not been met with open arms by the medical community. The major counterargument against our interpretation of supply-sensitive care is that illness is the cause of the variation. Chapter 9 guides the reader through our studies, which show that differences among regions in the prevalence of chronic illness do not explain variation in the frequency of physician visits, hospitalizations, and other forms of supply-sensitive care. The same is so for demographic factors such as age, sex, and race. While black patients with chronic illness tend to get more supply-sensitive care than other racial groups, black patients living in regions with low overall use of supply-sensitive care receive less care than nonblack patients living in high-use regions. The factor lurking behind these patterns of utilization is the capacity of the system—the number of hospital beds and physicians per capita.

The bottom line question is whether more is better. In the absence of clinical research, supply-sensitive care is perhaps best described as a black box, or mystery medicine. There is no corpus of scientific evidence that can be marshaled to answer the question of whether or when more care is better. Chapter 10 describes our epidemiologic research that looked into the marginal impact of increasing the intensity of supply-sensitive care on survival and on patient satisfaction. In both cases, we find evidence that, at least for Medicare enrollees in traditional fee-for-service medicine, more is not better; indeed, it may be worse. In other words, the problem is the overuse of care in high-intensity regions, not the rationing of care in low-intensity regions.

This is not merely a problem at community hospitals. Overuse also plagues patients who are cared for in the hospitals that are considered the nation's best. But when it comes to managing chronic illness, it is not necessarily those who have the best reputation, including such recognition as high ratings from *U.S. News & World Report (USN&WR)*, who are doing the best job. Chapter 10 examines the management practices of prestigious academic medical centers to show that, despite their reputations as bastions of medical science, their practice patterns show about as much variation as other hospitals across the United States. However, some hospitals are, in fact, better. Organized systems of care such as the Geisinger Clinic and Intermountain Healthcare are typically more efficient in the way they manage chronic illness, providing high-quality care at lower costs.

There are compelling reasons why the nation needs to challenge the way chronic illness is managed in the United States. Variation in the intensity of care, particularly the use of acute care hospitals, is the major cause of the more than two-fold variation in Medicare per capita spending among regions. It is not the prices, it is the use of care—the volume—that matters more. Given the lack of coordination between sectors of care, what logically seem to be sensible strategies for reducing inpatient care—building skilled nursing home beds or encouraging home health care, for example—simply do not pay off. The overuse of care by the chronically ill is getting worse everywhere but more so in regions that already are at the top in care intensity. The problem is not just in Medicare; variation and overuse affect those under 65 years of age and appear to be highly correlated with variation in Medicare, which is not so surprising, given the importance of local capacity in influencing utilization. Reducing the volume (overuse) of care in high-use regions will benefit taxpayers and patients and families by reducing the subsidies from more efficient regions to help pay providers in less efficient regions and high copayments by patients living in high-cost regions. It will also reduce the medicalization of death.

8

Understanding Supply-Sensitive Care

Our work in Vermont and Maine focused mainly on surgical procedures, but lurking in the background was another form of care that showed a very different pattern of variation. We found that surgical procedures displayed unique signatures in each location in Maine and Vermont. The rates of tonsillectomy and hysterectomy might be high and that of back surgery low in one place, and vice versa in another region, and a third region might show a low rate for all three—and this surgical signature was remarkably stable over time. Admission rates for nonsurgical care, however, appeared to be another matter entirely. It looked as if the rates in a community followed a consistent pattern: a region with high admission rates for one medical (nonsurgical) condition tended to have high rates for other medical conditions. We also had early evidence that the supply of medical resources, such as hospital beds and physicians, was related to the rates of hospitalization for medical conditions and to the use of imaging tests and electrocardiography. But our hypothesis was difficult to test in the early 1970s, because the myriad overlapping diagnostic codes hampered our ability to know with any precision which patients were admitted for medical conditions.

This limitation disappeared in the early 1980s, when the Health Care Financing Administration implemented the diagnosis-related group, or DRG, payment system, which reimbursed hospitals a set amount for each individual diagnosis, regardless of how long the patient stayed in the hospital.

The DRG system of coding the cause of hospitalization offered us a new tool for studying practice patterns. Using this system, we were able to group the literally thousands of diagnoses physicians use to classify their patients into clusters of related conditions. Moreover, because every patient who was admitted to the hospital was assigned a DRG, we were now able to study the entire population of hospitalized patients according to clinically meaningful causes for being hospitalized and according to whether they were medical or surgical patients. Because of the assistance of the Maine Health Information Center, we obtained access to hospitalization data covering a three-year period, from 1980 through 1982.

Our DRG research revealed that admission rates for virtually every medical condition varied to a remarkable degree.[1] We compared admission rates among thirty hospital service areas in Maine and used certain common surgical procedures as benchmarks for evaluating variation. Not one medical condition exhibited the low variation pattern seen for hospitalization for a fractured hip, the condition for which the admission rate closely follows the incidence of the condition itself. Indeed, the dial on our variation gauge was telling us that supply factors were likely playing a role in determining utilization rates for all medical conditions, some more than others. Only three medical conditions—heart attacks, strokes, and bleeding from the stomach or intestine—were moderately variable: they showed less variation than the admission rates for hysterectomy. The admission rates for over 90% of medical conditions were classified as "high variation medical conditions": they exhibited greater variation among Maine hospital service areas than hysterectomy, and about 40% were more variable than back surgery.

We realized that understanding the pattern of variation in admission rates was critical to health care policy—that "to be successful, cost-containment programs based on fixed, per admission hospital prices will need to assure effective control of hospitalization rates." It was also important for clinical reasons. By focusing on specific medical conditions, we hoped to be able to connect our epidemiology of variation, which we were measuring at the level of populations, to the clinical experience of physicians, and to interest them in working to reduce unwarranted variation. But while our results gained the attention of physicians in Maine, they did not seem to make much of a stir elsewhere. Skepticism was particularly evident among physicians in the nation's teaching hospitals, who found it all too easy to dismiss the findings from this largely rural state as having no relevance to modern scientific medicine. My counterattack was to take the study of practice variation to the citadels of America's academic medical centers.

The Boston–New Haven Studies

Boston and New Haven occupy a special place in my portfolio of small area analyses for illuminating the supply-sensitive care phenomenon. These two communities are served by some of the nation's finest teaching hospitals, and most patients who are hospitalized there go to the principal academic medical centers of Yale University, Harvard University, Boston University, and Tufts University. Moreover, Boston and New Haven are remarkably similar in the demographic characteristics of their populations that predict the need for health care. Yet how different is the amount of acute hospital resources allocated to those populations! Over the years and until very recently, the number of acute care hospital beds per 1,000 used by residents for Boston has exceeded that of New Haven by about 55%. The number of hospital employees per 1,000 serving Bostonians generally ran about 90% higher, and hospital expenditures per capita in Boston were about twice those of New Haven.

My curiosity about the clinical purposes for which these "extra" acute care resources in Boston were used was first aroused by a small area study we conducted using data for 1978. This study, which I published in 1984 in *Health Affairs*, showed that residents of Boston used 4.4 beds per 1,000 residents, while New Haven residents used 2.7—a difference of 1.7 beds per 1,000.[2] At that time, we could not distinguish between surgical versus medical admissions, because the data we had did not include a diagnosis. By the mid-1980s, however, we obtained hospital discharge information similar to the Maine data, allowing us to use the DRG classification system to study the situation in some detail for hospitalizations that happened in 1982. We found that the physicians in Boston used 739 more hospital beds per 1,000 in 1982 in treating their patient populations than predicted by the New Haven benchmark.[3] As predicted by the Maine DRG study, most of those beds (71%) were used to care for adult patients with medical conditions. Seven diagnoses, all of them for chronic conditions, accounted for about 30% of the excess bed use for medical conditions: low back pain (not treated surgically) accounted for the largest portion, followed by gastroenteritis, congestive heart failure, pneumonia, diabetes, cancer of the lung (not treated surgically), bronchitis, and asthma. Five percent of the beds were used for pediatric patients with medical conditions; 12% for minor surgery (the kind of surgery that today is mostly done in the outpatient setting); and 12% were for major surgery.

For those patients hospitalized for medical conditions and minor surgery, the difference in bed use between the two communities was explained largely by a higher rate of admission to hospitals for Boston patients, not by longer lengths of stay in the hospital. By contrast, rates of admission were the same in both communities for major surgery, so the difference in bed use in that case was explained entirely by the Boston hospitals' longer lengths of stay. Once again, beds per 1,000 exerted a powerful influence on medical admission rates, but it had little effect on rates of admission for surgery, with the exception of minor surgery, which was more often performed in the inpatient setting in Boston than in New Haven.

Evidence for a Subliminal Effect of Capacity

By the time we began studying New Haven and Boston, we already suspected that more beds led to higher hospitalization rates for medical conditions. The question was, were physicians aware of it? Before the results of the study were published, I sought interviews with physicians who practiced in Boston and New Haven. I wanted to learn whether the physicians who were actually making the decisions to hospitalize were aware that their practice patterns were different in the two communities and that the availability of beds seemed to be influencing their decisions. I was particularly interested in learning whether, in supply-constrained New Haven, physicians sensed that beds were scarce—whether they ever felt a need to hospitalize patients but could not, because all the beds were full. In short, w*ere they consciously rationing hospital care because of a lack of hospital beds?*

What I learned from these interviews helped me gain insight into the largely *unconscious* nature of demand induction for supply-sensitive treatments. At first, I did not show the physicians our results, but simply asked them if they were aware that there were differences in the rates of hospitalization between the two communities. They were not. Indeed, a number of New Haven physicians I talked with who had previously practiced in Boston said that they did not think local practice styles were different, or that they had changed when they moved to New Haven. The clinicians of New Haven denied that they were rationing care, and once I informed them about the relative differences between Boston and New Haven, they seemed to take pride in their more conservative practice style.

The study, which was published in *The Lancet* in May 1987, bore the rhetorical title: "Are hospital services rationed in New Haven or over-utilized in Boston?" The study showed conclusively that even among communities served by famous academic medical centers, there were large differences in population-based hospitalization rates. Moreover, for the care that we were calling supply-sensitive, physicians with strong academic credentials were quite unaware that they practiced differently or that they might actually change their practice styles, depending on the number of hospital beds available.

A Look at Outcomes

Toward the end of the 1980s, our research group acquired access to Medicare data for New England, allowing us to search more closely for evidence that differences in the supply of resources might be leading either to rationing or overuse of health care. We revisited Boston and New Haven to compare hospital use and mortality, and to see if the difference in utilization was associated with a difference in overall population mortality rate.[4] First, we confirmed that the chance of being hospitalized still varied substantially between the two locations. It did. In 1982, 21% of the Medicare population living in Boston was hospitalized at least once compared to 16% for New Haven, and 33% of the hospitalized patients in Boston were readmitted one or more times within the study year compared to 25% for New Haven. We then looked at overall population mortality—all deaths that occurred in the hospital plus all deaths that occurred elsewhere—and found that Medicare death rates for Boston and New Haven were virtually identical.

Might New Haven patients have lived longer had their physicians admitted more of them to the hospital? We could not know from this study, but at least this much of the outcomes puzzle was becoming clear: the lower rate of hospital use in New Haven was not associated with a *higher* overall mortality rate.

The study also provided further insight into how hospital capacity may influence utilization rates. A common hypothesis ran something like this: clinicians hospitalize patients based on *sickness*. The sickest get hospitalized first, then the next sickest, and so on until beds are exhausted. Regions with fewer beds per capita run out first, so in these regions the "case-mix" of hospitalized patients will include a greater proportion of the severely ill than the mix in regions with more beds. We tested this theory by comparing the population-based hospital statistics for Boston and New Haven. We found that on an annual basis, a greater proportion of Medicare patients were admitted once or more to hospitals in Boston than those in New Haven which had fewer beds, suggesting that capacity influences the decision to admit, leading to more hospitalizations for those who were less severely ill in Boston. The lower case-fatality rates in Boston hospitals were also consistent with this interpretation.[5] On the other hand, the bed effect also seemed to influence the hospitalization rate for those who were the most severely ill: on a population basis, Boston patients were much more likely to die in the hospital than someplace else, such as at home or in hospice care. For Bostonians, 40% of all deaths occurred in the inpatient setting, compared to 32% for New Havenites. It was as if Boston hospitals were a giant vacuum, hoovering patients of varying levels of sickness into beds, but not necessarily making a difference in their outcomes compared with New Haven.

A New Way to Study Practice Variations

We conducted yet another test of our theory that in Boston the clinical threshold for admitting patients was lower for a broad spectrum of medical conditions when compared to New Haven. This study, published in 1994 in the *New England Journal of Medicine*, used a new method for measuring practice variations based on a cohort design.[6] It focused on patients who all experienced a specific clinical condition, and followed them over time. (See Box 8.1 for a description of the advantages of cohort studies.)

The first part of the study was conducted on residents of Boston who were hospitalized for one of the handful of clinical conditions that are more or less uniformly diagnosed, and for which, once the diagnosis is made, virtually all physicians recommend hospitalization. To become part of the study, a resident of Boston or New Haven had to have been hospitalized for one of these "index events," a hip fracture; a surgical procedure for cancer of the colon, lung, or breast; an acute myocardial infarction; a stroke; or gastrointestinal bleeding. For these conditions, the hospitalization rates were about the same for residents of Boston and New Haven (because the rates of the conditions were about the same for the two cities). The goal of the study, however, was not to compare the rate for the initial hospitalization among Bostonians and New Havenites—we already knew that they were pretty much the same. Rather, we were interested in comparing the pattern for *subsequent* hospitalizations, to test the hypothesis that Bostonians with identified chronic illnesses were being hospitalized much more frequently than similarly ill patients in New Haven. To do this, we first identified all patients hospitalized for an index event over a two-year period, and then linked the initial record for each patient to all subsequent hospitalizations that occurred for that patient during a period of time that extended up to three years. We then analyzed the records for each of the six cohorts (groups of patients with hip fractures, cancer, etc.) to calculate the admission rate for each six-month period of follow-up.

The results confirmed our hypothesis. Overall, the risk for *subsequent* hospitalization following the index event was 1.6 times higher for patients

Box 8.1.   *The Advantages of Cohort Studies*

While very useful for studying patterns of variation, cross-sectional geographic studies are less useful for studying outcomes of care, particularly questions concerning the impact of treatment on specific types of patients—say the survival of heart attack patients who receive (or do not receive) a particular drug. For such questions, epidemiologists typically use cohort studies, which "enroll" patients who experience a given event and observe what happens to them subsequently, depending, say, on the medical community where they live. An important advantage of the cohort approach is that it can include everyone with the disease, and not just those accepted into the conventional randomized trial. (Often randomized trials exclude patients with complications, or older patients.) Furthermore, the use of cohort studies allows for far more patients—often in the thousands—which increases the statistical precision of the results. Cohort studies do lack pure randomization, but we have found that populations of heart attack patients, for example, tend to be similar regardless of where they live. Furthermore, the Medicare data allows for adjustment for comorbidities (other conditions the patient may have had during the index hospitalization), as well as demographic factors, such as age, sex, and race, that may affect the individual's level of illness and outcome. This allows us to compare the outcomes of similar patients (apples to apples!) who live in different regions and experience different intensity of care.

living in Boston compared to New Haven—an almost exact replication of our study published in *The Lancet*, which used the classic small area analysis design showing that population-based rates of hospitalization were different between the two cities. Moreover, as predicted by our previous small area variation studies, the large majority of the readmissions were for medical, not surgical conditions. A patient who had been first admitted for a heart attack, for example, might be readmitted for congestive heart failure. The effect of bed capacity on clinical decision making seemed about equal for all cohorts. In other words, *the effect did not depend on the initial diagnosis*; for the cancer cohorts, the risk of subsequent admission for Bostonians was 1.6 times greater than for New Havenites; when the initial condition was a hip fracture, it was 1.6 times greater; and for acute myocardial infarction and for stroke, it was also 1.6 times greater.

Indeed, the threshold effect of beds worked to influence the risk of hospitalization for all patient subgroups. Women in the Boston cohorts (regardless of initial diagnosis) were 62% more likely to be hospitalized than their counterparts in New Haven. For men, the rates were 67% higher; for white patients, 66% higher; for nonwhite (mostly black) patients, rates were 43% higher; for older patients (75 years of age or older), 69% higher; and for younger Medicare patients (aged 65–74), rates were 54% higher. As predicted by previous studies, the threshold effect influenced primarily medical and minor surgery cases, rather than major surgery. Virtually every acute and chronic illness diagnostic group was affected.

Evaluating Hospital-Specific Performance

The second part of our study broke further ground in advancing the methods for evaluating patterns of care. The cohort method was adapted to provide hospital-specific estimates, allowing, for the first time, an investigation into the rates of admission according to the hospital most often used by the patient, rather than the region as a whole. (See Box 8.2.) We uncovered considerable differences in the risks of hospitalization for individual teaching hospitals within Boston. Compared to the most conservative teaching hospital, the Yale-New Haven Hospital, the rates of admission were substantially higher for all Boston teaching hospitals. Some were below the increased risk factor of 1.6 measured for the area as a whole, while others were well above it.

Armed now with hospital-specific data, I once again sought the opportunity to see if clinicians in Boston teaching hospitals, whose decision making was responsible for determining which patients were hospitalized, were aware that their practice styles varied according to where they practiced. Keeping the identify of each Boston teaching hospital hidden, I first showed them data comparing the admission rates of the six major teaching hospitals in Boston to the Yale-New Haven Hospital. For these institutions, admission rates were between 50 and 98% higher than Yale-New Haven. Here are the ratios compared to Yale-New Haven:

Hospital A	1.98
Hospital B	1.86
Hospital C	1.62
Hospital D	1.61
Hospital E	1.57
Hospital F	1.50
Yale-New Haven	1.00

Box 8.2. *Measuring Hospital-Specific Performance*

If each Boston hospital were like a prepaid, staff model HMO, such as Kaiser Permanente, we would know from the enrollment files the exact size of the populations they serve. The cohort method provided us with a way of estimating the population at risk for the vast majority of U. S. providers, who were not (and still are not) organized in this way. We assigned patients to the hospital where the index event occurred: the hip fracture, cancer surgery, etc. We then analyzed the data to determine which hospitals were used for subsequent admissions. There was a high degree of loyalty among the Medicare patients, as most subsequent hospitalizations occurred at the same hospital as the initial one. (Among the 11 hospitals in the study, between 62% and 90% of readmissions were to the index hospital.) Thus, we could calculate the rate for subsequent hospitalizations—using the number of patients with hip fractures, cancers, and so on as denominators—with assurance that the clinical decisions that led to hospitalization were primarily made by clinicians associated with specific teaching hospitals. It thus became possible to compare the rates for specific hospitals in Boston and New Haven.

I then asked them to guess, based on their personal experience, where their own institution was in the spectrum of variation, and to name the other Boston hospitals. None were aware of their own, much less any other institution's, relative frequency of hospitalizing patients. Many guessed that Hospital A, with admission rates 1.98 times greater than Yale-New Haven, was the Massachusetts General Hospital. As it turned out, Massachusetts General was Hospital F, the Boston hospital that was closest to New Haven in its rate of admission, though it still exceeded the Yale-New Haven Hospital's practice pattern by 50%.

The most interesting case concerned the admission rates for Hospitals A and C. One is Boston City Hospital, the hospital serving the indigent of Boston; the other is Boston University Medical Center. At the time of this study, these two "hospitals" were in fact a single building separated into two separate hospital wings, each with its own complement of beds relative to the size of the population it served. The physicians attending at the Boston City Hospital also served the Boston University Medical Center and vice versa. The data showed that the rate of admission for patients loyal to Hospital A was significantly higher (statistically and clinically) than for Hospital C. I asked them to guess which hospital was which. Although some were onto my game by then, most guessed that Hospital A, with the highest rate of admission per 1,000 had to be Boston City Hospital, primarily because it served the poorest—and therefore the sickest—segments of the Boston population. They were wrong. The admission rate at Boston University Medical Center (Hospital A) was the highest of all Boston teaching hospitals, almost twice that of Yale-New Haven, and 22% greater than the admission rate among patients loyal to Boston City Hospital, suggesting that the complement of beds available for the insured population was greater than the complement of beds for the indigent. This natural experiment provided important insight into the subliminal, yet powerful effect that bed supply exerts on physician decisions. *The physicians were simply unaware of the changes in their own practice styles that occurred when they crossed the firewall dividing the two wings of the hospital complex.* (The assumption that poverty—and illness—is the most important determinant of variation in admission rates persists, and it was raised again in 2009 during the debate over health care reform, as discussed in subsequent chapters.)

What about the outcomes of care? An important advantage of the cohort methodology is its ability to measure survival following an initial admission event such as a heart attack or hip fracture. Using this method, we could directly address important questions about health care rationing that could not be answered by small area correlation studies. Were New Haven physicians keeping patients out of the hospital that would have lived longer had they been admitted? To answer this question, we followed our heart attack, stroke, hip fracture, cancer, and intestinal bleeding patients for up to three years. While Bostonians with these conditions received about 60% more hospitalizations, they did not live any longer. The overall mortality for the cohorts during the entire period of follow-up was essentially the same in the two cities. The implications of this finding were both clear and arresting: for these two cities—and their constituent academic medical centers—the extra care delivered to patients in Boston did not appear to improve life expectancy. The variation in supply-sensitive care appeared to be a case of overuse in Boston, not rationing in New Haven.

The Invisible Hand of Capacity

The idea that the supply of resources "causes" an increase in utilization of services is not a new one. Indeed, in the health care policy world, it is often held as the truism known as "Roemer's Law," named for Milton Roemer, who concluded in the 1960s that a hospital bed, once built and available, will be used no matter how many beds there are.[7]

With the completion of the first round of Dartmouth Atlas studies in the 1990s, we were able to conduct the first national study of the association between available hospital beds and hospitalization rates. Among the 306 Dartmouth Atlas regions, as predicted by our earlier studies, hospitalization rates for hip fracture showed virtually no relationship with hospital bed capacity (R^2 = .06). By contrast, having more hospital beds was directly associated with higher hospitalization rates for patients with acute and chronic medical conditions. Indeed, the association between beds and admission rate was quite strong. More than half—54%—of the variation was associated with bed capacity (Figure 8.1).

The pattern makes medical sense. When, as in the case of hip fracture, the incidence of disease is the most important determinant of variation in hospitalization, the supply of resources is not closely associated with the utilization of care. The market is "cleared" of need, as every case of hip fracture has a priority claim on hospital beds, no matter what the per capita supply of beds. For most medical conditions, however, the clinical decision to hospitalize

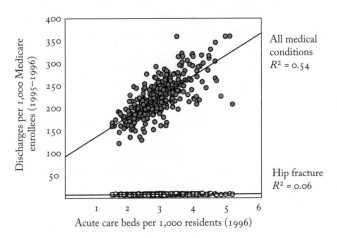

Figure 8.1.   The association between hospital beds (1996) and discharges for medical conditions and for hip fracture (1995 through 1996) among hospital referral regions. (Source: Wennberg, J. E., and E. S. Fisher, eds. 2006. *The Care of Patients with Severe Chronic Illness: A Report on the Medicare Program by the Dartmouth Atlas Project. The Dartmouth Atlas of Health Care 2006.* Hanover, NH: The Center for the Evaluative Clinical Sciences [online].)

a patient is not so clear-cut and the "supply" of cases that current medical practice labels as appropriate for admission nearly always exceeds capacity. In other words, there are nearly always more sick people than there are beds. For most acute and chronic illnesses, the diagnosis is not in itself sufficient grounds for hospitalization. The clinician is forced to make decisions on the hospitalization of individual cases that have a place on a spectrum of severity—to distinguish between shades of grey, not the binary black-and-white hip fracture decision. Physicians make these decisions within the context of available beds. The key idea here is that when a physician faces uncertainty concerning medical prognosis, the dominant cultural bias is to err on what is perceived to be the side of safety—to prescribe hospitalization when a bed is available. Moreover, under fee-for-service Medicare, economic incentives are squarely in sync with the "more is better" assumption, even when the physician does not directly benefit financially from the decision to hospitalize.

In the absence of explicit theory and useful rules of thumb, decision making is often guided by a general assumption that when in doubt, more health care is better. Both doctors and patients assume that the acute hospital setting, with all of its resources and concentrated medical skills, is a better place to deal with sick patients with guarded or uncertain prognoses than are other settings, like the patient's home or even the nursing home, where care is seemingly less organized and there are fewer physicians and nurses available. Under such an assumption, the availability of beds becomes critical. Among teaching hospitals in Boston and New Haven, the occupancy rates were all quite high, but beds were always available for the "low variation" conditions like hip fracture, or cancer patients needing surgery, cases that everyone agrees require hospitalization. But these conditions comprise only a small proportion of patients using beds—even in regions with constrained beds per 1,000 people. Thus, at any given point in time, the patient population of the hospital with medical diagnoses is composed mostly of patients with acute and chronic illnesses that are susceptible to the threshold effect of capacity. And when there are more beds per capita, there are more opportunities to place the patient in the "safer" inpatient environment.

The reader will recall that our studies in Maine found that each hospital service area had a surgical signature, its own peculiar pattern of surgical rates for different conditions—high rates for some, low rates for others. Moreover, the overall rate of surgery (the total discharge rate) is not closely correlated with the rate for any given surgical procedure. By contrast, the rate of hospitalization for a specific high variation medical condition tends to be closely associated with total discharge rates; and within a given region, hospitalization rates tend to be more or less uniform across all high variation medical conditions. The medical signatures for Boston and New Haven, as reported in the 1998 Atlas, are illustrated in Figure 8.2.

We found a similar pattern when we looked at the frequency of physician visits. Patients had more physician visits per capita in regions where the per capita supply of physicians was higher, particularly for physicians that spend most of their practice time on older, chronically ill patients, such as general internists and cardiologists (Figure 8.3). This association between supply and utilization makes sense in the outpatient setting, given what is known about the way patients are scheduled for follow-up visits. Most physician visits are revisits, scheduled by the physician (or, more likely, their office personnel), who typically fill most available hours with established patients. Most patients with chronic illnesses are assumed to need monitoring, and the only real question the physician faces in rescheduling is the relative need among the individual patients for whom he routinely provides care. (The sicker ones, of course are seen more often.) But if physicians have fewer patients in their patient population, the frequency of revisits will be higher for all patients with chronic illness—the sickest and less sick as well.

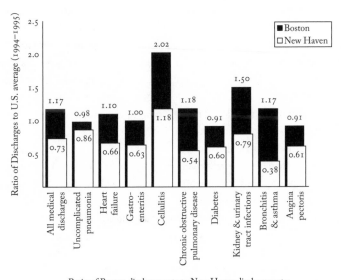

Figure 8.2.   The medical signatures of the Boston and New Haven hospital service areas (1994 through 1995). (Source: Wennberg, J. E., and M. M. Cooper, eds. 1998. *The Dartmouth Atlas of Health Care 1998*, Chicago, IL: American Hospital Publishing.)

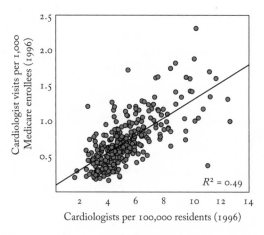

Figure 8.3.   The association between cardiologists and visits to cardiologists among hospital referral regions (1996). (Source: Wennberg, J. E., and E. S. Fisher, eds. 2006. *The Care of Patients with Severe Chronic Illness: A Report on the Medicare Program by the Dartmouth Atlas Project. The Dartmouth Atlas of Health Care 2006.* Hanover, NH: The Center for the Evaluative Clinical Sciences [online].)

It's tempting for some to believe that physicians are acting as self-serving, even cynical inducers of demand, hospitalizing patients and scheduling revisits so that they can make more money. But this cannot be the explanation, as there are no normative scientific standards for rescheduling or hospitalization to be transgressed. Astonishing as it may seem to many patients and even some health care policy analysts, medical science provides no guidance on what the best practice interval between visits should be or when to hospitalize. There is remarkably little medical theory and almost no medical evidence concerning the optimum frequency of interventions for supply-sensitive services. This was evident both through my personal interviews with academic clinicians in Boston and New Haven, and also in the lack of formal discourse in medical texts concerning best practices regarding the appropriate frequency of the use of supply-sensitive services. In the standard medical texts that inform the practice of both primary and medical specialty care, and in the practice guidelines that constrain clinical decision making, one searches in vain for even the briefest discussion concerning the criteria for admitting chronically ill patients to the hospital and to intensive care, or the optimal interval between revisits for patients with established disease.

The lack of guidelines, or evidence, or any form of normative scientific constraint on physician decision making for supply-sensitive care has a profound impact on the health care economy. The number of physician office hours available for monitoring and managing the care of the population living in a region is closely dependent on the supply of clinically active physicians per 100,000 residents. Take a hypothetical case. In region A, which has twice as many cardiologists as region B, twice as many hours will be available for a cardiologist to schedule. On average, region A's population will experience twice as many visits per person compared with region B, and the mean interval between visits will be about half that of Region B. Neither the patients nor the clinicians in regions A and B will be aware of the differences in practice style. The patients will assume that their medical need determines the schedule for revisits. Physicians will allocate their time to patients on the basis of relative illness, with the sicker patients experiencing more frequent visits. Most physicians in both communities will be working long hours, believing that the care they provide is necessary care, and totally unaware that capacity differs—or that capacity influences their clinical decision making. Only the epidemiologist, peering at health care from 30,000 feet, can see the patterns of practice and make the connection between capacity and utilization.

What Accounts for Variation in Capacity?

Understanding supply-sensitive care requires an understanding of why capacity itself varies so much from region to region (and from hospital to hospital). In my experience, satisfactory answers to the question, "Why do some hospitals in some regions grow more rapidly in relation to the size of the local population than do others?" do not emerge from the 30,000-foot perspective or statistical correlations. Epidemiology has in its book of methods what traditionalists call "shoe-leather" research—that is, getting out on the streets and looking for explanations that might solve a mystery. The most famous example remains John Snow's careful charting of the outbreak of cases in the London cholera epidemic of 1854, when he pinpointed contaminated drinking water supplied through the Broad Street pump by the Vauxhall Water Company as the source of contagion. Following in the footsteps of Snow, I have had the opportunity to undertake two shoe-leather investigations of the dynamics of hospital construction, both of which illuminated how the capacity of local health care markets became established.

Consider first the example of Boston and New Haven, where different regulatory regimes influenced the growth of hospital capacity. Consistently over the years, the capacity of the acute care hospital sector in Massachusetts exceeded that of Connecticut. For example, the number of acute care hospital beds per 1,000 allocated to the health of Bostonians exceeded that of New Havenites by about 55%; the numbers of hospital employees per 1,000 serving Bostonians generally ran about 90% more, and hospital expenditures per capita were about twice those of New Haven. These differences can be traced to the period shortly after World War II, when the hospital industry enjoyed a period of growth, stimulated in part by the Hill-Burton Act.

Passed in 1946, the act required states to develop "state health plans" on the need for beds, in order to receive federal subsidies for hospital construction. In many states, including Massachusetts, Hill-Burton grants were tied to a planning methodology designed to ensure that the occupancy of hospitals did not exceed a given level. Thus, the more pressure that was placed on available beds, the more "need" there was determined to be, independent of the actual numbers of hospital beds per 1,000 in the community or region.

As I learned from a 1987 interview with John Thompson, who had recently retired from his professorship in hospital administration at Yale, the evolution of the Hill-Burton planning process in Connecticut was quite different from Massachusetts. In Connecticut, the decision process was dominated to a large extent by the CEOs of the existing hospitals. Their basic strategy was to keep new competitors out of their local markets, using the state's Certificate of Need, or CON, legislation to thwart attempts to establish new hospitals. Thompson, who had been part of the process, believed that this was the primary reason why over the years Connecticut has been at the low end of the national spectrum in hospital beds per 1,000. He cited two specific examples of how the process responded to keep capacity low in the New Haven area. One was the reaction to a petition by several dissident physicians who wished to leave the teaching hospital to start a suburban hospital in a neighboring community. The other was a proposal to build a Jewish hospital. Both were turned down during the CON process (as were similar applications in other parts of the state).

The CON process in Massachusetts, by contrast, was much more open to the influence of various interests that wanted to expand the hospital industry. Thompson cited competition between Boston teaching hospitals as a major reason for the expansion of capacity in that region: each hospital required its full complement of services and obtained the needed approvals from the CON administrators (and capital from banks, bondholders, and federal subsidies) without difficulty. Growth of the hospital sector in the greater Boston area was also susceptible to the pressure for a place to practice medicine from physicians who did not win, or did not want, appointments at a Boston teaching hospital, but who stayed in the area and were welcomed on the staffs of community hospitals. This pressure was particularly strong in the Boston area because of the many academic training programs that produced new medical residents (who characteristically seek to practice medicine in the region where they train).

In other communities, hospital capacity is built up for different reasons. Take Augusta and Waterville, two neighboring communities in central Maine, where competitive dynamics and religious preference created the pressure to build more beds. The following facts emerged from our studies in Maine in the 1970s. At that time, Augusta and Waterville had about 50,000 persons each, but very different supplies of acute care hospital beds: about 3.5 beds per 1,000 for residents of Augusta and about 5.5 beds per 1,000 for Waterville. In Waterville, there were three hospitals: one an osteopathic hospital, the second an allopathic Catholic hospital, and the third nonsectarian and allopathic. (The Catholic hospital and nonsectarian allopathic hospital have since merged.) In Augusta, history produced but one nonsectarian hospital that, from the beginning, welcomed allopathic and osteopathic physicians as well as all religions. Having three hospitals netted 60% more beds per capita for Waterville—and higher per capita spending and utilization.

Why did the three hospitals in Waterville not come to some market equilibrium, with each taking care of its share of the population, and none building more beds than necessary? I have already made the case that the physician is ineffective as society's agent for constraining the overuse of supply-sensitive care, largely because he or she is almost entirely unaware of the effect of supply on his or her discretionary decisions, and because clinical science imposes no significant constraint on physician decision making in ways that might also place limits on their use of resources. One can be quite sure that in 1970, the administrators and boards of trustees of the three hospitals in Waterville, or anyone else in a position to influence decisions on capacity, were not at all concerned about the possibility of excess beds per capita in their community; it would never have crossed their minds, for any number of reasons. There was little recognition that supply could drive utilization, and a widespread assumption that more medical services led to better outcomes. In addition, several "system-level" factors were at work to reduce awareness of the consequences of any decision to increase capacity. First, key information was lacking: because population-based data on resource capacity was unavailable, administrators and boards of trustees of hospitals were unaware of hospital capacity relative to the size of the resident population in their own region, much less the number of beds their own hospital used in caring for its loyal population. Second, the capital for expanding the acute care sector was readily available, no matter how many hospital beds per capita there already were. During the 1970s and 80s, the federal Hill-Burton Act subsidized the construction of hospitals, but its planning methods were flawed. Again, the problem can be traced in part to lack of population data: the signal that planners relied upon for measuring scarcity of beds was the occupancy rate—the percentage of available beds that on average are filled. But the occupancy rate is an unreliable measure of the needs of the population, because it is largely uncorrelated with either prevalence of illness or the existing bed supply. In Vermont, for example, as we documented in our 1973 paper in *Science*, the use of this measure to determine need resulted in paradoxical decisions on the part of the state health planning agency, calling for additional bed construction in regions that already had a high per capita number of beds.

Finally, there were no direct economic consequences to employers and individuals living in Waterville in terms of the price they paid for health insurance. Those who buy insurance are insulated from the true cost of care in their local communities, so they do not put pressure on hospitals to constrain utilization or the growth in capacity that can drive it. In the late 1970s, Blue Cross was the dominant provider of health insurance in Maine and the price Blue Cross charged for a policy was the same throughout the state, no matter what the actual level of per capita utilization, and thus spending, was in a given region. Furthermore, hospitals are viewed as desirable to the community, both in generating local jobs and in attracting new residents.

In our Maine research, we documented striking differences in per capita reimbursements by Blue Cross in Maine and then compared how much the residents in different communities had paid out for insurance versus how much care they received. In 1979, Blue Cross paid the providers in Waterville $221 per subscriber on average, 1.46 times greater than the $151 it paid per subscriber in Augusta, meaning that the 22,800 Waterville subscribers received nearly $1 million worth of care more than they (or their employers) paid to Blue Cross. Residents of Augusta, by contrast, received $750,000 less care than they paid for.[8] One has to wonder, if the price of health insurance had been adjusted to reflect local market per capita costs, would the citizens of Waterville have come to a different conclusion concerning the need for three hospitals, and taken steps to reduce their excess capacity? These may seem like small numbers today, but given the dramatic increase in the cost of health care, both in terms of utilization and price per unit of service, the magnitude of dollar transfers from low to high cost communities now reaches into the billions of dollars. (In Chapter 12, I provide an estimate of the amount of transfer payments under traditional Medicare.)

The Patterns of Practice Today

The pattern of practice for supply-sensitive care today is very much the same as it was when I first began my studies in New England some 30 years ago. In preparing this chapter, I repeated as closely as I could the 1980–1982 Maine study of variation in medical conditions discussed earlier in this chapter, using Medicare data from 2005. I looked at the pattern of variation in discharge rates among the 306 Atlas hospital referral regions for 59 medical conditions identified through the DRG coding system. With one exception, the story across the nation in 2005 is essentially the same as it was in Maine in the 1980s. Back then, 90% of medical discharges in Maine were high variation—as variable or more so than hysterectomy; in 2005, most Medicare patients in the country—88% of Medicare discharges for medical conditions—were hospitalized with high variation medical conditions—more variable than knee replacement.[9]

Figure 8.4 illustrates the pattern of variation for eight medical conditions, selected because they are the most common in terms of frequency of hospitalization: each accounts for about 250,000 or more of patients hospitalized for medical DRGs in 2005 among Medicare recipients. Together, the eight conditions account for 40.9% of all medical conditions. Discharge rates for stroke and bleeding from the gastrointestinal tract exhibit moderate variation among the 306 regions, with a coefficient of variation that lies between hip fracture hospitalizations and knee replacement. The discharge rate for

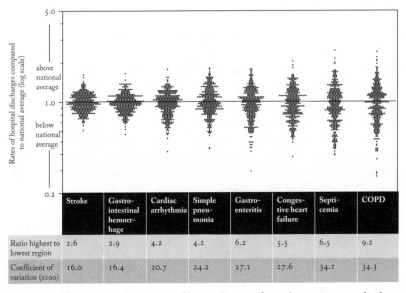

	Stroke	Gastro-intestinal hemorr-hage	Cardiac arrhythmia	Simple pneu-monia	Gastro-enteritis	Conges-tive heart failure	Septi-cemia	COPD
Ratio highest to lowest region	2.6	2.9	4.2	4.2	6.2	5.5	6.5	9.2
Coefficient of variation (x100)	16.0	16.4	20.7	24.2	27.1	27.6	34.1	34.3

Figure 8.4. The pattern of variation of hospitalization for eight common medical conditions among hospital referral regions in 2005. (Source: Dartmouth Atlas Project database.)

cardiac arrhythmia is on the boundary between high and medium variation, with a coefficient of variation similar to knee replacement. Discharge rates for patients with pneumonia, gastroenteritis, and congestive heart failure are more variable than knee replacement; discharge rates for chronic pulmonary obstructive disease and septicemia are more variable than back surgery.

The exception was the change I noted in the pattern of variation for patients with acute myocardial infarction. In the Maine study, heart attack discharge rates followed the moderate variation pattern. In the 2005 Medicare study, however, heart attacks classified as medical conditions were highly variable, in fact more variable than the rates for knee replacements. The increase is explained in part by the DRG coding convention. The Maine study was conducted before the advent of percutaneous coronary intervention, or PCI—a procedure involving using a catheter to expand a coronary artery, such as stents. By 2005, heart attack victims were often treated with PCI and thus, under the DRG convention, they became classified as "surgical patients." But this is not the only reason why variation increased. Diagnostic practice also changed. In the 1980s in Maine, the diagnosis of a heart attack was made primarily on the basis of a blood test and changes in the electrocardiogram caused by damage to the heart muscle. By 2005, the availability of methods to improve blood flow and prevent damage to the heart muscle, and more sensitive blood tests, had led to earlier interventions, often in patients for whom the diagnosis of acute myocardial infarction is less certain. Depending on how hard they look, more patients will be diagnosed with a heart attack in some hospitals than in others.[10]

Recent years have brought about some interesting changes in discharge rates for medical conditions in New Haven. Across the United States, discharge rates for medical conditions rose from 224 per 1,000 in 1995 to 244 per 1,000 in 2005, a 9.0% increase. During the same period of time, discharge rates for residents of Boston increased 6.5%—a roughly similar increase. New Haven rates, however, rose dramatically. In 1995, the discharge rate was 166 discharges per 1,000; by 2005, the rates had risen 41.4% to 234 per 1,000. The high rate of growth in utilization among New Haven hospitals went a long way to closing the Boston-New Haven gap: in 1995, discharge rates in Boston were 59% higher than New Haven; by 2005, they were only 20% higher.

At the time of this writing, we are still investigating the question of why, after years of stability, the New Haven profile changed so dramatically. Between then and now, New Haven built more beds, increasing its capacity by about 5.6%, even though the Medicare population did not grow. The New Haven increase in discharge rates was associated with a 29% decline in length of stay. (The drop in lengths of stay in essence released beds that were then used for new admissions.) The changes in traditional Medicare were also associated with a striking rise, and then a fall, in Medicare HMO enrollment in the intervening years, rising from essentially zero in 1995, peaking at 30% of the Medicare population in 1999–2000, and falling back to 9% by 2003–2005. Unfortunately we do not have records for hospitalizations for the HMO population, nor for the patient population under 65, which are likely essential for fully understanding the sudden shift in practice patterns.

* * *

By the end of the 1980s, our research projects were well on the way to building the factual basis for understanding practice variations for supply-sensitive care. Beginning with the Vermont survey, we saw that while illness obviously influenced patient behavior in seeking medical care—and sicker patients on average got more care than the less sick—illness did not explain the variation in the amount of care patients received in different regions of the state. In Maine, we saw that hospitalization rates for conditions such as hip fractures, which clinicians all agree need to be hospitalized, showed little variation. On the other hand, hospitalizations for conditions such as pneumonia, chest pain, and congestive heart failure varied substantially, much more than seemed plausible on the basis of differences in lung or heart disease.

We continued these studies in Boston and New Haven, where we followed patients when they were hospitalized for heart attacks, hip fractures, and a few other conditions for which the initial hospitalization was considered mandatory. Although it was unlikely that Bostonians with these conditions were sicker than New Havenites, they nonetheless experienced 60% more hospitalizations over a three-year period of follow-up after the index hospitalization, mostly for such medical conditions as pneumonia, chest pain, and congestive heart failure, for which there is no guidance for physicians about when to hospitalize.

We also accumulated evidence that patients living in regions with fewer resources and lower utilization of hospitals were not experiencing worse outcomes. In Vermont, we found no correlation between hospitalization or medical spending and mortality; in Boston and New Haven, mortality rates were similar, even though hospitalization rates were much lower in New Haven. And when we followed victims of heart attacks, stroke, hip fracture, gastrointestinal bleeding, and colon cancer for up to three years, we found no differences in survival between Boston and New Haven patients, despite dramatic differences in their hospitalization rates for high variation medical conditions.

More recently, thanks to the Dartmouth Atlas Project, the scope of our research has expanded. Our findings, summarized in the next two chapters, confirm that the prevalence of illness plays only a minor role in driving practice variation across the United States; that patient preferences do not explain care intensity; and that patient survival, patient satisfaction, and quality of care tend to be worse in regions where care is more intense.

9

Chronic Illness and Practice Variation

The idea that the supply of medical resources can influence utilization is not new—Milton Roemer said it in the 1960s—yet it has proved to be one of the most contentious aspects of our research. Physicians are often deeply threatened by the notion that the supply of everything from hospital beds to slots in their appointment books can influence their day-to-day decisions about their patients, decisions they prefer to believe are grounded in rational medical judgment and sound science. Hospital administrators and boards of trustees do not want to acknowledge that their expensive expansion plans may not always be in the best interests of patients, or society. Nor have economists always been receptive to the specter of systematic market failure resulting from a mismatch between the supply of medical resources and the medical needs and wants of patient populations.

The principal argument made against our characterization of the role of supply factors in influencing utilization has been that regions and hospitals that deliver more services do so because they have sicker patient populations, or they have more demanding patients than regions and hospitals that deliver fewer services per capita. It is certainly possible that residents of a region like, say, Los Angeles want more care than residents of San Francisco. But can patient demand explain the extraordinary variation in utilization that we see between regions? And it is true that sicker patients access the health care system more frequently than less sick patients. This has been evident since the

1960s, as shown in the research by Andersen and Newman[1] at the University of Chicago. Jack Fowler's study,[2] reported in Chapter 2, confirmed this to be the case in Vermont.

But what matters most in terms of the utilization and costs of care is what happens to patients after they access the system, as with, for example, patients from Boston and New Haven who have heart attacks and hip fractures. As we have extended our studies to the national Medicare program, we have found that similarly ill patients use vastly different amounts of care, depending on where they live and the providers they use. Variations in utilization, resource capacity, and costs among regions are only loosely linked with the prevalence of illness.

In evaluating how the needs and desires of patients influence the utilization of acute hospital care, it is useful to view the question from three perspectives. How much care do those who are similarly ill get, depending on where they live or the providers they use? (This question addresses the amount of services consumed, conditional upon illness.) How much illness is there in a patient population—or what is the prevalence of illness—and how does this influence utilization? Finally, do those who get more care, particularly at the end of life, actually want more care—and do they get the care they want? This chapter looks at how we answer these three questions, and it builds the case that illness and patient preference do not explain the variation we see in supply-sensitive care.

How Much Care Do Similarly Ill Patients Get?

This turns out to be a difficult question to answer, because it is hard to adjust for severity of illness. The strategy we hit upon for addressing this question was to compare the patterns of services received by chronically ill Medicare enrollees during fixed intervals prior to death. There were several reasons to use this method. First, virtually all chronically ill Medicare patients are quite sick in the months leading up to death. This is the nature of chronic disease; patients grow sicker and sicker over time, and while some may die relatively rapidly from one disease or another—a catastrophic stroke or heart attack, for example—most patients with chronic illness experience an inevitable worsening of symptoms and gradual decline in functional status that ultimately leads to death. Second, the chronically ill by necessity access the health care system in the months prior to death. They are sick and in distress. They suffer acute exacerbations of their conditions that may leave them unable to breathe, or eat, or walk. That means we are able to capture the health care experience of virtually all patients in a given region who die in a given period of time. Third, by restricting the cohort to those who died, every patient in the sample population is identical along at least one very important measure of health status: all are dead at the end of the period of observation. Fourth, by adjusting for age, sex, race, and type of illness—factors known to be associated with the utilization of care—we remove the possible contribution of differences in the frequency of these factors to variation in care intensity.

Here is how we constructed our cohorts. First, we searched Medicare records to identify all Medicare patients who died within a given period of time (most often, over a calendar year). Then we measured their utilization based on the bills that Medicare paid for the services they had incurred over fixed intervals of time prior to death—the last six months of life, for example. By further restricting the cohort to patients who succumbed to one or more of nine chronic diseases[3] and adjusting for age, sex, race, and the type of chronic illness, we believe it is very unlikely that variations in severity of illness from place to place would remain a likely explanation for the variations in the use of acute care hospital and physician services observed during this period of time.

Using this population, we found wide variation in the intensity of care Medicare enrollees received according to the region where they lived. To illustrate, I will use the Dartmouth Atlas Project's measure for hospital care intensity, called the hospital care intensity index (HCI index), which reflects both the amount of time spent in the hospital and the intensity of interventions delivered during hospitalization (Box 9.1). As shown earlier in Figures 8.2 and 8.3, variation in hospital utilization and physician visits is highly correlated with the supply of hospital beds and physicians.

We found *a four-fold* variation in inpatient care intensity among the 306 hospital referral regions for services provided during the last two years of life. Inpatient care intensity was greatest in the Newark, New Jersey, region, where the HCI index was nearly double the national average. Patients living there averaged almost five weeks in the hospital and experienced on average 76 inpatient physician visits over their final two years of life. In Los Angeles and Miami, the HCI indices were about 80% above the national average; Medicare enrollees spent about 28 days in the hospital over the last two years of life and incurred more than 70 inpatient physician visits. The index for Detroit was about 25% above average, and patients there experienced 23 days in the hospital and 49 physician visits. For Cleveland, Boston, San Francisco, and Baltimore, it was near the national average; patients living there averaged about 20 days in hospital and about 34 inpatient physician visits per patient. The index for Denver and Minneapolis was about 28% below the national

Box 9.1.   *How the Hospital Care Intensity (HCI) Index Is Constructed*

The HCI index is a summary measure of the intensity of inpatient care. It is based on two supply-sensitive utilization measures: the average number of days patients spent in hospital and the average number of physician visits patients experienced. These are highly correlated with hospital beds, physician supply, and Medicare spending but are not biased by differences across regions in prices or in the way Medicare pays for its services. The index is computed as the average of two ratios: the ratio of the number of inpatient days in a region or hospital cohort, compared to the national average, and the ratio of the number of inpatient physician visits per patient, also compared to the national average. The HCI index can be calculated for any cohort of patients and for any fixed interval of time. In the examples in this chapter, the HCI index is constructed for cohorts of chronically ill patients during six-month intervals prior to death and during the last two years of life.

average, and patients spent on average 15 days in the hospital and incurred about 24 physician visits. Health care in Portland, Oregon, and Salt Lake City, Utah, was at the low end of the care intensity spectrum: the HCI index was, respectively, 46% and 49% below the national average, and on average, patients spent about 12 days in the hospital and experienced 16 inpatient physician visits during the last two years of life.

Were residents of Newark being given more care because they were sicker? Certainly a large segment of the city's population is impoverished, uninsured, and black, three characteristics that often go hand in hand with poor health outcomes. And while mortality rates were higher in Newark than in other parts of the country, remember that we were comparing only the people who died. Even people who live in Grand Junction, Colorado (one of the healthier regions of the United States), who were suffering from chronic illness in the two years leading up to their death were very sick indeed. Furthermore, everyone in our sample had at least the basic Medicare insurance coverage, and we adjusted for racial, age, and gender differences and differences in the frequency of chronic illness in our calculations, allowing us to compare utilization measures across diverse regions.

Evidence to support our contention that these differences in the intensity of care delivered are not a reflection of regional differences in illness in the population can be seen in the fact that it does not matter which specific chronic illnesses patients have. The pattern is consistent across virtually all chronic illnesses in any given region compared to another. As we saw in the last chapter, for nearly three decades hospitalization rates for a number of chronic illnesses in high-bedded Boston were uniformly elevated over the rates for low-bedded New Haven, creating the medical signature. In other words, consistent with our theory regarding the threshold effect that capacity exerts on clinical decision making, a region's pattern of care for one type of patient—such as cancer patients—tends to be similar for other types of chronic illness, such as congestive heart failure (CHF) or chronic obstructive pulmonary disease (COPD). This turns out to be a general phenomenon, typical of health care across the entire United States. Among the 306 hospital referral regions, those with a low HCI index for one chronic condition have low HCI indices for other chronic conditions, and vice versa. In the case of Newark, for example, patients with cancer were as likely to experience more days in the hospital with multiple physician visits as patients with chronic heart failure. In Minneapolis, just the opposite was the case.

The national pattern of variation for patients with common chronic illnesses is illustrated in Figure 9.1. It does not matter which chronic condition a patient has—in a given region (and hospital), the propensity to use inpatient care in managing severe chronic illness is the same, as illustrated by the strong correlation between the HCI index for patients with cancer and

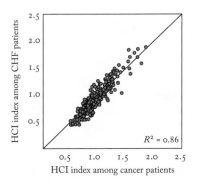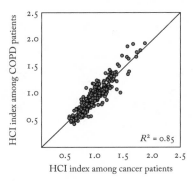

Figure 9.1.   The association between the intensity of inpatient care measured by the HCI index for patients with selected chronic illnesses during the last two years of life among hospital referral regions (deaths occurring 2001 through 2005). CHF, congestive heart failure; COPD, chronic obstructive pulmonary disease. (Source: Dartmouth Atlas Project database.)

patients with CHF, and for patients with cancer and patients with COPD. The same is true for other chronic illnesses. For example, the HCI index for COPD and CHF is highly correlated (R^2 = 0.93).

The same story holds for patients with different socioeconomic characteristics. Just as we had seen in the 1980s for Boston and New Haven, the pattern of variation indicates a systems-level or regional-level effect that influences the amount of care, independent of factors associated with the level of illness. Blacks consistently receive more care than others living within the same region, even after adjusting for age, sex, and illness. For example, blacks in Newark, Los Angeles, Detroit, Baltimore, Atlanta, and Minneapolis all spend 43% to 55% more days in the hospital and incur 28% to 66% more inpatient visits than do those of other racial backgrounds (Table 9.1). But the table makes two other important points. First, the intensity of inpatient care for blacks varies substantially among major metropolitan areas. This is so even for cities that have a high proportion of blacks such as Newark, Detroit, Baltimore, and Atlanta. Blacks in Newark spent 55% more days in the hospital than their counterparts in Detroit, 71% more than in Baltimore, and 87%

Table 9.1.   Use of Acute Care Hospitals by Blacks and Nonblacks Living in Selected Hospital Referral Regions During the Last Two Years of Life

Region	Percent Black	Days in Hospital		Inpatient Visits	
		Black	Nonblack	Black	Nonblack
Newark	21	48	31	113	74
Manhattan	17	44	34	111	71
Los Angeles	10	39	27	94	72
Miami	7	37	28	67	54
Philadelphia	15	33	24	67	57
Chicago	35	32	26	57	59
St. Louis	10	29	20	51	33
Baltimore	20	28	19	49	35
Atlanta	16	26	18	44	31
Cleveland	12	25	19	44	30
Boston	3	25	20	40	34
San Francisco	10	24	18	40	33

Days in hospital per 1,000 and inpatient visits per patient; data are for chronically ill patients who died 2001 to 2005 and are age, sex, and illness adjusted.
Source: Dartmouth Atlas Project database.

more than in Atlanta. Second, the same pattern of variation is occurring for those of other racial backgrounds (the majority of whom in most regions are white[4]). Nonblacks living in Newark spent 41%, 63%, and 75% more days in the hospital than those in, respectively, Detroit, Baltimore, and Atlanta. Indeed, the regional differences are so pronounced that nonblacks in Newark and Los Angeles receive more care than blacks in Atlanta.

Nationally, a consistent pattern was seen among the 306 hospital referral regions (Figure 9.2). The HCI index for blacks tended to be about the same as it was for the other segments of a region's population (as indicated by the clustering of dots along the 45-degree line), even though within a given region, blacks tended to use about 45% more inpatient care. The same pattern was seen for Medicaid (low-income) patients compared to non–low-income patients living in the same region.

Finally, as diseases progress, the pattern of care delivered in different regions is *consistent over time*. As I showed in Chapter 8, when we followed patients with hip fracture, heart attack, and colon cancer over six-month periods of time, hospitalization rates were consistently higher for residents of Boston during each six-month period of follow-up after discharge from the initial hospitalization. We now have data to show that consistency over time in the relative intensity of care for supply-sensitive care is typical of the entire nation. Using Dartmouth Atlas Project data, we followed patients with chronic illness back in time from death in six-month intervals and

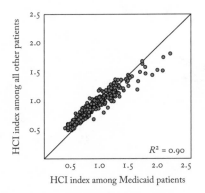 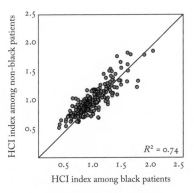

Figure 9.2. The association between the intensity of inpatient care measured by the HCI index for Medicare patients according to poverty status (Medicaid buy-in patients versus all others) (*left*) and race (black versus all others) (*right*) during the last two years of life among hospital referral regions (deaths occurring 2001 through 2005). (Source: Dartmouth Atlas Project database.)

correlated the HCI index in months 0 through 6 preceding death with the HCI index in months 7 to 12, 13 to 18, and 19 to 24. We found a strong correlation within regions in their patterns of care between each six-month interval, even though patients who were further from death were, on average, less severely ill. Figure 9.3 illustrates the close correlation between frequency of care among regions during the last six months of life (measured by hospitalization and inpatient physician visits) and frequency of care between months 19 and 24 before death. That patients were less ill during this earlier period is reflected in the fact that hospitalization and physician visits were roughly 3 to 4 times lower than during the last six months of life. But the variation in rates among regions was striking during both periods of time, and it was highly correlated.

Physicians and hospital administrators have found it difficult to accept that similarly ill patients can receive such different amounts of care, depending on where they live, and some argue that the variation must somehow be explained by differences in illness, despite all our efforts to account for that possibility. I will address this argument shortly. But first I want to examine a criticism made by Peter Bach and his colleagues in a 2004 article in the *Journal of the American Medical Association*.[5] Studying care received before death, write the authors, "can lead to invalid conclusions about the quality

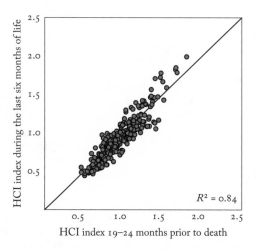

Figure 9.3.   The association between the intensity of inpatient care measured by the HCI index 19 to 24 months prior to death and during the last six months of life among hospital referral regions (deaths occurring 2001 through 2005). (Source: Dartmouth Atlas Project database.)

or type of care provided to dying patients." Follow-back from death studies, they point out, are case-series studies—studies that begin with an event, in this case death, and reconstruct what happened previously by moving back over fixed periods of time. The gold standard to which they compare the follow-back from death case series is the cohort study, a method that begins with an enrollment event—such as the diagnosis of colon cancer—and then follows the patient forward in time. They rightly point out that these two approaches can lead to different conclusions based on the same patient population, and that patients who die soon after the time of diagnosis will show lower rates of utilization of care than patients who linger on for months or years. (See Box 9.2 for a more detailed explanation of their criticism.)

Box 9.2.   *How a Follow-Back from Death Study Can Result in a Biased Estimate of Utilization and Costs of Care for Patients Dying from Cancer*

The problem arises because patients with the same cancer but of different ages have different life expectancies. In their article, Bach et al.[5] provide an example: a typical patient 85 years of age who is newly diagnosed with advanced (stage 4) cancer of the colon lives about five months after diagnosis. Spending calculated according to the cohort method yields an accurate estimate of the cost of managing dying patients because it is calculated by measuring per capita spending per patient month of survival after diagnosis. This is a much higher estimate for the cost of dying from stage four cancer of the colon over time than would be case if spending were based on the last year of life, where only five of the twelve months of follow-back would be for the time when the patient was actually sick with cancer. By contrast, the typical patient with the same diagnosis who is 65 years of age lives longer—the authors estimate eleven months—so their accumulated expenditures over the last year of life are considerably greater, not necessarily because they were treated more intensely during the year preceding death, but because they lived longer after being diagnosed. Thus studies using the follow-back from death method might erroneously be interpreted as showing age-related bias: much lower spending for older patients that in reality reflects life expectancy differences, not care intensity differences.

How do we defend the Dartmouth use of follow-back from death studies? First and most important, our results adjust for the diagnosis of the patient, which can affect prognosis, as well as age, sex, and race. If in some regions people are more likely to die from diseases with a very poor prognosis (which could mean that they are sick and in need of treatment for a shorter portion of their last two years), then our measures of utilization and spending are adjusted for those differences. Finally, it is important to note that when we use the "gold standard" cohort method to follow patients with heart attacks, hip fracture, colon cancer, and other conditions for which we are reasonably certain we can identify the initial (index) hospitalization, we find virtually the same pattern of variation in utilization among regions over three years of follow-up as we do using the follow-back from death method.[6]

What Is the Prevalence of Chronic Illness, and How Does This Influence Regional Variation in Per Capita Utilization and Spending?

Let me now turn to the question of the role of illness as a driver of variation in utilization and spending among regions. The Fowler interview studies in Vermont established that patient-reported illness rates were not very different from one Vermont community to another, and that illness was therefore not likely to be an important factor in the two-fold or greater variation in rates of health care utilization in Vermont. When we extended the scope of our study to a national scale, we used the Medicare Current Beneficiary Survey (MCBS), which asks patients to rate their health care along a scale from poor to excellent. In a study reported in the 1999 Dartmouth Atlas,[7] we found that sicker patients used more hospital care; those reporting poor health status spent 2.7 times more days in hospital on average than those reporting themselves to be in excellent health. But what was interesting was that, just as we saw in Vermont, there was little correlation between the percentage of Medicare enrollees who reported they were in poor, good, or excellent health, and the number of hospital beds in their regions. Finally, we estimated the "need" for hospital beds in a region according to how sick patients were.[8] There was virtually no difference in the predicted need for hospital beds among the different regions based on reported level of illness of Medicare enrollees. But there was a lot of variation in both the supply of beds and the rates at which they were actually used. Survey respondents who lived in the lowest-bedded regions (less than 2.9 beds per 1,000), had, based on illness level, a predicted use of 2.2 hospital days per person, and an actual use of only 1.6 days. Those living in the highest-bedded regions (more than

3.9 beds per 1,000) had the same predicted use—2.2 days per 1,000—but an actual use of 2.6 days, 1.6 times greater than those living in the lowest-bedded region. This is not meant to suggest that average utilization rates are the same as optimum utilization, since there's virtually no science to show which rate is right. What these differences do say is that the supply of beds has a powerful effect on hospitalization, regardless of how sick patients are.

What about Medicare spending per capita, hospital care intensity, and the prevalence of chronic illness? Not surprisingly, spending goes up when utilization and intensity of care go up. Spending in 2005 varied more than 2.7-fold among the 306 hospital referral regions, from an annual average of $5,281 in Rapid City, South Dakota, to $14,359 in the Miami, Florida, region. The variation in spending was essentially uncorrelated with the rates of such preference-sensitive services as elective surgery. The primary clinical driver of variation in overall Medicare spending among regions is the intensity of the use of supply-sensitive care, particularly the use of acute care hospitals for patients with chronic illness. Inpatient care intensity for those with chronic illness, as measured by the HCI index during the last two years of life, explains about 67% of the variation in per capita Medicare spending, at least for fee-for-service patients (Figure 9.4, left).

By contrast, the *prevalence* of chronic illness explains very little of the variation in Medicare spending. In the 2008 edition of the Dartmouth Atlas,[9] we showed that the prevalence of severe chronic illness, measured by the

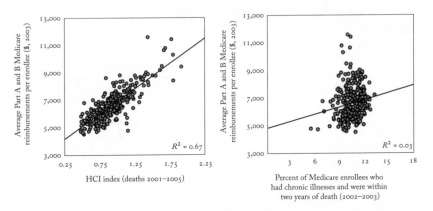

Figure 9.4. The association between per capita spending under traditional Medicare (2003) and the hospital care intensity (HCI) index measured over the last two years of life (*left*) and the prevalence of severe chronic illness (2002 through 2003) (*right*). (Source: Dartmouth Atlas Project database.)

percentage of Medicare enrollees who were in their last two years of life, varied substantially from region to region, ranging from 5.4% of Medicare fee-for-service enrollees living in Honolulu, Hawaii, to 13.6% for those living in Slidell, Louisiana. Sicker regions tend to spend more: prevalence of chronic illness accounts for about a $1,500 per capita difference in spending between regions where patients are the sickest compared to regions where patients are the healthiest. *But only a small proportion of the 2.7-fold variation in Medicare per capita spending in 2005—about 3%—was associated with variation in the prevalence of chronic illness* (see Figure 9.4, right). In other words, sickness does not explain the variation in spending.

Do Those Who Get More Care Actually Want More Care?

None of the studies reviewed so far in this chapter have addressed directly the question of patient preferences for care at the end of life—the desire of patients and families for a peaceful passing, as free from pain as possible, on the one hand, or to have everything possible done to postpone death. In considering the issue of intensity of end of life care, it is important to realize that such care is managed very differently from one region to another. For example, for deaths among patients with chronic illness occurring in 2005 among the 306 hospital referral regions, the intensity of terminal care, measured by the percentage of patients whose death was associated with a stay in an intensive care unit, varied more than 2.5-fold, from 12% in Minneapolis, Minnesota, and Des Moines, Iowa, to 30% in Los Angeles, California, and New Brunswick, New Jersey.

Such differences raise a number of questions of profound importance to patients and their families. Do patients and families want more care? Do they want physicians to exhaust all remedies as the patient approaches death? Or would they rather die at home or in some other familiar place with lots of family support? Perhaps most important, do patients get the care they prefer?

The answer to this last question is that they may not. For me, the most convincing evidence comes from a large-scale intervention study funded by the Robert Wood Johnson Foundation that became known by its acronym, as the SUPPORT study.[10] The level of care intensity that patients preferred at the end of life was less than the amount actually provided, even after an extensive effort was made both to establish how intensely individual patients with a high probability of dying actually wanted to be treated and to ensure that providers knew their patients' wishes.

Here are some of the details. In the early 1990s, health services researchers Bill Knaus and Joanne Lynn organized the SUPPORT study to improve end of life care at five major teaching hospitals (located in five different hospital referral regions). The first phase of their study documented shortcomings in clinical care at these hospitals. Patients often experienced unnecessary pain and their physicians were often unaware of patients' preferences with regard to end of life care, including cardioresuscitation. Advanced planning for end of life care was clearly inadequate. The second phase of the study consisted of an intervention to improve care.[11] The hypothesis was that providing patients and families with information about patient prognosis and improving communication among patients, physicians, nurses, and family members would lead to end of life care decisions that promoted patient preferences and autonomy.

The study results were deeply disappointing. Knaus' and Lynn's conclusion, published in November of 1995 in *the Journal of the American Medical Association*, came as a shock to many advocates for the reform of end of life care:

> The...intervention failed to improve care or patient outcomes. Enhancing opportunities for more physician-patient communication, although advocated as the major method for improving patient outcomes, may be inadequate to change established practices. To improve the experience of seriously ill and dying patients, greater individual and societal commitment and more proactive and forceful measures may be needed.

One mark of failure was the study intervention's lack of impact on improving compliance with the patient's preference to die at home. Among the patients who indicated that they preferred to die at home, the majority, 55%, actually died in the hospital. At the same time, those who wanted to die in the hospital often did not; less than half (46%) of those who preferred to die in the hospital actually did.[12] But the chances of dying in the hospital varied strikingly among the five teaching hospitals, ranging from 26% to 66% of deaths.

In a subsequent analysis, Rob Pritchard and his Dartmouth colleagues provided an explanation for the variation.[13] In multivariate analyses, they showed that the supply of hospital beds in the region where the hospitals participating in the SUPPORT study were located was highly predictive of the chance that a patient participating in the SUPPORT would die in the hospital, even after elaborate steps had been taken to ensure that patient preferences were respected. (This was especially the case when they measured the actual use of these beds based on the average number of occupied beds or patient days of care.) In other words, the capacity effect seemed to dominate clinical decision making, despite patient preferences. The association between patient days of care and place of death is evident in Figure 9.5.

It is of course quite possible that patient preferences as stated at one point in time in the course of a serious illness might change; once death is near, a patient might become a strong advocate for the "more is better" assumption. At the minimum, however, we learned from the SUPPORT study that patient preferences for place of death, stated at a point in time when they were already seriously ill from a condition that soon proved fatal, did not predict the actual place of death.

Given the supply-sensitive nature of such care, it is hard to address the question of end of life care outside of the general context of how intensely physicians use the acute care hospital in managing chronic illness. As we have seen, care during the terminal phase of life is part of the overall pattern

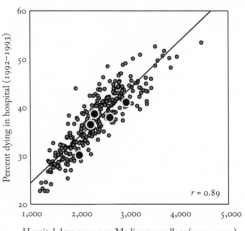

Hospital days per 1,000 Medicare enrollees (1992–1993)

Figure 9.5.   The association between overall use of hospitals measured by hospital days of care and the percentage of deaths in the region that occurred in hospitals. The five large circles indicate the regions in which the five hospitals participating in the SUPPORT clinical trial are located. (Source: Pritchard, R. S., E. S. Fisher, J. M. Teno, et al. 1998. Influence of patient preferences and local health system characteristics on place of death. *Journal of the American Geriatrics Society* 46:1242–1250. Reproduced with the permission of the *Journal of the American Geriatrics Society*, John Wiley & Sons Ltd., publishers.)

of use of inpatient care in managing chronic disease. The time of death cannot be predicted very accurately, so even if patients and physicians agree in theory on the course of terminal care, those using hospitals with a habitual pattern of higher care intensity will die more often in an intensive care unit than those using hospitals with lower care intensity, simply because of difficulties in knowing when death is likely to occur. The Pritchard reanalysis of the SUPPORT data supports this interpretation. *Reducing exposure to high intensity, futile care at the end of life will require paying attention to reducing the overuse of acute care hospitals in managing acute and chronic illness over the course of the patient's illness, not just at the end of life.*

* * *

These findings—that patient wishes are trumped by practice patterns and the supply of resources—have profound implications for both health care policy and for patients' lives. In Chapter 10, I will discuss evidence that appears to show that greater care intensity may not only be wasteful but also be harmful. This would suggest that patients with chronic illness should be encouraged to seek care from hospitals with low care intensity scores on the HCI scale; with good technical quality measures; and with high satisfaction ratings from those who use them. As we will see in subsequent chapters, the waste and harm in the current system behoove policy makers to come up with reforms that will spur providers with evidence of overuse to achieve the benchmarks for efficiency of such hospitals.

10

Is More Better?

For patients with chronic illness, geography matters. Depending on where they live, and which hospital or health care organization they are loyal to, they receive very different levels of care. The level varies with the availability of resources. Supply-sensitive care provided to chronically ill Americans—primarily visits to physicians, hospitalizations for medical conditions, use of extended care facilities, and home health agency services—accounts for well over 50% of Medicare spending. Variation in the use of acute care hospitals by those with chronic illness is the primary reason for the more than two-fold variation in spending among regions of the country in Medicare per capita. This much we know.

But is more care better? Do Medicare patients living in regions with higher per capita spending that deliver greater amounts of supply-sensitive care have better outcomes than those living in regions where they receive less care? Do they live longer because they receive more services? Is the quality of their care better? Are they more satisfied with their care?

Economists would say that these are all questions about marginal value, and one way to think about the marginal value of the increased use of health care is with a graph. Figure 10.1 will be instantly familiar to health care policy analysts. Suppose that all regions of the United States could be described by an association between health care inputs (on the horizontal axis) and health outcomes (on the vertical axis). In the conventional viewpoint, spending

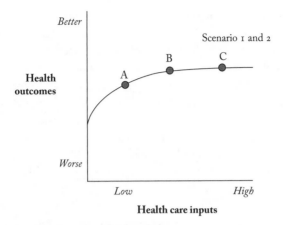

Figure 10.1. Relationship between health care inputs and health outcomes: hypothetical curve I.

more gets us better health. Let's call this Scenario 1. So if we compare, say, Minneapolis (which might fall on the curve at Point A) and Miami (Point B), we should observe better health outcomes—longer survival, better functioning, and greater satisfaction—in Miami. While we might see diminishing marginal returns for each additional health care dollar spent, as long as spending is cost-effective on average, we would expect that the higher spending in Miami (Point B) would be worth it in the sense of providing additional health benefits at a reasonable cost. Furthermore, the implication for health care policy would be that valuable health care is being withheld or rationed in Minneapolis, even if the clinicians there are not aware of it.

An alternative scenario, let's call it Scenario 2, is that Minneapolis is located at point B, and Miami is located at point C. Now, Miami still provides more care for similarly ill patients. Under this scenario, there is no rationing of valuable care, but incremental increases in care intensity (and spending) bring no gain in health outcomes. This might occur, for example, because the potential gains from increased rates for hospitalizing chronically ill patients are offset by adverse events such as a serious hospital-acquired, drug-resistant infection. This scenario corresponds to what Alain Enthoven, the Stanford University health care economist, has called "flat of the curve" medicine—the incremental health gains from spending more on health care are essentially zero.[1] The associated policy prescription is that simply cutting back on health care utilization in high-cost regions like Miami would yield substantial cost savings, and at no cost to patient outcomes.

The problem with Scenarios 1 and 2 is that neither seems to fit the facts.

As I describe later, there is growing evidence of a small but *negative* association between health care intensity and health outcomes measured in terms of survival. Under Scenario 3, physicians do not knowingly expose their patients to harm, yet the incidence of medical errors and other unintended consequences of increased treatments exceed any benefit from increased care intensity. Figure 10.2, which is not so familiar to health policy analysts, allows for negative marginal returns from the increased use of health care. Under Scenario 3, Minneapolis might be at point C, and Miami at point D—where more care indicates worse outcomes and higher costs. In this case, the policy prescription is a no-brainer—by reducing the intensity of care in high-rate regions, we could reduce the risk for iatrogenic illness by lowering the exposure of the population to hospitalization and other interventions prone to medical error.

My colleague Jonathan Skinner has drawn my attention to another interpretation of the observed negative correlation between expenditures and health outcomes: that is, at any given point in time, two regions are on different production functions (Scenario 4). Thus, in Figure 10.3, Point E corresponds to Minneapolis on PF(1), and Point F to Miami on PF(2). What is meant by a different production function? In its simplest form, it might be that people in Miami are intrinsically sicker than their elderly counterparts in Minneapolis; thus, for a given level of spending, we would expect to find those in Miami to fare less well because they suffer from (let's say) more chronic disease. However, Dartmouth studies have been careful to control for this source of bias, whether by focusing only on people with heart attacks or hip fractures and controlling for comorbidities and other factors that would affect their level of sickness at baseline or by controlling for the type and nature of chronic illness.

There could be another reason for high-intensity, poor-outcomes regions to be on a lower production curve where it takes many more inputs to achieve more benefit: the *organization* of health care in Miami may be less efficient. Providers may be neglecting to provide low cost but highly effective treatments, or patients may be subjected to errors of omission or commission because of poorly coordinated care. For example, one recent study found that most of the hospital-level difference in survival following a heart attack could be explained by differences in the use of inexpensive yet highly effective treatments such as beta-blockers and aspirin.[2] Thus, regions or hospitals with higher spending rates could experience worse outcomes not because of the higher utilization per se but rather because they underuse effective care— they neglect to provide the aspirin or beta-blockers in the first place. To put

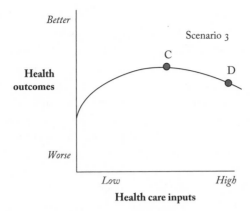

Figure 10.2. Relationship between health care inputs and health outcomes: hypothetical curve II.

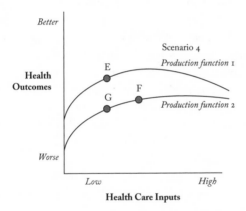

Figure 10.3. Relationship between health care inputs and health outcomes: hypothetical curve III.

it in the language of social sciences, high spending levels and poor outcomes may be the consequence of a *third* factor—poor organization and systemic coordination failure, which we know are endemic in our health care system. We need not take a stand on what causes what—whether poor coordination leads to an oversupply of resources, or oversupply leads to poor coordination of care. Both can be happening at the same time. An oversupply of hospital beds and interlocking networks of specialists could combine to generate both complex and overlapping health care treatment strategies, coupled with poorly organized health care and worse outcomes.

The important distinction between this new Scenario 4 and Scenarios 2 and 3 lies in what it implies, were high-intensity regions to cut back on services. In the earlier scenarios, we can simply curtail health care utilization and gain better outcomes, or at least no worse outcomes, while saving money and reducing the incidence of medical errors and other iatrogenic events by reducing exposure to too much medical care, a win-win situation. But in this fourth scenario, cutting back on spending in Miami at Point F, on the lower production function, would not suddenly turn disorganized Miami providers into highly organized group practices like the Mayo Clinic. (I will talk more about the effect that organization of health care delivery has on the patterns of practice and utilization in future chapters.) Instead, health outcomes would likely decline, perhaps to Point G. In practice, the various scenarios are not mutually exclusive—we could observe that our third scenario indicates a consistent failure to provide effective care to heart attack victims, say, while Scenarios 2 and 3 indicate the overuse of supply-sensitive care, particularly inpatient care, for those with acute and chronic illnesses.

Our research finds support for both hypotheses: greater care intensity is associated with higher mortality rates and poorer objective measures of process quality; and organized care systems are associated with lower care intensity and higher quality. Let me now turn to some of the evidence that suggests where the United States currently sits on our hypothetical production function curves with respect to the marginal and average value of health care spending.

Care Intensity and Mortality

When physicians deliver supply-sensitive care, particularly inpatient care, their principal clinical objective is most often a reduction in mortality. Of course that is not always the case. They also deliver care to relieve suffering and improve the quality of life. But most of the time they are trying to help their patients live as long as possible. (Preference-sensitive care, by contrast, is often aimed at reducing morbidity—improving the quality of life.) Consequently, our team's research has concentrated on evaluating the marginal impact of supply-sensitive services on survival. The strategy has been to exploit the natural experiments afforded by the apparent randomness in the frequency of use of supply-sensitive services, using measures for which a strong a priori argument can be made that the differences are not due to differences in illness.

Supply-sensitive care during the last six months of life has proved to be a reliable measure. By definition, these patients are similar across regions in one primary indicator of health status—all are dead at the end of a six-month period of observation. There is great variation among hospital referral regions in the intensity of supply-sensitive services delivered to patients during this period of their lives. Obviously, the amount of care cannot be used to make inferences about the outcomes for these patients—all are dead. Instead, measures of intensity of care—per capita Medicare spending, physician visits, hospitalizations, and intensive care unit admissions—can be used to define where each region is located along a spectrum of care delivery that is not explained by illness differences. Think of these indicators as a gauge measuring the propensity of the providers in a region to deliver supply-sensitive care, regardless of how ill patients are. In view of the high correlation in care intensity among regions over different periods of time prior to death (see, for example, Figure 9.3 in the previous chapter), we consider care intensity during the last six months of life an illness-independent indicator of a region's tendency to deliver more or less care, not just to its dying patients but in fact to all patients with severe chronic illness.

One of our research goals has been to evaluate the power of supply-sensitive services to decrease the mortality rates of the resident population. We have undertaken several studies whose results consistently show that, at best, the United States is on the flat of the hypothetical production function curves. None of our studies have offered evidence in support of the conventional wisdom that more spending and more utilization of services is better, at least among the insured. My early research, which compared population-based mortality in Vermont,[3] and subsequent studies comparing Boston and New Haven,[4] showed no evidence that care intensity was associated with population mortality rates. Another study found essentially no association between spending and outcomes; the researchers estimated these effects by comparing outcomes for regions experiencing both high and low levels of health care intensity, as measured by physician visits and intensive care unit days in the last six months of life and spending for heart attack patients.[5] This study controlled for a battery of possible factors that might confound the results such as disability, poverty, and the underlying incidence of illness as measured by hospitalizations for hip fractures, heart attacks, colon cancer, and other conditions whose rates of hospitalization vary little, regardless of the supply of beds.

The strongest evidence to date rests in a study by Dr. Elliott Fisher and his colleagues, who used the cohort method to evaluate survival up to five years after an initial hospitalization for hip fracture, colon cancer resection, or heart attack.[6] By linking claims over time, patient comorbidity at the time of enrollment in the study could be controlled for, and the interval to death ascertained for those patients who died within five years. It thus became possible to study patients with specific diseases and to evaluate the marginal effect of increasing care intensity on survival while controlling for morbidity at the patient level.

In this study, the researchers used a measure of care intensity they called the "End of Life Expenditure Index," which is a price-adjusted estimate of Medicare spending for hospitals and physician services over the last six months of life. For each of the three cohorts, the researchers found a higher mortality rate in high spending regions. For example, compared to the lowest 20% of regions in per capita spending, survival in the regions ranking in the top 20% was worse: mortality for patients who had hip fractures was 1.9% higher; and for colon cancer and heart attack patients, it was 5.2% higher. Fisher and his colleagues could find no compensating improvements in the quality of life or functional status as measured by the Medicare Current Beneficiary Survey, even though Medicare spending per capita in the high-cost regions was 1.62 times that of the low-cost regions.[7]

How should these associations be interpreted? First, it is important to recognize the limitations of observational studies, even when conducted using cohort methodology. Observational studies designed to evaluate the relationship between medical treatments and outcomes are, by their nature, subject to the criticism that the results could be explained on the basis of an "omitted variable"—some unrecognized but nonetheless important factor related to outcomes that the researchers failed to take into account. The ideal study design for dealing with this problem is, of course, the randomized clinical trial (RCT).[8] RCTs are designed to test well-specified medical theories and outcomes—for example, whether there is a reduction in five-year mortality from breast cancer due to a new cancer treatment compared to "usual practice." But we could not very well conduct a classic RCT of supply-sensitive services. For one thing, medical theory regarding the appropriate frequency of use is vague at best, so there is no clear hypothesis to be tested. For another, the evaluation problem involves estimating the marginal impact on life expectancy of varying levels of frequency of care. It would be very difficult, to say the least, to randomize patients to a control and treatment group when the "group" is defined by location along a continuum of varying intensity and where membership in a group is based on geographic location.

To get over these limitations while simultaneously adhering as closely as possible to the logic of experimentation, our strategy has been to look for natural experiments, to evaluate the outcomes of care among regions (and hospitals) where care intensity varies and where care intensity (the "treatment") is not correlated with illness. Jon Skinner's skill in the statistical methods used by economists to define and evaluate natural experiments has proved invaluable to our progress. He has shown that care intensity during the last six months of life meets the critical criterion for a "good" treatment variable, although in some studies at the area level, modest correlations were found with predicted mortality.[9] It is certainly possible that the evidence in support of Scenario 3 (where more spending results in a decline in health outcomes) may be affected by undetected differences in illness among regions, although the consistency of the finding of a positive association between higher care intensity and higher mortality (and the strength of the patient level cohort method) remains disturbing, even if the magnitude of our findings is slightly off. I do believe, however, that our findings tell us that the conventional wisdom is wrong. Greater care intensity does not decrease mortality for those with chronic illness. Given the conservative nature of our methods, it seems highly unlikely that the hypothesis that greater intensity decreases mortality has been mistakenly rejected because of the influence of unmeasured factors associated with patient illness. For this to happen, the distribution of unmeasured illness would have to be largely, if not almost entirely, uncorrelated with the array of illness variables we have used in our analyses. In other words, we would have to have ignored a variable that has a very large impact on levels of illness in a population but which also shows no correlation to variables that are widely recognized to affect health. For these reasons we are confident in our conclusion that, when mortality is the endpoint of care, the United States is, at best, on the flat of the curve.

Is the Quality of Care Better in High-Cost States and Regions?

Over the last fifteen or so years, concerns about the quality of U.S. health care have focused on the underuse of effective services—evidence-based interventions such as lifesaving medications for heart attack victims. Several members of our research group became interested in looking at the association between Medicare spending and underuse: Do patients living in areas (or using hospitals) with greater Medicare spending and more resources such as medical specialists score better on objective process quality measures that quantify provider proficiency in delivering effective care? The first two studies, undertaken by Katherine Baicker and Amitabh Chandra, compared performance among the fifty states, and among the 306 regions.[10] The results in both studies were essentially the same; both states and regions with higher levels of Medicare spending had worse quality scores on measures of effective care. Spending more seemed to lead paradoxically to greater underuse. Moreover, states and regions with a predominance of medical specialists compared to primary care physicians tended to have worse scores. As I will show, such regions also have higher acute care hospital intensity as measured on the hospital care intensity (HCI) index, as well as higher costs.

As the quality movement has evolved and the patient choice movement has taken hold, the Centers for Medicare & Medicaid Services (CMS) has led the way to ensure that quality measures are available to the public, in the hope that patients will be influenced by such information in choosing where to seek care. Beginning in 2005, CMS has posted hospital-specific quality scores on its website for heart attack, pneumonia, and congestive heart failure patients. Recently, one of our graduate students, Laura Yasaitis, working with several faculty members, linked this information to the Dartmouth Atlas Project database to conduct another examination of the association between Medicare spending and quality—this time at the individual hospital level.[11] The results confirmed the previous finding; hospitals with higher per capita spending, as indicated by their spending level in managing chronically ill patients during the last two years of life, had worse quality scores for patients suffering from heart attack and pneumonia. I will discuss why this could be so a little further along in this chapter.

What About the Patient's Experience?

Thus far, we have not considered the quality of care from the perspective of the patient. Are people living in high-cost regions, where they are likely to receive high-intensity care, getting the care they want? What about patients who live in lower cost regions? Do patients in high-cost regions have better access to specialists when they need them? Are they happier with their treatments, even though, as we have shown above, objective measures of both quality and outcomes—including survival—may be worse? Our research group recently undertook two studies that directly measure the patient experience. The first, by Jack Fowler and his colleagues, was a national interview study to examine the relationship between Medicare spending and patient perceptions of the quality of their care.[12] The second used the results of a national survey of the patient's experience to examine the relationship between the patients' perception of the quality of their hospital experience and the intensity of inpatient care as measured by the HCI index.[13] Both studies suggest that more care is not producing more satisfied or happier patients. Here is a summary of what these studies show:

The Fowler study, published in the *Journal of the American Medical Association* in the spring of 2008, interviewed over 2,500 Medicare enrollees, asking them to rate their care as to its quality. Responses to two of the three rating questions showed no correlation with regional spending. However, the study uncovered a significant inverse relationship between Medicare spending and the patients' *global* rating of their care. For example, 63% of respondents living in regions where Medicare spent the least gave their care a high rating (a score of 9 or 10), compared with 55% of those living where Medicare spent the most. In reporting their results, Fowler and his colleagues reached the following overall conclusion: "No consistent association was observed between the mean per capita expenditure in a geographic area and the perceptions of the quality of medical care of the people living in those areas." In other words, from the patient's point of view, for most of the factors measured, health care in the United States was on the flat of the curve. More care certainly was not associated with greater satisfaction with that care, at least among Medicare recipients.

The researchers also asked questions concerning the patients' perceptions about unmet need for specialist care and found an *inverse* correlation between spending and access: 8% of respondents in the highest per capita spending regions reported unmet need for specialists compared to only 3% of those who lived in the lowest spending regions. The greater perception of scarcity was occurring in the high-cost regions, even though there were many more specialists available on a per capita basis. Sound familiar? As reported in Chapter 2, the earlier Fowler interview study documented much the same phenomenon: Vermonters living in Burlington, where the per capita number of medical specialists was high, reported greater difficulty in getting to see a physician when they wanted to. Now, on a national basis we see evidence that having more physicians does not necessarily mean greater access to care or greater perceptions on the part of patients that their medical needs are being fulfilled. As I will discuss in Chapter 15, policy makers need to resist the temptation to treat the symptoms of pseudo-scarcity of physicians by churning out more doctors.

The Dartmouth Atlas Project looked further into the hypothesis that, from the perspective of the patient, the United States may even be on the descending arm of the benefit-utilization curve. Concentrating on the use of acute care hospitals, we used the HCI index, which reflects both time spent in the hospital and the intensity of physician intervention during hospitalization for Medicare patients, and measures of the patient's experience of hospital care that came from a new database posted on the CMS website on March 28, 2008, the Hospital Consumer Assessment of Healthcare Providers and Systems (HCAHPS) survey, conducted by the CMS.[14] The survey, because it is designed to be a report card on how adult patients experience care in their own hospitals, requires a very large sample of recently hospitalized patients. The initial CMS study was based on over 600,000 discharged patients from 2,473 acute care hospitals. Patients answered questions about ten aspects of their experience, one of which was to provide a global rating of their satisfaction with their inpatient experience on a scale of 0 (most dissatisfied) to 10 (most satisfied), similar to the approach Jack Fowler used in his study. CMS then calculated for each hospital the percentage of patients who gave the hospital a low, intermediate, or high rating for each aspect of care. We further aggregated the data to the regional level.

What did we find? First, there is an eight-fold range among the 306 regions in the percentage of patients who gave their hospital a low global rating (a score of 6 or less). It varied from 4% of patients hospitalized in the region with the fewest dissatisfied patients to 30% in the region with the most dissatisfied patients. We then tested the hypothesis that greater intensity of use of hospitals was associated with greater patient dissatisfaction with care, based on the global rating patients gave. The association was positive (R^2 = 0.26; p <.001). Indeed, patients living in the regions with highest care intensity tended to rank their hospitals less favorably on all aspects of care, including the communication between physicians, nurses, and the patient; pain control; providing help when needed; cleanliness of rooms and quietness at night; discharge planning; and willingness to recommend the hospital they had used to others.

We then looked at the association between care intensity, low overall rating of hospitals, and the objective quality measures for patients with heart attacks, congestive heart failure, and pneumonia that CMS also posts on its website. Just as predicted by Laura Yasaitis' study, we found that regions with greater care intensity tended to have lower quality. But we also noticed a correlation between quality measures and patient ratings: regions with lower patient ratings of hospitals tended to have worse quality, as measured by CMS quality scores (R^2 = 0.16, p < .001).

Why should these two dimensions of care quality be correlated at all, because the events that go into the hospital's technical quality scores are generally not observable by the patient? After all, patients are not rating their hospitals on the basis of whether they received a pneumonia vaccine on admission or antibiotics within a specified amount of time. The correlation suggests the possibility of an overlapping causal pathway: chaotic, disorganized care results in less attention to patient needs and wants along the several dimensions measured by the HCAHPS survey. At the same time, care that is delivered by multiple physicians, with no one person in charge, also leads to substandard care, excess services, and worse performance on technical quality measures. Organized care, by contrast, pays more consistent attention to "patient-centered" care and is able to coordinate services to better achieve therapeutic goals, including those that are measured in the CMS quality scores.

We do indeed find an association between organized care, higher technical quality, and lower care intensity. The health care markets in many of the regions that rank in the bottom 20% on the HCI index are dominated by organized systems of care—large group practices or hospital systems. Minneapolis, Sacramento, Seattle, Portland, Oregon, and Salt Lake City are examples. In these regions, well-established organized systems of care dominate the health care landscape. The group practice model is also prevalent in other regions with low HCI scores, including the Mayo Clinic (Rochester, Minnesota, and LaCrosse, Wisconsin, regions), the Geisinger Clinic (Danville, Pennsylvania, region), the Billings Clinic (Billings, Montana, region), the Marshfield Clinic (Marshfield, Wisconsin, region), the Duluth Clinic (Duluth, Minnesota, region), the Scott and White Clinic (Temple, Texas, region), the Dartmouth-Hitchcock Clinic (Lebanon, New Hampshire, region), the University of Iowa Clinic (Iowa City region), and the University of Wisconsin and the Dean Clinics (Madison, Wisconsin, region). With a few exceptions, (for example, the Henry Ford Clinic in the Detroit region and the Ochsner Clinic in the New Orleans region), large group practices are notably absent in regions with higher HCI scores.

I will return in later chapters to suggest that organized care with a low HCI index should serve as "best practice" benchmarks for evaluating the efficiency of health care organizations in delivering care for those with chronic illness. To give the reader a heads-up on where the discussion is going, however, let me call attention to the practice patterns in regions in the lowest 20% of the HCI index, compared to the regions in the highest quintile when it comes to caring for chronically ill patients during the last two years of their lives (Table 10.1).

As the reader can see, the bottom 20% of regions—those often dominated by organized care systems—and the top 20% of regions are very different in terms of the amount of resources they use and the care patients with similar types and severity of illness experience. The health care providers serving high-intensity regions spend much more money per patient and use many more hospital beds and many more physicians—primary care physicians as

Table 10.1.   Practice Patterns in Managing Chronic Illness in Regions that Ranked in Highest and Lowest Quintiles on the Hospital Care Intensity (HCI) Index

	Hospital Care Intensity (HCI) Quintile		
	Lowest	Highest	(Ratio)
HCI index score	0.67	1.46	(2.17)
Resource inputs during the last two years of life			
Medicare spending per patient	$38,300	$60,800	(1.59)
Physician labor inputs per 1,000 patients			
All physicians	16.6	29.5	(1.78)
Medical specialists (MS)	5.6	13.1	(2.35)
Primary care physicians (PC)	7.4	11.5	(1.55)
Ratio PC/MS	1.34	0.88	(0.66)
Hospital bed inputs per 1,000 patients	40.0	70.8	(1.77)
Terminal care			
Patient days per patient, last six months of life	8.5	15.6	(1.83)
Inpatient visits per patient, last six months of life	12.9	36.3	(2.82)
Percent seeing 10 or more MDs, last six months of life	20.2	43.7	(2.16)
Percent of deaths with ICU admission	14.3	23.2	(1.63)
Percent enrolled in hospice	30.1	30.2	(1.00)

ICU, intensive care unit; MD, physician.
HCI index is based on last two years of life, from 2001 to 2005; the lowest and highest quintiles contain approximately equal numbers of patients. Rates are adjusted for age, sex, race, and chronic conditions.
Source: Dartmouth Atlas Project database.

well as medical specialists—in providing care. Medical specialists tend to dominate practice, as evidenced by the ratio of primary care physicians to medical specialists. Patients in high-intensity regions spend much more time in the hospital and incur many more physician visits; many more physicians are involved in their care; and they are much more likely to experience a stay in the intensive care unit at the time of their deaths. In reviewing these facts, it is good to keep in mind that, on average, the outcomes and quality of care tend to be better, and patients are better able to access physicians and are more satisfied with care in low-intensity regions.

* * *

From work that began in Vermont, Maine, Boston, and New Haven, and more recently from our research for the Dartmouth Atlas Project, my colleagues and I have concluded that illness explains only a small fraction of the variation in the practice of medicine for the chronically ill that we see in different parts of the country. Acute care hospital use is closely associated with acute care hospital capacity and physician supply. The amount of supply-sensitive care provided is not governed by strong medical theory, much less by valid medical evidence. Physicians are generally unaware of where they or their hospitals stand on the spectrum of care intensity. In a medical environment where both physicians and patients believe implicitly that more care is better, the variation seems best explained by the effect that capacity exerts on the clinical decision making that lies behind the frequency of services.

However, for supply-sensitive care, more is not better. In regions with high care intensity, cohorts of patients with hip fractures, colon cancer, and heart attacks receive more services and they have higher mortality rates over the years following their initial index event than those in low-intensity regions. Patient satisfaction with hospital care is worse in high-intensity regions, as is the quality of hospital care, as measured by using CMS published data for the treatment of heart attacks, pneumonia, and congestive heart failure. These findings are consistent with Scenario 3, introduced at the beginning of this chapter, the hypothesis that the United States is on the wrong side of the utilization-benefit curve, at least in terms of our use of acute hospital care for the chronically ill. They are also consistent with Scenario 4, the idea that high spending levels and poor outcomes are a consequence of a third factor—inefficiency resulting from poor organization and systematic coordination failure in the health care system.

II

Are "America's Best Hospitals" Really the Best?

Finding solutions to unwarranted variation and overuse of care requires leadership from academic medicine, the institutions on which the nation depends to ensure that medicine is based on valid clinical science. Yet even among the select few academic medical centers that reside at the very top in terms of their national reputation for excellence, there is little evidence that clinical practice is based on a scientific consensus on the best way to practice medicine. Academic medical centers appear to vary as much as other hospitals in the United States in terms of the quality of the care they deliver, in the various ways they spend Medicare's money and use resources, and in the experiences they provide their patients. Mobilizing academic medicine to assume responsibility for improving the science of health care delivery is a major task facing those who want to reform health care in the United States.

Academic medical centers also vary substantially in the way they organize their health care delivery "systems" or, in many cases, nonsystems. Many appear to share in the general chaos of American medicine, exhibiting little evidence that their medical staffs provide coordinated care for their chronically ill patients. A few are formally organized as large, multidisciplinary group practices and, as I show in this chapter, the regions served by these organized academic medical centers tend to be relatively efficient: their method of delivering services costs Medicare less, uses less physician labor and resources, and subjects chronically ill patients to a much lower intensity and more "conservative" pattern of practice. If the rest of the nation were to achieve the benchmarks of these institutions, the nation would need many fewer hospital beds and physicians. This chapter will examine these issues, and in doing so it will challenge the nation's academic medical centers to step up to the plate and take on the task of improving the efficiency of their own care, so that they might serve as an example to the rest of the nation.

America's Best Hospitals?

Each year, many of America's academic medical centers figure prominently at or near the top of the list in *U.S. News & World Report*'s (*USN&WR*'s) "Best Hospitals" issue. Using a method that relies to a large extent on professional reputation,[1] the magazine tells readers which hospitals represent a patient's best bet for several specific chronic conditions, including heart disease, cancer, and lung disease, and which rank best on overall performance. Being designated as a "best hospital" is a prized distinction and hospitals that attain it proudly display their rank in advertisements and adorn their buildings with banners proclaiming their excellence.

But what do these ratings tell us about the relative efficiency of care and the patient experience? The Dartmouth Atlas Project method for evaluating performance in caring for those with chronic illness (described in detail in the Appendix) results in three reports: the Medicare Spending Report, the Resource Allocation Report, and the Patient Experience Report. Our ratings offer a very different picture—and one that as yet has not motivated hospitals to advertise their ranking.

Take the five hospitals at the top of the *USN&WR* honor roll list for 2008: the University of California, Los Angeles Medical Center (UCLA); Massachusetts General Hospital (MGH); Johns Hopkins Hospital; the Cleveland Clinic Foundation Hospital; and St. Mary's Hospital, the principal hospital of the Mayo Clinic in Rochester, Minnesota. These hospitals enjoy consistently stellar reputations, not just in the pages of *USN&WR*, but also among patients, physicians, and policy makers. Yet what is remarkable about our evaluation of these hospitals is the extraordinary lack of consistency in how they actually treat patients.

These five hospitals show wide variation in the intensity of the care they give to the chronically ill. They also vary in terms of relative efficiency— the resources they use to treat similar groups of patients and the per capita amount Medicare spends on those patients (Table 11.1).

Table 11.1. Routine Performance Reports for Managing Chronic Illness During the Last Two Years of Life (Deaths from 2001 through 2005) for Highly Ranked Academic Medical Centers

	Johns Hopkins Hospital	Mayo Clinic (St. Mary's Hospital)	UCLA Medical Center	Cleveland Clinic Foundation	Massachusetts General Hospital
Rank among best hospitals	1	2	3	4	5
Medicare spending per patient, last two years of life					
Total Medicare spending	$85,729	$53,432	$93,842	$55,333	$78,666
Inpatient site of care	$63,079	$34,372	$63,900	$34,437	$43,058
Outpatient site of care	$13,404	$7,557	$14,125	$8,906	$11,509
Skilled nursing/long-term care	$3,287	$7,114	$6,891	$5,101	$15,149
Home health care	$1,813	$662	$3,994	$2,194	$4,718
Hospice care	$2,217	$2,054	$1,649	$2,485	$1,503
All other care	$1,929	$1,673	$3,283	$2,210	$2,729
Resource inputs per 1,000 patients, last two years of life					
Physician labor					
All physician FTE labor	25.7	20.3	38.5	26.1	29.5
Medical specialist FTE	8.9	8.9	21.2	10.6	11.7
Primary care physician FTE	10.0	6.8	9.6	8.8	11.5
Ratio of medical specialist to primary care labor inputs	0.89	1.30	2.20	1.20	1.02

Hospital beds					
All beds	78.2	58.2	85.8	65.5	79.2
High-intensity ICU/CCUs	11.8	16.4	13.8	14.3	15.0
Intermediate-intensity ICUs	8.2	2.0	24.3	4.8	1.0
Medical and surgical beds	58.2	39.8	47.7	46.4	63.2
Patient experience, last six months of life					
Hospital days per patient	16.5	12.0	18.5	14.8	17.3
Physician visits per patient	28.9	23.9	52.8	33.1	39.5
Percent seeing 10 or more physicians	44.6	41.0	52.9	48.2	53.5
Terminal care					
Percent of deaths in hospital	36.5	30.2	43.2	38.6	44.5
Percent of deaths with ICU admission	23.2	21.8	37.9	23.1	22.5
Percent enrolled in hospice	35.2	29.1	28.8	36.6	23.8
Average co-payment per patient last two years of life	$3,390	$2,439	$4,835	$3,045	$3,409

CCUs, coronary care units; FTE, full-time equivalent; ICU, intensive care unit.
Source: Dartmouth Atlas Project database. Ranking of hospitals is by *U.S. News & World Report* "Best Hospitals" for 2007.

Medicare Spending

Let's look first at how much Medicare spends per capita on chronically ill patients in the last two years of life at these five hospitals. These estimates are based on deaths that occurred from 2001 through 2005:

- Medicare spending for all services was nearly 76% more on a per capita basis for patients loyal to UCLA Medical Center, compared to the Mayo Clinic's St. Mary's Hospital patients and 70% more than the Cleveland Clinic Foundation Hospital patients.
- Pulling out just inpatient care, Medicare spending was about 85% greater on a per capita basis for patients using UCLA Medical Center and Johns Hopkins compared to the Mayo Clinic's St. Mary's Hospital and the Cleveland Clinic Foundation Hospital.

Per capita spending in other sectors also shows striking variation:

- Medicare spending at UCLA Medical Center for ambulatory care (outpatient facilities and physician offices) was 87% greater than at St. Mary's Hospital.
- Massachusetts General patients incurred almost three times as much spending for skilled nursing facilities and long-term care hospitals as patients at the Cleveland Clinic Foundation Hospital.
- Home health care spending for Massachusetts General patients was seven times greater on a per capita basis than for St. Mary's Hospital patients.
- Hospice spending varied about 65%, with the highest spending rate for Cleveland Clinic Foundation Hospital patients and the lowest for Massachusetts General Hospital.

It is important to remember that most, although not all, of this variation in per capita spending is accounted for by differences in the volume of services—the number of days patients spend in the hospital or extended care facilities, or the number of visits that physicians make to hospitalized patients and office visits that patients make to their providers. Differences in price per unit of service have far less effect on spending. For example, compared to St. Mary's Hospital, UCLA Medical Center's 84% higher rate in per capita Medicare spending for inpatient care resulted from the fact that UCLA Medical Center patients spent 47% more days in the hospital per capita than the Mayo Clinic's patients. The price of care, by contrast, or the average reimbursement per day in the hospital, was 25% higher. For physician visits, where Medicare price controls are even more effective in keeping prices consistent across the country, the 125% higher UCLA Medical Center per capita Medicare spending was explained mostly by the high volume of physician visits per capita—which exceeded the Mayo Clinic's visit rate by 99%. Average reimbursements per visits, on the other hand, were only 13% higher.[2]

Physician Labor

The nation's five "best" academic medical centers differ widely in how they use physician labor in treating patients who are essentially similar in their needs. The UCLA Medical Center used 90% more full-time equivalent physicians per patient than the Mayo Clinic. Massachusetts General Hospital used 45% more; the Cleveland Clinic Foundation Hospital, 28% more; and Johns Hopkins, 27% more.

There are also remarkable differences in the mix between medical specialists and primary care physicians among the different hospitals. The workforce managing chronically ill patients loyal to the UCLA Medical Center is oriented toward medical specialists, while Johns Hopkins tends to favor primary care. The UCLA Medical Center used 2.4 times more medical specialist labor than Johns Hopkins. The ratio of medical specialist to primary care labor was 2.2 at UCLA Medical Center and 0.89 at Johns Hopkins.

This list of statistics suggests that there is little science behind the way academic medical centers deploy physicians in caring for their patients. And yet, these institutions have apparently reached a consensus on the need to expand the physician workforce and, in particular, the need for more specialists. But our data suggest that more physicians, and especially more medical specialists, will exacerbate the overuse of high-intensity care. (See Chapter 15 for further discussion.)

Hospital Beds

America's "best" hospitals also differ widely in how many beds per 1,000 patients they use for managing chronic illness over the last two years of life:

The UCLA Medical Center stands out for its overall high level of bed inputs and its emphasis on intensive care unit (ICU) beds, especially intermediate-intensity beds. (Ironically, the hospital recently was reconstructed and more ICU beds were added!) The UCLA Medical Center used on a per capita basis 47% more total beds and *twelve times* more intermediate "step-down" ICU beds than the Mayo Clinic. The UCLA Medical Center also had 20% more medical and surgical unit beds compared with the Mayo Clinic (but fewer high-intensity ICU beds). Looking at the total bed inputs, the Massachusetts General Hospital used 36% more than the Mayo Clinic, Johns Hopkins used 34% more, and the Cleveland Clinic Foundation Hospital used 13% more, largely because of their higher use of medical and surgical unit beds.

The Patient Experience

America's best hospitals differ in the intensity of care they deliver to their chronically ill Medicare patients—and the experience they provide their patients at the end of life. During the last six months of life (for deaths from 2001 through 2005), care intensity was lowest for patients loyal to the Mayo Clinic and highest for those using the UCLA Medical Center:

- Mayo Clinic patients averaged twelve days in the hospital and incurred twenty-four visits to physicians, and 41% of patients were seen by ten or more physicians.
- UCLA patients averaged 18.5 days in the hospital (1.55 times higher than the Mayo Clinic's) and incurred fifty-three physician visits (2.21 times the Mayo Clinic), and 53% of patients saw ten or more physicians.

At the time of death:

- Of patients loyal to the Massachusetts General Hospital and UCLA Medical Center, 44.5% and 43.2%, respectively, died while in the hospital, compared to 30.2% at the Mayo Clinic, 36.5% at Johns Hopkins, and 36.6% at the Cleveland Clinic Foundation Hospital.
- At UCLA Medical Center, 37.9% of deaths involved a stay in intensive care, compared to about 22% at the other four academic medical centers—a little more than half the rate at UCLA Medical Center. (As noted earlier, the high rate of use of ICU beds at UCLA Medical Center is for intermediate-intensity beds.)

Finally, for Medicare copayments, on average, those with progressing chronic illness using the UCLA Medical Center could expect copayments of nearly twice the amount paid by patients at the Mayo Clinic, 59% more than the Cleveland Clinic Foundation Hospital, and about 42% more than those using the Massachusetts General Hospital or Johns Hopkins.

The Extreme of Variation in the Patient Experience

These profiles in variation among America's best hospitals strike me as quite extraordinary. They represent the state of care delivered at academic medical centers, the bastions of American medical science. Patients go to these hospitals expecting to be cared for by highly skilled physicians using the most advanced medical knowledge, yet there appears to be little agreement among these institutions as to how best to care for patients with the most frequently encountered of diseases. And the five academic medical centers profiled here do not even represent the most extreme ends of the curve. Seven major teaching hospitals, all affiliated with medical schools, have patterns of practice that are even more aggressive than the UCLA Medical Center; fifteen are actually more conservative than the Mayo Clinic.

New York University Medical Center (NYU), Cedars-Sinai Medical Center, and the Robert Wood Johnson University Hospital (RWJ) are at the top of the care intensity score for U.S. hospitals, providing a very aggressive pattern of care in managing chronic illness during the last six months of life (Table 11.2). NYU is the most aggressive and shows evidence of poor care coordination: its patients average more than a month in the hospital and experience seventy-eight visits to physicians. Numerous physicians are involved in the care of any given patient, such that 65% of patients are cared for by ten or more physicians. All three of these hospitals provide a particularly aggressive brand of terminal care: 50% or more of deaths occur in hospital; 35% to 40% of deaths involve a stay in an ICU.

By contrast, care intensity in managing chronic illness ranks around the bottom 10% of U.S. hospitals for patients cared for at the Scott & White Memorial Hospital (the teaching hospital for Texas A&M Medical School), the University of Wisconsin Hospital, and New Mexico's teaching hospitals. Patients in these academic medical centers average ten to eleven days in the hospital and about twenty physician visits. Compared to the most aggressive patterns of academic practice, many fewer physicians are involved in the care of these hospitals' patients during the last six months of life, especially at the University of Wisconsin Hospital, where only 25% of patients saw ten or more physicians. Terminal care is much less intensive: about 30% of deaths occur in the hospital; ICUs are used much less often—only 13% of deaths

Table 11.2. The Patient's Experience of End of Life Care by Patients Cared for by the Three Highest and Three Lowest Ranked Academic Medical Centers on the Hospital Care Intensity (HCI) Index

	Top Three Hospitals Ranked on HCI Index			Bottom Three Hospitals Ranked on HCI Index		
	NYU Medical Center	Cedars-Sinai Medical Center	Robert Wood Johnson University Hospital	University of Wisconsin Hospital	University of New Mexico Hospital	Scott & White Memorial Hospital
HCI index percentile rank among U.S. hospitals	99.8	99.2	98.0	11.9	11.5	9.1
Patient experience, last six months of life						
Hospital days per patient	31.2	24.4	23.7	11.1	10.0	9.6
Physician visits per patient	76.9	79.3	66.1	18.4	19.5	20.6
Percent seeing 10 or more physicians	64.8	59.3	62.7	24.9	31.9	30.8
Terminal care						
Percent of deaths in hospital	50.5	52.9	50.3	27.4	32.6	29.3
Percent of deaths with ICU admission	35.1	40.0	37.2	16.1	25.3	13.0
Percent enrolled in hospice	20.1	19.6	27.0	40.5	43.1	45.3
Average co-payment for physician care per patient during last two years of life	$5,550	$6,500	$4,800	$2,050	$2,150	$2,200

HCI, hospital care intensity; ICU, intensive care unit.
Source: Dartmouth Atlas Project database; data are for deaths from 2001 to 2005.

among patients using the Scott & White Memorial Hospital are associated with an ICU stay, well less than half of the number for the top-ranked hospitals. On the other hand, hospice use at Scott & White Hospital is much greater: about double that of the more aggressive hospitals, with 40% or more of deaths associated with hospice care.

High-intensity care comes at a high price, for both Medicare and patients. Out-of-pocket copayments during the last two years of life for patients loyal to NYU average $5,550; for Cedars-Sinai, $6,500; and for RWJ, $4,800. These amounts were more than double the amount for patients using the three lowest intensity academic medical centers, where copayments were between $2,050 and $2,200.

Academic Pushback

Not surprisingly, many of the physicians and administrators who work in academic medicine have found our data difficult to swallow. Perhaps because several of our papers, as well as a chapter in the 2008 Dartmouth Atlas, focused on health care in Los Angeles, the administrators there have been particularly vocal. A July 27, 2009, opinion piece in the *Los Angeles Times* by John Stobo, MD, senior vice president in charge of the five University of California teaching hospitals, and Tom Rosenthal, MD, the chief medical officer of the UCLA Medical Center and associate vice chancellor of the David Geffen School of Medicine at UCLA, provides an example.[3] The authors, both physicians, dispute the "theory that the medical care in L.A. is inefficient or wasted" and argue that the principal cause for high utilization in Los Angeles is poverty, citing statistics that "more than 38% of L.A. County citizens live below the poverty line, 57% are black or Latino, and 24% are uninsured."

The Stobo-Rosenthal illness hypothesis simply does not fit the facts. I have already shown (see Chapter 9) that poverty and race are not adequate explanations for the variation in utilization and Medicare spending among regions. Not surprisingly, what holds for regions holds for individual academic medical centers. While some academic medical centers allocate more care per capita to their low-income populations compared with their high-income patients, others do just the opposite. What really matters in determining the amount of care used is the academic medical center where the patient is treated (See Box 11.1). Race and poverty also do not explain the variation in utilization among academic medical centers

Box 11.1   *The Poverty Hypothesis and Academic Medical Centers*

There is yet another way to evaluate the importance of income level in explaining the variation in spending and utilization. Using information from the year 2000 census, we grouped patients into quintiles according to the median household income in the zip code where they lived. We then studied the relationship between income level and the use of inpatient care according to the academic medical center the patients used. Figure 11.1 shows the relationship between the use of care for patients living in low-income communities—those living in the lowest quintile for median income—and those living in high-income communities, which fall into the highest quintile.

The figure makes it clear that the most important factor affecting variation in cost and utilization is not income level, but rather the specific academic medical center that patients use. However, there are some interesting differences in the relative amount of care that different academic medical centers deliver to their low-income and high-income patients: some academic medical centers deliver more hospital days and spend more per capita on patients from high-income communities, while others do just the opposite. For example, low-income patients using UCLA spend nearly 20% more time in the hospital during the last two years of life than do high-income patients—35.3 days versus 29.8. Johns Hopkins uses 17% fewer hospital days per patient when treating those from poor neighborhoods compared with its treatment of those from high-income communities—26.3 versus 31.6; and low-income and high-income patients using the Cleveland Clinic are hospitalized at about the same rate— 23.9 patient days per capita versus 23.6.

The high degree of correlation between patients from low-income and high-income communities across academic medical centers is best explained by the capacity hypothesis; the threshold effect that capacity exerts on the frequency of use of supply-sensitive care. But what about the strange pattern of variation within the same hospital? The differences between low-income and high-income patients using the same hospital may also be an effect of capacity. Let me return for a moment to the story of Boston University Hospital, told in Chapter 8, where we found that the admission rate for indigent patients was much lower than for everybody else. We traced this difference to fact that these two patient populations used different wings of the same hospital, and the reason for the variation, we suggested, was that there were fewer beds available per capita for caring for the poor (the Boston City Hospital wing) than for insured patients, who used the other wing of the hospital.

I suspect that a similar explanation fits the variation that we observe among the nation's best hospitals. The limits on hospitalization rates are set by the limits on the number of available hospital beds per capita. For hospitals that assign specific beds to patients based on income or insurance status, the per capita beds available to each population will likely differ, as they did for Boston University Hospital. For example, as I learned during my residency training at Johns Hopkins, poor, mostly black patients were treated on the Osler ward, a separate part of the hospital with a fixed number of beds. Given what we know about the effect of capacity, and the different rates of hospitalization for low-income and high-income patients at Johns Hopkins, I would predict that the number of beds available per capita on the Osler ward is lower. Further insights into differences such as these will require some "shoe leather" epidemiology, on the ground inquiry to map out how academic medical centers allocate their resources among various segments of their patient populations.

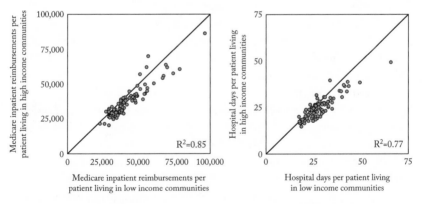

Figure 11.1   The relationship among selected academic medical centers between per capita Medicare reimbursements for patients from low-income and high-income communities (*left*); and between hospital days for patients from low-income and high-income communities (*right*) during the last two years of life. Academic medical centers that fall above the line have higher rates for patients living in high-income communities; those below the line have higher rates for those living in low-income communities.

Table 11.3.   Percentile Ranking on Hospital Care Intensity (HCI) Index Among U.S. Hospitals, Percentage of Hospitalized Medicare Patients Who Are Black and in Medicaid, and the Number of Hospital Days Per Patient by Black, Nonblack, and Medicaid Patients During the Last Two Years of Life for Selected Academic Medical Centers

Hospital	HCI Percentile	Percent Black	Percent in Medicaid	Days in Hospital per Patient		
				Blacks	Nonblack	Medicaid
Cedars-Sinai	99th	8.8	31.8	29.8	23.8	28.5
UC-Los Angeles	90th	8.1	20.6	20.6	18.2	21.6
UC-San Diego	44th	5.1	27.6	15.0	13.6	14.3
UC-San Francisco	39th	10.1	41.5	14.1	13.4	14.2
UC-Davis	27th	14.1	46.1	13.9	11.7	11.2

HCI, hospital care intensity; UC, University of California.
For chronically ill patients who died 2001 through 2005; data are age, sex, and illness adjusted.
Source: Dartmouth Atlas Project database.

located in Los Angeles, nor among the major academic medical centers belonging to the University of California System (Table 11.3). Judging by the percentage of patients who are black or on Medicaid, the University of California in Sacramento (UC-Davis) has the sickest patients: 14% are black and 46.1% are "dual eligible," that is, they are enrolled in both Medicare and Medicaid. Yet UC-Davis has the lowest HCI index and the lowest number of days in hospital for all of its patients—blacks, nonblacks, and low-income patients. At the UCLA Medical Center, where only 20% of Medicare patients are enrolled in Medicaid and 8% are black, patients spend much more time in hospital than their counterparts at UC-Davis. UCLA Medical Center's black patients average 48% more days in the hospital; Medicaid buy-in patients, 93% more; and nonblacks, 56% more. A scan of the table reveals that the University of California, San Francisco Medical Center also has proportionately more black and low-income patients than the UCLA Medical Center or Cedars-Sinai but UC-San Francisco uses many fewer hospital resources in managing chronic care for each segment of its patient population. Cedars-Sinai stands out as the most aggressive in the use of inpatient care: black, low income, and nonblack patients all spend about twice as many days in the hospital as those using UC-Davis, UC-San Francisco, or the University of California, San Diego Medical Center.

At the other end of the country, the Massachusetts Hospital Association, defending its teaching hospitals, has released a statement attacking the

Dartmouth Atlas because it ignores "cost of living differences" and the "added costs of educating the next generation of physicians." Cost of living differences do exist, and they are reflected in the payments that Medicare makes to hospitals. However, as I discuss in Chapter 12, the volume of care—the number of days in the hospital and physician visits per capita—is more important than regional differences in price in determining per capita Medicare spending. Moreover, when we adjust for differences in price, the variations in per capita spending among major academic medical centers change very little. Some of the cost of educating resident physicians is indeed folded into the payments Medicare makes to teaching hospitals, but this should not account for differences in spending among major teaching hospitals such as UCLA, Johns Hopkins, and Cleveland Clinic. Finally, as I discuss in Chapter 15, it is far from clear that our current workforce policies governing postgraduate medical education are in the public interest. They are producing a workforce that is more suited to the needs of acute care hospitals than to the care of the chronically ill—far too many specialists and not enough primary care physicians.

Another explanation we often hear is the threat of malpractice. Physicians, even those in academic institutions, overtest and overdiagnose to avoid the risk of being sued should something be missed or some disease arise in the future that might have been diagnosed earlier, if only a test—for example, a PSA exam—had been made. While the threat of legal liability may alter the baseline propensity to treat—raising costs everywhere—defensive medicine has yet to be shown to be an explanation for regional variation in spending and utilization. Katherine Baicker, Elliott Fisher, and Amitabh Chandra have shown an interesting association between an increase in the use of supply-sensitive care—namely, physician visits and consultations and imaging exams—and an increase in per physician malpractice payments at the state level.[4] The causal direction, however, is not so evident. Do more lawsuits lead to defensive medicine, or does practicing high-intensity medicine lead to more lawsuits? The conventional wisdom would be that rising malpractice payments cause physicians to practice defensive medicine. However, increased care intensity itself, obeying medicine's perverse laws of demand and supply, may contribute to increased frequency of malpractice actions: as described in Chapter 10, patients using high-intensity hospitals tend to be less satisfied with their care and the quality of care is marginally worse. The pattern of care of chronically ill patients living in high-intensity regions may result in more causes for legal action because their increased use of hospitals and "high tech" care exposes them to greater risk of medical errors. Thus, there is the possibility for an iterative cycle in which increased care intensity leads to more errors and more lawsuits from dissatisfied patients, and to more defensive medicine and more overtreatment as physicians seek to cover their bases—and so on.

Yet another argument commonly made against our data is that "patient demand" accounts for the variation among hospitals. In considering this possibility, it is well to remember that here we are not talking about elective or preference-sensitive care such as knee or hip replacements, where the primary purpose is often to improve the quality of life and where patient demand for a specific treatment can be fueled by ads on television and by patient social networks. For supply-sensitive care, the patient demand argument is in effect saying that, compared with Medicare recipients using the University of California teaching hospitals in Sacramento, San Francisco, and San Diego, those using Cedars-Sinai and the UCLA Medical Center want to be hospitalized more—that they desire more days in the ICU and insist on more visits from physicians—and as a result, undergo more of the uncomfortable, if not painful, procedures and tests that being in the hospital routinely entails. Cultural differences certainly exist in different regions of the country, and those differences undoubtedly have an effect on the tendency of patients to desire and demand more or less care, especially at the end of life. But our previous work in Maine, Massachusetts, Connecticut, and Vermont, the SUPPORT trial (which found that bed capacity trumped patient wishes in determining place of death), and the sheer magnitude of the variation in end of life care all suggest that patient demand cannot account for much of the variation we see among academic medical centers.

The bottom line, of course, is that more is not better. As I have pointed out in previous chapters, greater intensity of care is not associated with higher quality of care, greater patient satisfaction, or longer life. At the margin, on the basis of available data, for the population of chronically ill patients, the high-intensity pattern of care is futile; it is the flat of the curve at best and, as such, is inefficient and wasteful.

Organized Care as Benchmarks for Relative Efficiency

There is a better way to define "America's Best Hospitals," and that is according to the degree to which they provide organized care. I have pointed out that organized care systems—either large multispecialty group practices or integrated hospital systems—are the dominant form of medical practice in a number of the regions that rank in the lower 20% in the use of acute care hospitals in managing chronic illness. For any number of reasons, promoting the growth and further development of organized systems of care must be a high priority for health care reform, but one of the principal reasons for promoting their growth is because organized care systems tend to be relatively efficient compared to the rest of the delivery system. As such, they provide resource allocation benchmarks that, if widely implemented, would lead to dramatic reductions in the overuse of acute care hospitals and physician labor, at least in managing chronic illness. Or to put this another way, if other hospitals and physicians organized themselves along the lines of these efficient systems and used their resource allocation as models, the nation would save money and improve the quality of care.

The question is, how much physician labor and how many hospital beds are the right amount? Let's take a closer look at six regions where care is dominated by organized care systems and where the intensity of care is low. Three are home to integrated, multispecialty group practice academic medical centers: Rochester, Minnesota, which is served by the Mayo Clinic; Madison, Wisconsin, home to the University of Wisconsin and the Dean Clinics; and Temple, Texas, the region served by the Scott & White Clinic. The other three regions are served by large integrated hospital systems: Sacramento, California, has the Sutter Health system; Portland, Oregon, is served by Providence Health & Services; and the Salt Lake City/Ogden, Utah, region has Intermountain Healthcare.

Let's use the per capita resource allocation of these regions as benchmarks to make a national estimate of the percentage of reduction in resources needed if providers elsewhere were to achieve the efficiencies of these organized systems in managing chronic illness. The estimated percentage of savings in acute care hospital facilities and physician labor in managing chronic illness is based on resources used for patient populations in each region in the last two years of life. The savings vary according to which region we use as a benchmark, but all estimates point in the direction of significant overuse in many regions of the country.

Here is a summary of the range in estimated savings the nation would enjoy if all providers were as efficient as these benchmarks. The estimated reduction in hospital beds ranges from 23% to 42%; ICU bed reduction ranges from 16% to 55%; reduction in physician labor input for all physicians ranges from 18% to 35%; and medical specialists from 26% to 48%. The benchmarks even indicate a surplus in primary care physicians, with savings from 13% to 35%. For details, consult Table 11.4.

One important caveat must be noted: the variation in resource use among regions served by organized care is in itself substantial, suggesting that even greater reductions might be feasible if efficiency were further improved.

Table 11.4   Estimated Reduction in Resource Use in Managing Chronic Illness
During the Last Two Years of Life according to Benchmarks from Selected Regions
Served by Multispecialty Group Practices or Integrated Hospital Systems

Region	Estimated Percentage of Reduction in Resources in Managing Chronic Illness				
	Hospital Beds	ICU Beds	Total Physician Labor	Primary Care Labor	Medical Specialist Labor
Temple, Texas	23%	55%	27%	15%	43%
Sacramento, California	24	16	18	13	26
Rochester, Michigan	25	29	32	28	41
Madison, Wisconsin	29	53	34	25	48
Portland, Oregon	38	55	31	27	40
Salt Lake City/ Ogden, Utah	41	43	33	35	39

Most of the care in Temple, Texas, Rochester, Michigan, and Madison, Wisconsin, is provided by group practices; integrated hospital systems dominate care in Sacramento, California, Portland, Oregon, and Salt Lake City/Ogden, Utah.

The extent of variation also challenges the assumption that the care of the chronically ill in organizations such as these follows a defined and replicable model of care management that could be exported as a "best practice" strategy. Indeed, we do not find consistency even among different practice sites within a given system. We cannot find evidence for a typical Mayo Clinic "way" or a well-defined Kaiser "system." In Chapter 12, I briefly review the variation seen among different Kaiser Permanente care sites. The 2008 edition of the Dartmouth Atlas documents major differences from one Mayo site to another in care delivery over the last six months of life, suggesting that even this highly organized delivery system has not completely worked out what they are doing right or defined best practices for allocating resources. If they had, they would show more consistency among their various locations in Rochester, Minnesota; Phoenix, Arizona; Jacksonville, Florida; and Eau Claire, Wisconsin. Here are some examples of how care varied during this period among Mayo Clinic hospitals in these regions for deaths from 2001 through 2005:

- Patients using St. Mary's, the major Mayo Clinic hospital in Rochester, Minnesota, spent an average of twelve days in the hospital, and four days in an ICU, and incurred roughly twenty-four physician visits per person over the last six months of life.

- Jacksonville Mayo (St. Luke's Hospital) patients spent on average twelve days in the hospital, and six days in ICUs, and incurred nearly forty-two physician visits per capita.
- Phoenix Mayo Hospital patients spent nearly ten days in the hospital, and two days in intensive care, and experienced on average twenty-seven physician visits per capita.
- Eau Claire Mayo (Luther Hospital) patients spent nearly nine days in the hospital, and one day in an ICU, and incurred twenty-three physician visits.

* * *

The extent of variation among academic medical centers in the way they manage chronic illness is incompatible with the hypothesis that these institutions share a common clinical science that informs their everyday practice. Like most other providers, their delivery of medical services is highly idiosyncratic. Per capita spending among academic medical centers for managing Medicare's chronically ill patients varies more than 2.5-fold; they use strikingly different amounts of physician labor and hospital facilities in managing similarly ill patients. Not all academic medical centers are alike, and regions where care is dominated by academic medical centers that are organized as multispecialty group practices or as integrated hospital systems tend to be relatively efficient compared to the rest. They use fewer resources while achieving high-quality care by available measures. These observations lead to one of the four goals of health care reform: *public policy should support the growth of organized systems as a means of controlling cost while improving quality.*

However, the patterns of practice even among academic medical centers that are organized care systems demonstrate considerable variation, even when we look at different sites within a single system. Given the poor state of clinical science, this should not be surprising. This leads to the second goal of health care reform: *Improving the science of health care delivery in managing acute and chronic illness must be a major goal of comparative effectiveness research* (as I will discuss in Chapter 13). Organized group practices, integrated hospital systems, and academic medical centers need to be recruited to the task. But research grants alone may not be a sufficient incentive. Rationalizing the black box of health care delivery will likely change the patterns of practice, leading to greater efficiencies and reduced utilization—and reduced revenue under fee-for-service reimbursement. For research that fundamentally changes the patterns of practice, comparative effectiveness research should be linked to shared savings programs that compensate providers for the loss of revenue associated with improvement in efficiency. I will discuss this strategy further in Chapter 13. In the following chapter, I offer the top ten reasons for overhauling the fragmented, dysfunctional, and profoundly inefficient way the U.S. health care system cares for the chronically ill.

12

The Top Ten Reasons
Why We Need to Reform the Way
We Manage Chronic Illness

I believe the arguments in the last few chapters build a strong case for challenging the way chronic illness is managed in the United States. The United States must take steps to reduce the overuse of acute care hospitals, which is bad for the nation's fiscal health as well as the welfare of its people. Here are the top ten reasons why we must rethink our investment in the acute care hospital sector and reform the way care is delivered.

1. An Overreliance on Acute Care "Rescue Medicine" for America's Chronically Ill Does Not Work

This strategy is simply not paying off. It is being pursued under the assumption that greater care intensity results in better survival and better quality of life and that patients view any small gain in life expectancy as worth the suffering and loneliness that accompany the technology-driven deaths so many of them experience. This assumption is wrong on two counts. Many patients with chronic illness and their families recognize the inevitability that life must end, and they value a higher quality of death over a short gain in length of life. All too often, that gain in life can be measured in mere days, many of which are spent suffering through the indignity and pain of being in the hospital. Moreover, for patients with chronic illness, greater intensity of hospital care does not even produce a net gain in life expectancy. While it may rescue some, it appears to hasten death for others.

2. Sutton's Law: If We Are Looking for Ways to Save Money, Hospitals Are Where the Money Is

Willie Sutton, who once robbed banks because "that's where the money is," might be surprised to find that robbing hospitals these days might be more profitable than robbing banks. Nearly a third of Medicare dollars is devoted to treating chronically ill patients during the last two years of life, with about 55% of this money going toward care delivered in an acute care hospital. An additional 15% is spent on skilled nursing and other long-term care institutions—spending that is also linked to an episode of acute care hospitalization because, under the payment rules of traditional Medicare, patients must pass through the hospital first before being admitted to long-term care.[1]

It is not just spending in the last two years of life about which we are concerned. Variation in hospital utilization for the chronically ill is what correlates most closely with the more than two-fold variation in overall Medicare spending seen among the three hundred 306 Atlas regions. A good way to illustrate this association is to show the correlation between total Medicare spending—spending for all services and all care sectors covered under traditional Medicare—and the hospital care intensity (HCI) index. (As described in Chapter 9, the HCI index combines two measures of acute care hospital utilization, inpatient physician visits and days spent in the hospital, into a single per capita measure of the volume of inpatient care delivered over the last two years of life.) The HCI index neatly summarizes care intensity over the period of time when chronic illness is rapidly progressing. It places states, regions, and individual hospitals on a spectrum ranging from the most conservative pattern of care to the most aggressive. As it turns out, about 65% of the variation in Medicare spending among regions is associated with the HCI index, the intensity with which patients with progressive chronic illness are treated (see Figure 9.4).

By contrast, the volume of preference-sensitive surgery—the combined utilization rate for the procedures discussed in Chapter 4—is *uncorrelated* with total Medicare spending in different regions (R^2 = 0.00). This may seem surprising, but I believe the idiosyncratic nature of the pattern of local variation in surgery is at work here. The reader will recall the surgical signature phenomenon discussed in Chapter 5, in which each region shows its own characteristic pattern of utilization of various surgical procedures. In any given region, one type of surgery can be delivered at a high rate and another at a low rate. When it all gets added up, both regions with high and low overall spending for Medicare have, on average, about the same aggregated rates for common surgical procedures.

We also find that spending more is not associated with better technical quality of care. We found no association between overall Medicare spending and the use of effective care: underuse is as common (or, according to some studies discussed in Chapter 10, more common) in high-cost regions as it is in low-cost regions. What this suggests is that higher spending does not purchase the infrastructure needed to ensure that providers follow the standards of practice dictated by evidence-based medicine. Or to put it another way, the care delivered in many hospitals is simply too chaotic to make certain that patients get what they need.

The bottom line: *In designing strategies to reduce geographic variation in overall Medicare spending, the overuse of acute care hospitals for the chronically ill is where the money is.*

3. It's the Quantity, Stupid

Paying attention to the overuse of hospitals means paying much greater attention to the volume of care, that is, to the utilization of hospital beds and physician services. This is because volume is actually more important than price in explaining overall differences in how much Medicare spends on similar patients in different regions or hospitals. This phenomenon helps explain why Medicare's ongoing attempts to contain physician and hospital costs by controlling prices have not succeeded in containing overall per capita spending. The fact that differences in utilization rates of inpatient care among regions contribute more than average prices to variation in per capita spending is something we first learned during our Vermont and Maine studies. We also see it in today's Medicare data.

Figure 12.1 shows that Medicare spending on physician visits to hospitalized patients during the last two years of life is more strongly related to volume (visits per patient) than to price (reimbursements per visit). Spending per patient varied almost four-fold among the 306 Dartmouth Atlas hospital referral regions, and the physician visit rate more than three-fold. According to the R^2 statistic, 90% of the variation in spending was "explained" by the average number of visits physicians provided. By contrast, price (the average reimbursement per visit) varied much less (only 1.6-fold), reflecting the partial success of Medicare's policies to standardize prices for physician services.

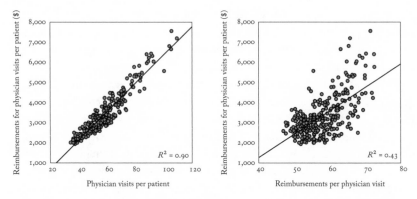

Figure 12.1. The relationship between Medicare reimbursements for physician visits and visits per patient (*left*) and average reimbursements per visit (*right*) during the last two years of life among hospital referral regions (deaths occurring 2001 through 2005). (Source: Dartmouth Atlas Project database.)

Even so, price was also rather strongly associated with per capita spending (R^2 = 0.43), probably because physician visits in high-rate regions are more likely to be provided by medical specialists, whose fees are higher than primary care physicians.

The same pattern of association can be seen for payments to hospitals for inpatient care[2]: among the 306 regions, reimbursements to hospitals per patient varied more than 3.8-fold during the last two years of life (Figure 12.2). Our measure for volume of care, per capita patient days in the hospital, also varied more than three-fold, while price (calculated as the average reimbursement per day in the hospital) varied 2.5-fold. Most of the variation in spending was associated with days in the hospital (R^2 = 0.56), not average price (R^2 = 0.17).

Volume is more important than price, not only for inpatient care and Medicare spending but also for other sectors and providers:

- Medicare reimbursements per capita over the last two years of life for skilled nursing facilities (SNFs) varied from less than $2,000 in some regions to more than $9,000 in others. Volume (days per patient in SNF) varied even more, while price (reimbursements per day in SNF) varied much less. The R^2 of association between volume and per capita reimbursements was 0.66; for price, it was 0.26.

- Hospice payments per patient varied from less than $600 to more than $7,000 according to region of residence. The number of days of hospice

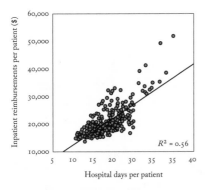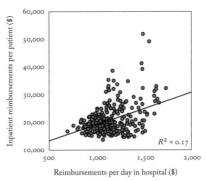

Figure 12.2.   The relationship between inpatient reimbursements and hospital days per patient (*left*) and average reimbursements per day in hospital (*right*) during the last two years of life among hospital referral regions (deaths occurring 2001 through 2005). (Source: Dartmouth Atlas Project database.)

care provided explained more than 86% of the variation in per capita spending per patient, while price (reimbursements per day in hospice care) accounted for less than 5%.

- Home health agency payments varied from about $500 to more than $5,800 per patient with chronic illness over the last two years of life. The number of visits per capita, which ranged from five to seventy-two among regions, explained 87% of the variation in spending; price differences (payment per visit) between regions were relatively slight, ranging from $73 to $207, and were essentially uncorrelated with total spending.

What this all means is that the volume, or amount of care delivered per patient, is generally more important than the price of each unit of care when it comes to addressing variations in Medicare spending—in all sectors of care, not just acute care hospitals. Medicare has repeatedly tried to rein in spending by controlling prices. And it has been successful up to a point: if it had not constrained price, the differences in prices would no doubt contribute more to explaining per capita spending variation and the variation might be even greater. But in a fee-for-service world, controlling prices without addressing volume will have only a limited effect on Medicare's per capita spending or, for that matter, any other insurer's spending. *Given the importance of the supply of medical resources in generating volume, reducing the overuse of acute care hospitals will require a strategy for dealing with capacity.*

4. More Skilled Nursing Facilities, Outpatient Care, and Home Health Care Will Not Cut Inpatient Hospital Use

Medicare's other strategy for controlling hospital spending—making non-hospital, lower-cost sites of care available—has also met with limited success. Over the years, policy makers have argued that the way to reduce unnecessary hospitalizations is to make care in other settings more readily available, so patients who are no longer acutely ill but who still need careful management can receive their care in less intensive—and less expensive—settings. This would not only allow earlier discharge from the acute care hospital, it would also, by further stabilizing the course of chronic illness, reduce the need for readmission to acute care facilities. And if hospice care were more widespread, fewer patients would be subjected to high-tech deaths in an intensive care unit (ICU). Or at least that is how the thinking goes. Based in part on these assumptions, Medicare has added benefits over the years for home health care, hospice, and SNFs, all in an effort to reduce the rates of hospitalization and spending.

It has not worked out very well. It turns out that simply making other kinds of care more readily available does not necessarily lead to a decline in hospitalizations or inpatient spending. Early in our research in Vermont, we saw no evidence that greater use of nursing homes and physician office visits was associated with lower rates of hospitalization. Today, the Dartmouth Atlas tells a similar story. Among the 306 hospital referral regions, higher utilization and spending in ambulatory settings, SNFs, and home health care were associated with *higher* utilization and spending for inpatient care. The association between inpatient spending and spending for SNFs and home health agencies is particularly strong (see Figure 12.3).

Hospice care was the only setting that showed an inverse association with inpatient days in the hospital and inpatient spending, and this effect of hospice is restricted to reducing the use of non-ICU beds. The sad truth is, *seeking care from a hospital that uses more hospice care does not reduce your chances of experiencing a "high-tech" death—one associated with admission to an ICU.*

What can account for these paradoxical findings? Why do physicians not make use of these alternative sites of care in a way that helps their chronically ill patients, many of whom are frail and suffering already, avoid the acute care hospital? There are several reasons.

First, payment policy makes it a requirement that Medicare patients be hospitalized in an acute care hospital before becoming eligible for admission to a skilled nursing home; thus, skilled nursing homes cannot serve as an

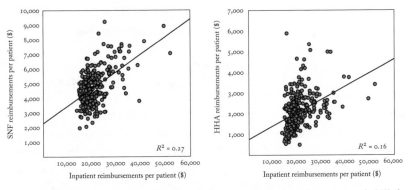

Figure 12.3. The relationship between reimbursements for inpatient care and skilled nursing facilities (SNFs) (*left*) and home health agencies (HHA) (*right*) during the last two years of life among hospital referral regions (deaths occurring 2001 through 2005). (Source: Dartmouth Atlas Project database.)

alternative to acute care hospitals, even though, as I discuss in Chapter 13, this might greatly reduce the use of acute care hospitals.

Second, under traditional Medicare, reimbursement between the sectors of care is not linked. Medicare pays for each type of utilization (e.g., inpatient, SNF, and home health) independently, without regard for the level of spending in the other sectors in caring for those with chronic illness. In the absence of an overall budget for managing care over time, there is no incentive to providers to work toward efficiency. *As I discuss in Chapter 15, it may become necessary to establish such an annual budget for managing chronic and acute illness if the nation is to deal effectively with the overuse of acute care hospitals.*

Third, as I argued in previous chapters, the culture of medicine itself ensures that available capacity is utilized. When patients experience an acute exacerbation of their underlying chronic illness(es), most physicians continue to believe that more intensive rescue care is better. In regions of the country where the acute care sector has been built up relative to the population served, the ready availability of inpatient beds makes the use of the hospital the path of least resistance, even when other sites of care are in place. Thus, the supply of hospital-based resources in the region where patients live influences how intensely they are treated.

Fourth, the positive association between the use of inpatient facilities and the use of skilled nursing homes and home health agencies makes clinical sense; these facilities are important in planning for the discharge of chronically ill patients from acute care hospitals. When more patients are hospitalized, more are discharged to other care sectors, creating "demand" for such services.

The tendency to rely on the acute care hospital is further exacerbated by the fragmented nature of much of the care that is delivered to chronically ill elderly patients. As the Institute of Medicine and others have pointed out, there is little coordination between primary care physicians and the many specialists the chronically ill often find themselves seeing; nor is there coordination of care between the various alternative sites where services can be delivered. Patients in nursing homes may be admitted for inpatient care for each crisis, leading to a hospitalized "high-tech" death, even when they have expressed strong preferences to avoid such an ending. Care transitions, or "hand-offs," can be particularly chaotic in health care markets where there is little coordination of care. Hand-offs between primary care and specialist physicians, between nursing homes and hospitals, between home health care and primary care, and between acute care and hospice and palliative care are often plagued with miscommunications about the patient's medical needs and care preferences, leaving patients in the wrong facility or receiving high-intensity care that will do little to alleviate suffering or improve outcomes. Often, the patient's advance directives—designed to guard against futile care that the patient does not want—are ignored in the heat of the moment. Similarly, patients with chronic conditions are routinely hospitalized during acute episodes of the underlying disease, episodes that often could have been controlled with better care management and coordination among physicians.

The key point here is that we as a nation have failed to recognize that our health care system is not self-regulating. We have left it to the "market," the patient, and his physicians to ensure that this highly technological and complex collection of services is delivered in a way that serves the patient. This strategy is not working. *Given the fragmented nature of the health care Americans now receive, reducing the overuse of acute care hospitals will require a strategy for coordinating the care of those with chronic illness.*

5. Overuse Will Not Go Away on Its Own—and It Is Getting Worse

An important reason for paying attention to the overuse of the acute care sector is that it is getting worse. The volume of services and intensity of care delivered to the chronically ill are increasing everywhere but especially in regions that already exhibit the most aggressive patterns of care.

We have examined changes in care intensity in managing chronic illness over the five-year period from 2001 to 2005 and found some alarming trends. Nationally, the per capita input per 1,000 patients of medical resources (beds, physicians, etc.) allocated to managing chronic illness during the last two years of life increased steadily each year (Table 12.1). By 2005, the nation's health care providers were using 15.3% more ICU beds than they did in 2001 for treating similar patients. The amount of physician labor used to manage chronic illness over the last two years of life also increased by 19.9% for medical specialists and 11.2% for primary care physicians.

Rates of utilization of ICUs and physician visits during the last six months of life also increased rapidly, *particularly among regions that at baseline (2001) were already providing the most care.* In other words, the disparity in utilization between high- and low-rate regions grew over the five-year period, because utilization rates are accelerating in the regions where utilization is already highest. In this study, regions were aggregated into five groups that were ranked on total Medicare spending per patient during the last two years of life among those whose deaths occurred in 2001 (Table 12.2). Each group had approximately equal patient populations. Average Medicare spending for deaths occurring in the lowest-ranked quintile was $30,709; in the highest-ranked quintile, it was $55,873 per patient, or 82% higher. Growth in utilization rates was proportionate to the baseline spending level; the greater the spending in 2001, the greater the percentage of increase in utilization over the five-year period from 2001 through 2005. For example, use of intensive care grew 18% in the highest-spending regions, 7.9% in the median-ranked regions, and 11.3% in the lowest-ranked regions. The range in variation in per patient days in ICUs increased from 2.16 for deaths occurring in 2001 to 2.29 for deaths that occurred in 2005. Medical specialist visits per patient grew 11.3% in the high-spending regions and 9.7% in the low-spending regions, with corresponding increases in the range in variation. The growth rate in primary

Table 12.1. Resource Inputs per 1,000 Chronically Ill Medicare Patients During the Last Two Years of Life by Year of Death, from 2001 through 2005

Resource	2001	2002	2003	2004	2005	% Increase 2001 to 2005
Intensive care beds	13.0	13.6	14.1	14.7	15.0	15.3
Medical specialists	7.7	8.1	8.5	9.0	9.2	19.9
Primary care physicians	8.5	8.7	9.0	9.3	9.5	11.2

Source: Dartmouth Atlas Project database.

Table 12.2. Increase in Utilization per Chronically Ill Medicare Patient During the Last Six Months of Life from 2001 through 2005 by Quintile of Per Capita Spending in Baseline Year 2001

Quintile	Patient Days in Intensive Care			Medical Specialist Visits			Primary Care Visits		
	% Increase in 5 Years	Ratio to Q5		% Increase in 5 Years	Ratio to Q5		% Increase in 5 Years	Ratio to Q5	
		2001	2005		2001	2005		2001	2005
1 ($55,873)	18.0	2.16	2.29	11.3	2.79	2.84	6.2	1.43	1.49
2 ($43,058)	16.0	1.72	1.80	7.0	1.97	1.92	6.6	1.21	1.26
3 ($37,179)	7.9	1.47	1.43	5.7	1.61	1.55	3.1	1.11	1.12
4 ($34,365)	11.6	1.27	1.27	5.1	1.35	1.30	4.3	1.09	1.11
5 ($30,709)	11.3	1.00	1.00	9.7	1.00	1.00	2.2	1.00	1.00

Q, Quintile.
Spending is for the last 2 years of life.
Source: Dartmouth Atlas Project database.

physician care visits per patient in the high-spending regions was 6.2%, almost three times that of the low-spending regions. The disparity between the highest- and lowest-quintile regions increased from a factor of 1.43 to 1.49.

In view of the evidence that more aggressive use of inpatient care appears to result in worse outcomes, *the fact that care intensity in managing severe chronic illness and end of life care is growing everywhere, and is growing at a faster rate in regions that already provide the most aggressive patterns of care, should be cause for alarm. We must focus our attention on reducing the growth of care intensity, particularly in regions where the intensity of care is already high.*

6. It Is Not Just a Medicare Fee-for-Service Problem

The overuse of acute care hospitals is not just a problem for Medicare, and it is not simply a phenomenon of fee-for-service reimbursement. It affects those younger than 65 years of age, those in preferred provider organizations (PPOs), those in managed care health maintenance organizations (HMOs) (the Medicare Advantage Program and commercial HMOs), and those in Medicaid. It does not seem to matter who is paying or how.

The fact that variation in the way chronic illness is managed is not just a problem for elderly Americans, aged 65 years and older, was evident early on in our Vermont and Maine data, which covered the entire population, not just those in Medicare. At that time, all physicians in New England were reimbursed through fee-for-service, and the patterns of care for older and younger patients were strikingly similar. The story is the same today. In a study of patients insured by Blue Cross in Michigan, Dr. David Wennberg (my son) and I documented striking variation in hospital discharge rates from one region of the state to another[3] (Figure 12.4). The rates for Michigan Blue Cross members varied more than three-fold and were highly correlated with rates for Medicare enrollees living in these regions, suggesting that the same factors influencing the utilization of acute hospital care of the elderly are also influencing the care of younger patients. The most important factor affecting the rate of hospitalization for the young as well as the old was the supply of hospital beds.

Similar studies conducted in Louisiana by the company Health Dialog show strong regional correlations between utilization rates not only for Medicare and commercially insured patients but also for patients covered by Medicaid.[4] The similarity between the experiences of these three different patient populations suggests *that the national Medicare data can be used as a*

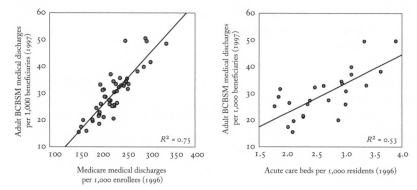

Figure 12.4.   The association between medical discharges for adult Blue Cross/Blue Shield of Michigan (BCBSM) enrollees (1997) and Medicare medical discharges (1996) (*left*) and acute care hospital beds (1996) (*right*) among Michigan hospital service areas with 100,000 or more residents. (Source: Wennberg, John E., and David E. Wennberg, eds., *The Dartmouth Atlas of Health Care in Michigan*, Hanover, NH: The Center for the Evaluative Clinical Sciences, Dartmouth Medical School, 2000).

provisional indicator of the way specific regions and hospitals treat all chronically ill patients, not just those covered under Medicare fee-for-service.

Nor is the overuse of acute care hospitals restricted to fee-for-service or PPO providers. This became evident in a recent study headed by Laurence Baker, a Stanford economist, who examined California hospitalization rates for patients enrolled in four different insurance plans: the Medicare Advantage Program (Medicare's capitated HMO plan); commercial HMOs (capitated plans, including Kaiser Permanente, available to those under 65 years of age); traditional fee-for-service Medicare; and PPO plans from private insurers. The study compared hospitalization rates on a hospital-specific basis for care provided to the chronically ill over the last two years of life, using the Dartmouth Atlas Project methodology.[5] The volume of hospital care—measured as days in hospital—showed extensive variation, even among patients in commercial HMOs. Moreover, *hospitals with high discharge rates for Medicare also had high discharge rates for the other three insured groups, and vice versa.* In other words, the likelihood of being admitted to the hospital varied in a similar way, independent of differing economic incentives embodied in these different insurance plans. However, the length of stay in the hospital was *lower* for patients enrolled in Medicare Advantage and commercial HMOs, suggesting that once hospitalized, HMOs work to get patients out of the hospital as soon as possible—an interpretation that is in line with the economic incentives providers face when caring for patients insured under a capitated reimbursement plan.

The overuse of supply-sensitive care and unwarranted variation in rates of surgical procedures is a problem affecting all payers and all patients, independent of economic incentives now built into standard reimbursement practices, including capitation. As I discuss in Chapter 15, developing regional or statewide all-payer databases to make variation transparent should become a goal of health care reform.

7. Organized Systems of Care Do Not Have All the Answers (Yet)

Many policy makers believe that organized care systems hold the key to health care reform and point to such large group practices as the Mayo Clinic and Kaiser Permanente or to hospital networks such as Intermountain Healthcare as "best practice" examples of care that should be emulated elsewhere. The Dartmouth Atlas Project provides evidence that group practices and organized hospital networks do indeed tend to use fewer resources, have lower spending, and offer higher-quality care, at least compared to the rest of the system, which is far less organized. As shown in Chapter 11, benchmarks from these organized group practices suggest large savings could be gleaned if high cost, poorly organized hospitals and health care markets were to achieve the efficiency of organized group practices. However, the care of the chronically ill in organized group practices does not as yet follow a defined and replicable model of care management.

I reviewed the data showing variation within the Mayo Clinic sites in Chapter 11. Here we review how hospital care intensity varies among populations enrolled in the Kaiser Permanente system. Recently, Mark Stiefel and Paul Feigenbaum of Kaiser worked with Elliott Fisher to examine hospitalization rates among thirty-eight Kaiser regions, of which twenty were located in northern California, twelve were in southern California, and six were in other states.[6] They found a more than two-fold variation in days in the hospital and a four-fold variation in days spent in intensive care units (ICUs) during the last six months of life for Medicare Advantage patients. Although Kaiser rates tended to be lower than those for the fee-for-service Medicare population in the corresponding medical communities, the Medicare fee-for-service and the Kaiser rates were highly correlated, with R^2 = 0.37 for patient day rates and R^2 = 0.61 for ICU use.

Quite frankly, I was surprised by this result. I had long subscribed to economist Alain Enthoven's point of view that the superior efficiency of

Kaiser derived from its commitment to what Alan called "private sector health planning." Kaiser, unlike fee-for-service organizations, knows precisely the number of Kaiser members in each of its geographic regions and thus knows its "denominator"—the size of the population it serves. I had assumed that Kaiser would therefore be able to manage hospital capacity throughout its various geographic locations, seeking to achieve more or less equal numbers of hospital beds per capita in each region (with some adjustments for levels of illness in the local population) and thus ensure that the utilization rates for patients with chronic illness would be about the same everywhere. This study makes clear that this is not the case: even in the Kaiser system, there is little consistency in the way capacity is distributed among different locations. The correlations between the rates of acute care utilization seen in the Dartmouth Atlas Medicare fee-for-service data and the Kaiser rates suggest that regional capacity affects the behavior of Kaiser physicians in a manner that is similar to how it affects providers reimbursed under fee-for-service Medicare.

Variation in the use of acute care hospitals is a problem affecting organized as well as disorganized systems of care. That said, organized systems of care like Mayo and Kaiser are still more efficient than most other providers. Developing replicable, evidence-based models of care management and resource allocation must become a goal of health care reform; as I discuss in the next chapter, organized systems must play a central role in achieving this goal.

8. It Isn't Fair: Reason No. 1

The overuse of acute care hospitals and the way Medicare is financed together create a problem of geographic inequity, in which taxpayers in low-spending states are subsidizing the care of citizens in high-spending states and patients (and employers) who buy health insurance in low-spending regions within states are subsidizing the price of insurance for those in high-spending regions in other parts of their states. These cross-market subsidies are sometimes very large. For example, assuming that Medicare spending continues to rise at a per capita inflation-adjusted rate of 3.5%, a typical 65-year-old in Los Angeles, California will receive over $72,000 more in Medicare-financed health care than a typical 65-year-old in Minneapolis, Minnesota, or about the price of a new BMW Series 5.[7] But the money does not purchase a sports car, which for Los Angeles residents would yield real pleasure. Nor, as we have shown, does it purchase elective surgery, including interventions that might improve the quality of life, such as knee replacements or the removal of cataracts.[8] On average, elective surgery rates are just about the same in low-cost Minneapolis; Portland, Oregon; and Salt Lake City, as they are in high-cost Manhattan; Los Angeles; and Miami. The transfer payments principally purchase more hospitalizations, more stays in ICUs, and more physician visits for those with chronic diseases.

This cross-market subsidization is the result of federal taxes and insurance premiums that are not adjusted for local spending patterns.[9] And local health care spending patterns are determined in large measure by capacity. The most important "system" factor (as opposed to a factor having to do with patients, such as the prevalence of illness) determining whether a community is a net importer or exporter of Medicare dollars is the size of its acute care hospital sector relative to the number of chronically ill patients who need treatment. Miami, Manhattan, and Los Angeles have overbuilt their hospitals; Minneapolis; Portland, Oregon; Sacramento; and Salt Lake City have been more frugal, using fewer hospital beds, less physician labor, and less expensive technologies such as ICU beds and medical imaging devices. It seems ironic that taxpayers in those regions are punished for the frugality of their health care providers by having to subsidize the care of Medicare recipients in regions like Los Angeles, Miami, and Manhattan.

The problem is only getting worse, because, as we have seen, care intensity for managing chronic illness is growing faster in regions that historically have been net importers of Medicare dollars. Financial disparity among regions, at least in terms of Medicare spending, thus can be expected to increase. Ironically, from the perspective of *clinical* equity, regions with less dependency on acute care hospitals appear to be better off; they tend to have better outcomes and less overuse of services.

Another reason for reducing the overuse of acute care hospitals is that it would substantially improve geographic equity in Medicare.

9. It Isn't Fair: Reason No. 2

Overuse imposes a second economic penalty, one that is unfair to patients who live in high-spending, high-use regions. In fee-for-service Medicare, patients are responsible for 20% of the cost for physician services and for medical equipment such as wheelchairs and oxygen treatments. While providers in high-cost regions are "winners" because the subsidies help pay for their overuse of care, the patients in these regions lose on two accounts. First,

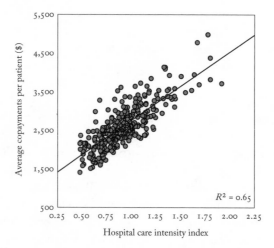

Figure 12.5. The association between hospital care intensity (HCI) index and average copayments per patient during the last two years of life among hospital referral regions (deaths occurring 2001 through 2005). (Source: Dartmouth Atlas Project database.)

because per capita spending is greater, they face higher copayments, which they must pay out of pocket unless they have supplemental insurance. For example, the average copayment over the last two years of life for patients living in Miami is $5,000, and in Los Angeles, it is $4,400; for those living in Minneapolis, it is $1,900, and in Portland, Oregon, it is $2,100. But Los Angeles and Miami residents lose on yet a second account; the increased payments are directly associated with the overuse of acute care hospitals, as is evident in the close association among the 306 hospital referral regions between the HCI index and copayments for which patients are responsible (Figure 12.5). The additional care they are receiving and paying for has no net marginal benefit. *Reducing the overuse of acute care hospitals will reduce economic costs to patients and would probably improve their outcomes , as long as providers also make the move from disorganized to organized care,*

10. Overuse Alters the Life Experience of the Patient for the Worse

Perhaps the most important reason for reducing the overuse of acute care hospitals is the penalty that it imposes on the lives of patients and their families. It is not just a matter of wasted resources; it is a matter of how Americans experience the inevitable decline in their health that ends in death. At the same time, it is equally important to remember that the overuse of care is not just a phenomenon at the end of life. Care intensity during terminal care and during the last six months of life is only part of a pattern; regions and hospitals that provide aggressive rescue care at this stage in the progression of illness also do so at earlier stages. If a high-tech death in the hospital were the price the dying must pay to make sure that those with progressing chronic illness enjoyed a longer life and a higher quality of life, then it might be viewed as the cost of medical progress. But the evidence indicates that this is not the case. Overuse involves the medicalization of death in an apparently futile effort to extend life expectancy.

The impact on Americans can be seen in the Dartmouth Atlas Project statistics: most Americans will die from chronic illness, but their experience of death will vary according to where they live. Among Medicare patients who die from chronic illness, 30% of those living in Los Angeles and 29% of those in Miami will experience a stay in an ICU at the time of death; in Minneapolis and in Portland, Oregon, only 14% will. The overuse of acute care hospitals imposes a burden on patients, which heretofore has occurred largely with little or no awareness on the part of patients, families, or their physicians.

Awareness on the part of patients and their families, and their physicians, of the pattern of practice in their own community and at their own hospital is an important step in the process of change. In subsequent chapters, I will discuss how patients, their families, and their physicians might use Dartmouth Atlas Project information to help patients receive the kind of care that most closely fits their preference.

* * *

There are compelling reasons for the nation to deal with the overuse of medical care, particularly the acute care hospital sector. But to take action, we need to identify inefficiency, estimate waste, measure the patient experience, and then reform the delivery system, so that it is more efficient and more focused on the needs and wishes of patients and delivers higher quality care and better outcomes.

PART IV

Pathways to Reform

My understanding of the sources of unwarranted variation and undisciplined growth in health care points to the importance of replacing disorganized, chaotic "systems" of care with organized systems; replacing delegated decision making and the doctrine of informed consent with shared decision making and the standard of informed patient choice; improving the science of health care delivery; and constraining undisciplined growth in health care capacity and spending.

The final section of my book sets forth some ideas and strategies for how these goals might be accomplished. The focus for Chapter 13 is on promoting the growth of organized care by providing economic incentives to providers who accept responsibility for caring for their population of loyal patients—not just in the acute phase but throughout the course of their illness, a strategy that seems particularly suited for chronically ill patients. The economic incentive is shared savings—the opportunity for providers who become more efficient to retain part of the savings to reinvest in care and reduction of debt. The shared savings strategy could result in large rewards for providers in high-cost regions who reduce their inpatient spending to the per capita levels of providers in low-cost regions. Academic medical centers are called on to undertake the necessary research to rationalize the clinical pathways for managing chronic illness—and to adjust their resource inputs toward the efficiency benchmarks that emerge from their research. Shared savings would be key to the completion of this mission.

Chapter 14 considers several approaches to promoting shared decision making and establishing informed patient choice, including changes in state laws governing malpractice to provide greater immunity to physicians who provide high-quality shared decision making, demonstration projects, economic incentives, and the assumption by primary care physicians of advocacy and professional accountability for ensuring informed patient choice as a standard of practice. Comparative effectiveness research along the lines discussed in Chapter 7 would make it feasible for primary care physicians to assume this role.

While the nation desperately needs to reengineer clinical practice, it cannot depend on reform of the delivery system as the primary means for controlling capacity and spending. In this upside-down economy, reform requires working from the top down as well as from the bottom up. In Chapter 15, I outline six steps that can be taken to place limits on capacity and spending and buy time for reform of the delivery system to take hold.

The final chapter summarizes the challenge of practice variation.

13

Promoting Organized Care and Reducing Overuse

Motivating providers to coordinate care and achieving savings from reductions in overuse will require new policies and new ways of thinking about chronic illness and how to organize and finance health care. The lion's share of Medicare spending goes toward caring for the chronically ill, patients who are treated as if they have acute (e.g., temporary) conditions. But chronic illness does not go away. No matter how successful "secondary prevention" may be, barring major breakthroughs in medical science, most patients with chronic illness are on a trajectory that usually lasts until death, with symptoms and functional decline becoming progressively more debilitating for the patient and more costly for families and for Medicare. For this patient population—the nation's most costly—Medicare is not an insurance plan intended to cover unforeseen risks; it is the payer for care over an extended period of time involving an inevitable decline in health and rise in costs. The relevant episode of illness is thus measured in months and years, and strategies to manage the patient's care must have a similar long-range focus.

The way chronic illness is managed differs markedly from region to region and from provider to provider within regions. A provider's pattern of practice in treating chronic disease extends throughout the course of the patient's illness, not just during its terminal phase. Hospitals that are overtreating in the last six months of patients' lives are overtreating them long before that. Moreover, overuse is driven in large measure by the influence that capacity (workforce and facilities) exerts on physician decisions made in the absence of medical evidence. Thus, the remedy for overuse and unwarranted variation must simultaneously focus on several variables at multiple levels—adjusting resource capacity relative to the size of the population of patients served, coordinating care efficiently across multiple caregivers and multiple settings over time, and ensuring the timely use of specific interventions as called for by the dictates of evidence-based medicine, all of which requires an organized system of care accountable to a defined patient population.

The current reimbursement system makes such reforms exceedingly difficult, if not impossible. It reimburses for utilization, not care management over time; rewards high-intensity inpatient care handsomely; pays relatively little for primary care and other components of care essential for population-based, communitywide management of chronic illness; rewards rather than punishes unnecessary duplication of services; does not compensate hospitals for losses associated with reduction in acute care capacity; and fails, for the most part, to make distinctions between high- and low-quality performance.

Ironically, a "Made in the USA" model for organizing care that is accountable to a defined patient population—and how to pay for it—already exists in the form of prepaid group practices such as Kaiser Permanente and Group Health Cooperative. So why has the model not spread? One reason is that it is extremely difficult to organize providers to become team members and coordinate care. But even when providers want to become organized, economic incentives work against them. People have been working on this problem for a long time. In the years leading up to the Clinton health reform proposal, I attended several meetings of the Jackson Hole Group, organized by Paul Ellwood and Alain Enthoven. Much of the discussion focused on how to create market incentives to "drive" providers into competing organized systems where health care workers and administrators work as a unified team to coordinate care across sectors, including hospitals, extended care facilities, nursing homes, and other community-based health facilities, and where care takes place within the constraints of an annual budget.

The plan for managed competition based on Enthoven's concepts went down with the Clinton health care plan. It became a target of proponents of a single-payer system who viewed it as a "last ditch" effort to preserve the insurance industry. Skeptics also emerged who did not believe that the "market" would adequately control prices. But it also died because of lack of relevance and appeal to Americans who did not live in urban settings. In many parts of the country, it is not feasible to divide providers into competing groups. Indeed, to sustain a fully competitive model along the lines proposed under the managed care initiative, we have estimated that a region would need a minimum of 1.2 million people.[1] In 1990, only 42% of the U.S. population lived in such regions. In less-populated regions, competition among providers makes less sense, and in rural, small town America, it makes no sense at all.

Shared Savings as an Incentive to Promote Organized Care

Prepaid group practices such as Kaiser Permanente or Group Health Cooperative remain a compelling American success story, and it is of interest that they did not get their start because of market competition. Some began primarily in rural regions to provide care where none existed; in small towns that expanded dramatically during World War II to provide care to shipyard workers; or, as in the case of Group Health Cooperative, as a consumer-owned cooperative to serve the needs of Seattle. Soon after the failure of the Clinton plan, my colleagues and I began thinking about how payment reform could be designed to give health care providers in Vermont and New Hampshire—where the population base of local medical markets falls way below the required population base for competition between integrated health care systems—the flexibility they need to address unwarranted variation. From my Vermont days, I was aware of the pattern of overuse in Randolph, a small town in the middle of the state. In the late 1960s, Randolph stood at or near the top of the distribution in per capita spending and utilization, primarily because of its high rate of admission to the town's one hospital for medical conditions. As Dartmouth Atlas Project data became available in the mid-1990s, Randolph continued to stand out as a high utilizer, and we thought it might be possible to devise a plan that would help the providers of Randolph become more efficient.

A few things had changed since Randolph first came to our attention. Many of the primary physicians living in the community had joined the staff of the local hospital, Gifford Memorial, as full-time, salaried employees. Salaried physicians employed by the Dartmouth-Hitchcock Medical Center—living either on site in Randolph, or in Hanover—were now providing most of the specialty care. Those two changes meant that Randolph had already come part of the way toward becoming an organized group practice. We suggested a plan to the provider community to pay for care on a per capita basis. Everyone, administrators and physicians alike, seemed to agree that this would help them deliver higher-quality care and provide better stewardship in managing costs and resources.

We worked with the providers to develop a proposal for a demonstration project to establish a budget for managing care for the population of Randolph, based on what we called "virtual capitation."[2] This was technically feasible because the claims data allowed us to associate the providers of care—the physician staff of the Gifford Memorial Hospital and the Dartmouth-Hitchcock Medical Center—with the population they served. We could then calculate how much money was spent for this population on an annual basis and use this to establish a prospective budget for the ensuing year. Payments would be made on a regular monthly basis. Savings obtained—for example, by reducing the capacity of the acute care hospital, which our data showed far exceeded the benchmark of other hospitals in the region—could thus be captured by the providers and reinvested in new services, including those not covered under fee-for-service at that time, such as anticholesterol statin drugs for high-risk patients, disease management programs, and community-based prevention programs. Our payment model was designed to give the Randolph health care providers the flexibility they needed to reallocate resources to more efficient purposes and to give Medicare (and other insurers, were they to join) the assurance that global (total per capita) spending could be controlled.

When we proposed a project based on these ideas to Medicare, we received only a lukewarm response, and after several years of going back and forth, the idea died of attrition (and exhaustion). But the concepts of shared savings, global budgets, and virtual capitation that did not require the formal enrollment of patients into a health maintenance organization (HMO) have lived on. In the early 2000s, Senator James Jeffords introduced legislation modeled after our failed efforts to reengineer health care in Randolph, which became law under Section 646 of the Medicare Prescription Drug Improvement and Modernization Act of 2003 (Pub. L. 108–173), as the Medicare Health Quality Demonstration Program.[3] The law allows providers to establish prospective budgets for managing care, freeing them to allocate resources toward caring for patients over time, rather than investing in whatever service line is supported by the fee schedule. The law allows the Secretary of Health and Human Services to waive regulatory provisions, including the Stark anti-kickback statutes, so that providers can participate in a share of the savings obtained by improving efficiency and quality of care.

More recently, my colleagues Dr. Elliott Fisher and Jonathan Skinner, together with Dr. Mark McClellan and others at the Brookings Institution, have proposed a national shared savings program.[4] Their proposal would encourage providers in virtually every medical community to take steps to become "accountable care organizations" (ACOs), integrated health care systems capable of meeting certain quality standards and improving the coordination of care. If they accomplish this, Medicare would then share part of the savings from improvements in efficiency with the provider. If successfully implemented, the ACO model could greatly facilitate the transition from disorganized to organized care throughout the United States.

It is important to emphasize that the effort to promote organized and accountable care through shared savings programs is quite different from the effort in the 1990s to force patients into managed care. First, these projects focus on maintaining and improving quality, using accepted, objective measures, many more of which are available today than in the past. Second, the Centers for Medicare & Medicaid Services (CMS) is dealing directly with providers, not insurance companies motivated to capture their share of the revenue stream. Third, the patient's freedom to choose their provider is the same as under traditional Medicare. They are not locked into using a provider for a year or longer, as they were under managed care. They can leave and go elsewhere for care at any time they want if they become dissatisfied.

In this chapter, I discuss how providers might respond to shared savings incentives to organize and coordinate care, strive to achieve the efficiencies demonstrated by organized group practices and integrated hospital systems, and, in the case of academic medical centers, undertake the necessary research to rationalize the "black box" of supply-sensitive care.

Organized Systems of Care

Multispecialty group practices and integrated hospital systems, because they are "shovel ready" systems, would be the most obvious candidates to become ACOs. They have already accomplished what for most providers will be the most difficult task: they are organized and their physicians are practiced in care coordination and team medicine. Even so, there is considerable room for improvement in these organized systems. As discussed in previous chapters, chronic care management among well-organized, large multispecialty groups does not as yet follow a well-defined and replicable model that could be exported as a best practice strategy, or model. To undertake the necessary restructuring of capacity and the redesign of the clinical pathways for managing care, organized systems, like all providers, need a reimbursement plan that creates a target budget for managing their patient population over time and pays in real time a share of the savings in fee-for-service spending made possible by reducing utilization.

Organized practices are perhaps ideally situated to take advantage of shared savings as a strategy for capitalizing growth into other geographic areas, or within their own markets. They could acquire inefficient hospitals or physician practices; reduce the acquired practice's overuse of care, particularly acute care hospitals; and invest the savings to build a community-based, and primary care–based, system for managing chronic illnesses. The savings from improving the efficiency of acute care hospitals are potentially quite large, as illustrated by the recent acquisition and subsequent reduction in capacity of South Wilkes-Barre Hospital by the Geisinger Clinic. According to the Dartmouth Atlas, the Wilkes-Barre, Pennsylvania, region has only three hospitals. But compared to the Danville region, the home base of the Geisinger Clinic, hospital utilization rates for acute and chronic illnesses in Wilkes-Barre were much higher. Our data indicate that Geisinger Clinic's decision to reduce acute care hospital capacity will result in large savings in health care spending—as much as $13.8 million per year for Medicare fee-for-service medicine alone. Systemwide savings of this magnitude, returned to group practices that participate in shared savings program, could provide a major source of capital for constructing the infrastructure of communitywide management of health care and a strong incentive for group practices to expand into new markets.[5]

Organized group practices may also extend their reach into new regions through growth in primary care and the use of physician extenders—nurse practitioners, physician's assistants, and case managers. The Kaiser Permanente health care system has shown how this can be done in Georgia, where Kaiser Permanente has expanded into new medical communities by deploying primary care physicians who are backed up by nurse coaches and selected medical specialist consultants.

Finally, individual hospitals and their associated physician staffs may become motivated to seek partnerships with large group practices or integrated hospital systems that already have the infrastructure and experience to help them through the transition from disorganized to organized systems of care.

Multihospital Networks

Hospital networks could conceivably serve as the nucleus for the rapid growth of organized care. The Sutter Health System in Sacramento and Intermountain Healthcare in Salt Lake City are models for how hospital networks can develop into coordinated care systems. Over the past few decades, a number of hospital systems have arisen around the country— some not-for-profit, some for-profit, some associated with academic medical centers, and others not. By 2005, fully 30% of traditional Medicare patients hospitalized for chronic illness during the last two years of life were treated primarily in hospitals belonging to networks with ten or more member facilities. There are striking variations among the hospitals belonging to these networks, suggesting that there is plenty of room for better management that would result in shared savings (Figure 13.1). For example, among the 139 Hospital Corporation of American (HCA) hospitals, Medicare reimbursements varied by a factor of 2.5, from about $38,500 per patient over the last two years of life to more than $95,000. There was even more variation among the hospitals belonging to the Tenet Healthcare Corporation (indeed, the highest per patient spending among all hospitals belonging to a network was seen at Tenet hospitals). Among faith-based networks, Catholic Healthcare West and Catholic Health East showed great variation.

The opportunity for significant savings is particularly high for providers in high-cost regions (Los Angeles, New Jersey, Miami, and downstate New York, for instance). This might motivate the management teams at hospital networks with facilities in both high- and low-cost regions to take aggressive steps to improve efficiency. Consider the opportunities for financial gain that would be available to Catholic Healthcare West, which in 2005 was comprised of thirty-three hospitals, of which five were located in the high-cost Los Angeles region and six in low-cost Sacramento. According to the Dartmouth Atlas routine reports, over the last two years of their chronically ill patients' lives, per capita Medicare spending for all sectors of care (not just inpatient care) was $90,662 for the five Los Angeles hospitals, whereas spending for similar patients treated in the six Catholic Healthcare West hospitals serving Sacramento was just over half of that, $49,157 per patient. Because they achieve better quality using fewer resources, the Catholic Healthcare West hospitals in Sacramento should serve as a relative efficiency benchmark for the system's hospitals in Los Angeles.

Here is an idea of the potential savings. Had the five Los Angeles hospitals and associated physicians learned to provide care at the Sacramento rate over the five-year period from 2001 through 2005, the cost of care for Catholic Healthcare West's patients in Los Angeles would have amounted to only $260 million in Medicare dollars. Instead, actual spending was $480 million. The difference between actual and predicted spending under the Sacramento benchmark—almost $220 million over five years—indicates the approximate amount that could become available if Catholic Healthcare West hospitals in Los Angeles were to successfully reach the Sacramento benchmark for relative efficiency in managing chronic illness. Note that these savings are only for care in the last two years of life and just for chronically

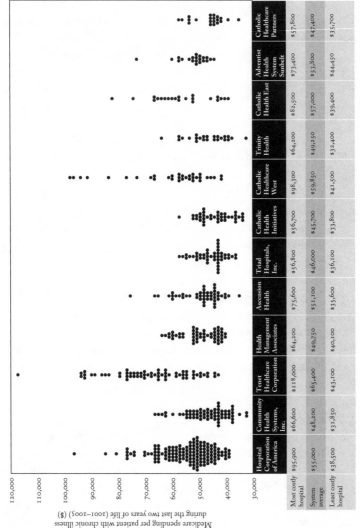

Figure 13.1. Medicare spending per patient during the last two years of life for patients with common chronic illnesses receiving most of their care from a hospital belonging to one of twelve hospital systems (deaths occurring 2001 through 2005). Each dot represents a hospital. (Source: Dartmouth Atlas Project database.)

ill patients, and thus this amount underestimates the total savings if Los Angeles Catholic Healthcare West providers were to reach the Sacramento Catholic Healthcare West level of intensity of care.

Physician Practice Networks

What about the prospects for a physician network—the so-called Independent Physician Associations (IPAs), which are particularly prevalent in California? Or a primary care network organized as a medical home that qualifies as an ACO? On the surface, the prospects seem quite good. As we have seen, even within a region such as Los Angeles, there is remarkable variation in Medicare spending for the chronically ill among patients loyal to a given hospital, mostly because of differences in intensity of inpatient care and the associated use of skilled nursing homes and long-term care hospitals. Assuming that the network's physicians are free to send patients to any hospital located within their community, the Dartmouth Atlas reports can point such organizations as IPAs toward the hospitals that have the lowest per capita spending for Medicare patients with progressive chronic illness. By merely transferring patients to the more efficient hospital, the physician network would likely realize a large reward for increased efficiency, without any apparent loss in the quality of care (Box 13.1).

From the point of view of Medicare and other payers, the overall impact may not be so favorable, unless strategies to reduce the overuse of acute care hospitals affect the capacity of the inpatient sector in a given *community*. Thus, increasing the efficiency of one hospital may turn out to be just another form of cost shifting, as the per patient intensity of care rises in the hospital that is losing patients. This is one reason why a shared saving strategy may need a big stick to keep overall spending under control on a hospital-specific as well as a regional basis. For example, Dartmouth routine reports would record any increases in per capita spending at St. Mary Medical Center above, say, the national average expected increase as determined by Medicare. This information could be used to tailor an overuse penalty (discussed in Chapter 14) to prevent any compensatory rise in overutilization that might occur as result of a decline in their patient population.

Academic Medical Centers

Academic medical centers, as shown in Chapter 11, exhibit striking variation in the intensity of care and the use of resources. As part of their responsibility

Box 13.1.   *How Physician Networks Might Benefit from a Shared Savings Program: The Long Beach, California, Example*

There are three hospitals in Long Beach, all within three miles of each other. Between 2001 and 2005, reimbursements to St. Mary Medical Center totaled $98,000 per capita over the last two years of life—22% more than the $81,000 that Medicare spent on similar patients using Long Beach Memorial Hospital. The third hospital in the community—Pacific Medical Center—spent $90,000 per capita, 11% more than Long Beach Memorial Hospital. By changing referral patterns to ensure that its patients with chronic illness are managed in conjunction with inpatient services provided by Long Beach Memorial Hospital, a physician network located in that community would realize a reduction in expected costs for managing chronic illness over the last two years of life of about $17,000 for patients transferred from St. Mary Medical Center and $9,000 for patients from Pacific Medical Center. In 2005, the quality of care composite scores for Long Beach Hospital were slightly better than those for St. Mary's; Pacific Medical Center did not report its quality results.

for the interface between clinical science and clinical practice, academic medical centers must be challenged to undertake the studies needed to establish a more scientific basis for managing acute and chronic illness over time. In addition to conducting comparative effectiveness research to test the efficacy of individual treatments and tests, making medicine more scientific requires the redesign and testing, and still further redesign and retesting, of care processes. If, as may well happen, academic medical centers end up providing fewer services in response to better evidence, the outcome will be a loss in revenue. Thus, a shared savings program may be an essential component of the incentive package academic medical centers will need to participate aggressively in the redesign of clinical practice. In other words, it will not be sufficient simply to pay them to conduct comparative effectiveness research. Medicare (and other insurers) must also offer the academic medical centers a financial bridge to greater efficiency.

For supply-sensitive care, care processes are pretty much a black box—the rate of services is driven primarily by available resources and a perverse payment system, unconstrained by medical theory and medical evidence. Very few health care organizations have a track record of accomplishments that provide a model of how this research and development might be conducted. Intermountain Healthcare, an integrated hospital network of fifteen hospitals located in western Utah and southeastern Idaho, is one of the few, and the research being conducted there serves as a window on the potential and pitfalls of reengineering the care of the chronically ill.

Inspired by the work of W. E. Deming, a guru of continuous quality improvement, Dr. Brent James and his colleagues at Intermountain embarked about fifteen years ago on a program to rationalize the way medicine was practiced across the Intermountain Healthcare system. Today, Intermountain is an impressive example of how comparative effectiveness research can reduce variation, improve care outcomes, and contribute to the science of clinical decision making. The clinical program for diabetes provides an example. Intermountain supports the care of more than 20,000 diabetic patients, delivered by more than fifty provider teams across the entire system. A key feature is the rationalization of the relationships between primary care and specialty care. The primary care physicians provide almost 90% of the care. Endocrinologists—the diabetes "knowledge experts"—work primarily in a consultative role to primary care, directly managing only the most difficult cases. A set of routine performance reports guide care management. The reports include a "Diabetes Action List"—a summary for each patient that a given team is managing—of crucial quality measures such as glycosylated hemoglobin, low-density lipids, retinal eye exams, and blood pressure. The report flags patients with unfavorable profiles. On the basis of these reports, specific steps are taken to address problems.

While useful in motivating members of the team to pay attention to outliers, the reports on comparative performance are primarily viewed as an opportunity to further examine the care pathways of high performing practices to learn why they are *comparatively more effective* than others. What is it that they are doing that others are not doing? In other words, the strategy is built around the principle that progress requires an organization that can learn from experience. Under the Intermountain approach, comparative effectiveness research is thus playing an important role in an iterative strategy to improve the scientific basis of clinical decision making.

The commitment to science and improvement in the scientific basis of clinical decision making underscores the Intermountain approach. The same infrastructure that results in the explication of clinical processes, tracking of outcomes, and linking together of care processes has positioned Intermountain Healthcare to undertake more traditional medical effectiveness research to evaluate clinical hypotheses using clinical trials or cohort studies that have been published in peer-reviewed journals.

When it comes to managing supply-sensitive care for chronically ill patients, the Salt Lake City region, where care is dominated by Intermountain Healthcare, is among the nation's most "relatively efficient" (see Chapter 11). For a number of conditions, Intermountain is moving beyond relative efficiency as a criterion for evaluating performance to evaluating health care delivery according to its cost-effectiveness—on "best practices" benchmarks that are based on real knowledge of the relationship between resource inputs and health outcomes. Thus, the resource input benchmarks and care processes documented in the case of diabetes represent a more reliable basis for understanding the content of "high value care," or care that delivers real outcomes, and how much it actually costs to deliver it.

Such information is critical for the long-term goal of basing reimbursement policy on the costs of delivering cost-effective care. To be sure, Intermountain has yet to complete the rationalization of "black box" care into clinical programs for a number of important chronic illness, and differences remain in the way medical resources are used in managing chronic illness from place to place within the Intermountain system. However, it has the infrastructure in place to turn its attention to these problems.

Outside of a few other organizations that have been willing, like Intermountain, to self-fund this research—the Geisinger, Marshfield, and Mayo Clinics come to mind—progress has been quite limited, even among organized practices that have the electronic medical record systems and infrastructure in position to carry out such research. An obvious reason is the lack of funding. Since the mid-1990s downgrade of the Agency for Health Care Policy and Research (and its metamorphosis into the Agency for Healthcare Research and Quality), federal funding for effectiveness research has declined to a few hundred million dollars annually, hardly enough to support a sustained assault on the lack of medical evidence.

But lack of research support is just one of the hurdles. The more significant constraint on conducting research that can fundamentally alter the pattern of practice is the threat that it may bring to the financial stability of the organization itself. Perhaps the most startling revelation yet to emerge is that even though Intermountain Healthcare is among the nation's most efficient health care organization in managing chronic illness, the rationalization of its care processes is leading to still greater efficiencies and recoveries of waste. As Brent James has discovered, no good deed goes unpunished, because streamlining Intermountain's delivery system and becoming more efficient is financially destabilizing. As their practice patterns became more efficient, fewer specialty services were needed; as care improved, hospitalization rates fell. While Intermountain was able to negotiate shared savings arrangements with some of its insurance companies, the net effect was a squeeze on revenue, a situation that naturally leads to troubling questions about how far improvement can be allowed to outpace the need for revenue.

Improving the scientific basis for managing chronic illness is critical to the reform of health care. To do it right, leading health care organizations from different parts of the country need to be recruited to this mission. Large group practices and integrated hospital networks are uniquely qualified to conduct research that depends on organized delivery systems, and research grants under the comparative effectiveness research agenda need to be targeted to bring such organizations on board. Teaching hospitals, particularly those like the University of California hospitals that exhibit strikingly different patterns of care, even while they belong to the same "system" of care, must also be recruited. Yet research grants will not be enough to ensure rapid implementation of this practice-changing research agenda. The redesign of care for the acutely and chronically ill, geared to improve efficiency and clinical outcomes, may fundamentally alter the resource requirements, changing the need for beds, physician workforce, and equipment—and disrupting the flow of volume of care–generated dollars essential for short-term financial stability. Progress in establishing cost-effective care as the standard of practice will occur at a snail's pace unless these organizations are at least partially shielded from major financial impacts associated with declining utilization rates. This is why the comparative effectiveness research agenda needs to be tied to a shared savings program such as Medicare's "Section 646" demonstration project.

Opportunities for Radical Redesign of Care for Aging America

A distinguishing characteristic of the American culture is its willingness to experiment to adapt to new challenges by figuring out what works, even when this means a radical departure from tradition. Over the past fifteen years, right here in Hanover, practically in the backyard of the Dartmouth-Hitchcock Medical Center, an example of radical redesign has taken place, but the implications for both the patient experience and health care costs have only recently become apparent. The experiment involves the evolution of a primary care–based approach to providing continuous medical care to the residents of a retirement community, located in Hanover, New Hampshire. Most of the 450 members of the community come from professional and business backgrounds, with many holding advanced degrees. As with most senior living communities, the members are sufficiently affluent to be able to purchase their home and also pay monthly fees. The security they purchase is lifetime care in the community. Once members, virtually all remain until death.

According to Dr. Dennis McCullough, the community's founding medical director, the approach to health care is based in a comprehensive discussion among caregivers and community members around medical care issues, including preferences for care at the end of life. Over time, a close collaboration between community members and care providers has created a "medical subculture" that embraces a remarkably conservative strategy for managing acute and chronic illnesses and care at the end of life. In addition to community participation and regularly repeated education on how the care system works, central elements include early family involvement in all recognized medical problems, promotion of a slowed pace for careful decision making for all chronic problems, and medical consultations as "advice consultations" (as opposed to transfer of patient management). These important elements were identified and implemented jointly with the community of elders. Many retired resident medical and nursing professionals (a number of whom had worked at the Dartmouth-Hitchcock Medical Center) were vital to the initial planning of the community's approach to health care. The approach to care developed by and for the community became the basis for "Slow Medicine," a philosophy and set of practices described in a book by the same name by Dr. McCullough.[6]

The care model is primary care-based, involving one full-time equivalent primary care physician and two nurse practitioners. As with many senior retirement communities, there are onsite facilities for dealing with progressing chronic illness, including a skilled nursing facility (SNF) that is qualified for Medicare reimbursement. The primary care team, composed of three or four people, is accountable for continuous care, on call 24/7, so use of the emergency department is generally avoided. The care team manages referrals to specialists and coordinates all admissions to the nearby Dartmouth-Hitchcock Medical Center. The use of the onsite SNF as a substitute for acute care hospitalization proved to be an important asset for accomplishing the goal of avoiding hospitalization. Even though Medicare does not reimburse the SNF for care unless the stay follows an acute care hospital admission, the members of the community and their providers are dedicated to avoiding acute care hospitalization, if at all possible. For example, patients who experience an acute problem, such as pneumonia or recurrence of congestive heart failure, are routinely monitored and treated in the SNF rather than being sent to the hospital. Physician and nurse practitioner fees are billed on a fee-for-service basis through Medicare. Care at the end of life, with rare exceptions, takes place within the community.

The success of the community's redesign of clinical practice in meeting the goals of the community for conservative management of chronic illness and supportive care at the end of life is reflected in the Dartmouth Atlas statistics. Measured over a ten-year period (1997 through 2006), the hospitalization rates were extremely low compared to the rates for the neighboring townspeople: only 5% of deaths occurred in the hospital compared to 22% of residents of similar ages living elsewhere in Hanover. (Nationally, about 32% of the deaths in the Medicare population occur in hospital; in some regions, such as McAllen, Texas, as many as 45% of patients die in hospital.) Community residents were hospitalized for surgical procedures at about the same rate as other citizens of Hanover, the greatest difference being in the use of hospitals for acute and chronic medical conditions. The admission rate for patients 75 years of age and older was only about one-third of that of others living in Hanover—68 admissions per 1,000, compared to 210 per 1,000. Emergency department use was similarly lower.

The potential for the radical transformation of the health care economy rests in communities and individuals coming to terms with preferences regarding the management of chronic illness and care at the end of life. Primary care is crucial to helping patients to both define and achieve their goals and support alternatives to acute care hospitalization. The story of what has happened at the Hanover retirement community provides an excellent example of what an ACO might look like: a defined system accountable for the continuous care of a population of patients, in a way that is responsive to their needs and their wishes. It is also an example of what is today widely advocated as the primary care medical home—a patient-centered or community-centered collaborative model for care, organized around a primary care team. It points to key features that should be supported under a shared savings program, including the organization of primary care as a full-time salaried team with 24/7 coverage and direct admission to an SNF without requiring a prior stay in an acute care hospital.

* * *

As the nation moves forward with health care reform, we must acknowledge the harms, both financial and physical, that overuse imposes on patients, especially the elderly. The goal of any health care system should be to promote health and to ease the suffering that comes with serious illness and dying. Much of our so-called "system" does neither. Yet there are models out there, examples of high-quality, high-value care and efficiency, that can and should lead the way toward a better, more just, more compassionate, and patient-centered way of doing business. This means that we have some, although not all, of the answers to the question of how to reengineer, streamline, and reform the way we manage chronic illness and care at the end of life. What remains to be seen is whether the nation has the will to experiment with different approaches and new ways of both reimbursing and organizing health care until we get it right.

14

Establishing Shared Decision Making and Informed Patient Choice

The democratization of the doctor-patient relationship—the replacement of delegated decision making by shared decision making and the doctrine of informed consent by a standard of practice based on informed patient choice—represents a transformation in the culture of medicine that will not be easy to achieve. That process was set back by the loss of funding for the Patient Outcomes Research Teams (PORTs) and the greatly diminished role of the Agency for Healthcare Research and Quality (formerly the Agency for Health Care Policy and Research). Nonetheless, shared decision making appears to be on firmer ground than ever before.[1] Patient decision aids have become available for an increasing number of clinical conditions, and their effectiveness has been established by more than fifty clinical trials—enough so that they have been subjected to review by the Cochrane Collaboration, an international network of researchers devoted to synthesizing and appraising medical knowledge through a systematic review of clinical data.[2] The review confirms that decision aids facilitate shared decision making; increase patients' knowledge of what is at stake; promote active engagement in decision making; reduce uncertainty on the part of the patient about which treatment to choose; and improve the agreement between the patient's values or preferences and the treatment option that is actually chosen.[3]

The availability of a growing library of patient decision aids makes feasible the broad implementation of shared decision making into everyday practice.

More and more providers are committed to ensuring that patients facing elective surgery have an opportunity to be fully informed and to share the treatment decision with their physicians, and decision aids are being integrated into everyday practice with increasing sophistication and efficacy. Legislators in several states appear to be on the verge of changing the legal standard for determining medical necessity, from informed consent to informed patient choice. And the nation, once again, may do something significant to improve economic incentives for the reform of the health care delivery systems. However, we still face significant barriers.

Getting to Shared Decision Making

Let me begin with a brief review of the history of the implementation of shared decision making at the Dartmouth-Hitchcock Medical Center, which illustrates some of the difficulties, as well as the successes, in bringing about cultural change. The first medical center to begin using decision aids in everyday practice was the Veterans Administration (VA) Hospital, which is in White River Junction, Vermont, just over the river from the Dartmouth-Hitchcock Medical Center in Lebanon, New Hampshire, and one of the teaching hospitals for the Dartmouth Medical School. In 1988, Mary LaBrecque, a respected nurse practitioner at the VA Hospital, teamed up with our research group to conduct the initial study of the benign prostatic hyperplasia (BPH) decision aid. She first used it as a kind of virtual "second opinion," showing it to about twenty-five patients who were on the waiting list for surgery for BPH. To everyone's surprise, nearly half of the patients who were waiting for surgery decided that they really did not want the surgery after all. Subsequently, Mary helped the VA to implement the use of the decision aid as part of a routine process for diagnosing patient preferences for BPH surgery. By all accounts the project was quite successful; patients were satisfied and physicians were adapted to increased patient participation in choice of treatment. And the project had a real effect on patient demand, resulting in significant savings to the VA as the rate of surgery dropped, just as it had in the HMO experiment discussed in Chapter 6. But despite (or rather because of) this success, the project was quite suddenly interrupted by the medical school's department of urology. It turned out that under shared decision making, the number of surgical procedures in the VA hospital dipped well below the level needed to ensure that urology residents performed enough BPH operations to meet the minimum required to qualify for board certification. Faced with this crisis, the needs of medical educators trumped patient preferences and the decision was made to end the VA experiment.

Shared decision making then found a new champion in 1996 in Dr. James Weinstein, who was recruited from the University of Iowa. A conservative surgeon by nature, Jim has long believed that patients need to be fully engaged in the decision about something as potentially life changing as surgery. Jim had already recognized the value of decision aids while he was at the University of Iowa, where he served as a member of the back pain patient outcomes research team funded by the Agency of Health Care Policy and Research. Soon after Jim came to Dartmouth, Health Dialog and the Foundation for Informed Medical Decision Making began the process of expanding the library of decision aids, and Jim saw to it that informed patient choice for orthopedic conditions became the standard of practice in his department. In 1999, Jim founded the Center for Shared Decision Making to coordinate the delivery of decision aids throughout the medical center, and shortly after that he recruited Kate Clay, a nurse and bioethicist, who still serves as program director. Annette O'Connor, a researcher from the University of Toronto and an expert in shared decision making, helped train Kate to support patients as they make decisions, a process that requires considerable clinical skill. With Kate as director, increasingly more patients have gone through the shared decision-making process, and she and Jim have been able to persuade more and more physicians at Dartmouth-Hitchcock to participate.

Breast reconstruction surgeon Dr. E. Dale Collins was one of the earliest converts, and she has helped to build a program that allows every breast cancer patient a chance to become fully engaged in the decisions that must be made about her treatment. As part of the shared decision-making process, each woman with early-stage breast cancer follows a defined clinical pathway, or sequence of visits with particular physicians and nurses, that begins with her initial diagnosis and ends with her treatment choice. Shortly after the diagnosis is made, she views a video-based patient decision aid, which explains the pros and cons of each treatment option. She then completes an online questionnaire aimed at probing the quality of her decision. Did she understand the video, and has she thought about how she feels about the alternatives? Finally, she discusses her options with Dale or one of the other surgeons, who uses the decision quality questionnaire as a reference point.

Let me illustrate how the shared decision-making process works with a real example. As an early-stage breast cancer patient, Mary Smith (not her real name) faced a choice. She had to decide between complete removal of her breast and lumpectomy, which involves local excision of her tumor, followed by radiation. Over the years, surgeons at Dartmouth-Hitchcock and researchers who study shared decision making have found that they can pre-dict with some accuracy which choice a woman will make, depending on how she feels about the tradeoffs between losing a breast versus having to worry about a local recurrence of her tumor. Some women are very concerned about loss of their breast and prefer lumpectomy and radiation; others wish to min-imize the possibility of local recurrence, and the need for ongoing surveil-lance as well as radiation, and therefore prefer mastectomy. Smith watched the patient decision aid, which described both procedures, the side effects of each, and the fact that the two are equally effective in terms of reducing her risk of dying of breast cancer. She also filled out a questionnaire designed to test her knowledge of the procedures and their different consequences, and her own values regarding keeping her breast versus not having to worry about a recurrence of her tumor. Smith decided on mastectomy.

The next step for Smith was an appointment with Dale, who is part of the multidisciplinary breast oncology program at Dartmouth-Hitchcock, a team that includes breast surgeons, oncologists, nurses, radiologists, and surgeons who specialize in reconstructive surgery. Before the appointment, Dale looked over the questionnaire that Smith had filled out and found that something was not quite right. The patient understood the tradeoffs between mastectomy versus lumpectomy, but she had indicated that she valued keep-ing her breast more highly than the peace of mind that she might gain by choosing mastectomy. That suggested to Dale that her patient should have chosen lumpectomy.

During the appointment, Dale discovered that her patient may not have understood her choice as well as she should have. Dale asked Smith to look at the patient decision aid again and think through her choice. After going through the process again, Smith told Dale that she had originally chosen mastectomy because that is what she thought her breast surgeon believed was best. After having her appointment with Dale and looking at the decision aid again, she realized that she really preferred lumpectomy. She understood that either surgery offered her an excellent shot at a cure, and perhaps most important of all, the choice was hers to make.

This patient's experience exemplifies everything that is right with shared decision making. She incorrectly intuited her surgeon's preference and would have undergone a major surgery, the loss of a breast, which she really did not want. Dale was able to probe Smith's decision with the help of the question-naire and a face-to-face interview. When she saw that the quality of Smith's decision was poor—it did not jibe with her values—the surgeon sent the patient back to the decision aid. Together, they were able to avoid a major medical error, a surgical procedure with lasting consequences that the patient did not want.

The questionnaire that measures decision quality is a key component of the process, ensuring that patients are making good choices for themselves, as the case of Mary Smith makes clear. These questionnaires are also important for auditing the overall performance of the breast cancer center. Reports are generated on a periodic basis to measure how well women score on the knowledge questions concerning risks and benefits, and the degree of agreement between the patient's own values and the treatment that was chosen. As I discuss later, high scores on decision quality measures could also be used to reward hospitals and clinics for doing well in implementing informed patient choice.

Getting to the point where shared decision making is widely practiced at Dartmouth-Hitchcock has taken a ten-year effort led by champions like Dale Collins, Jim Weinstein, and Kate Clay. It has been hampered by reimbursement systems that reward physicians handsomely for performing an operation but poorly for taking the time to learn what patients want. The culture of medicine has also been slow to change; physicians trained under the assumptions that it is the doctor's job to prescribe care and the patient's job to comply with medical advice need to learn and become comfortable with new roles, while patients have to come to understand that they face choices, and those choices involve tradeoffs on which only they can place value.

This chapter suggests three strategies for accelerating the cultural changes required to democratize the doctor-patient relationship. The first focuses on state legislators and state governments, and what they can do to change informed consent laws and otherwise promote the transition to informed patient choice as the standard of practice. The second involves payers, who can drive reform in parallel with the evolving legal environment, through changes in reimbursement policies. The third is for primary care physicians to become champions for shared decision making and informed patient choice.

Adopting Informed Patient Choice as the Legal Standard

Under current law, physicians who engage in shared decision making may expose themselves to malpractice suits. In a now famous case, at least among family practice physicians, a young resident named Daniel Merenstein helped a middle-aged patient decide whether he wanted to undergo a PSA test. The patient decided against the test, but when he subsequently went to another physician, he was given one without his knowledge. The test showed his PSA was high, and a subsequent biopsy found advanced prostate cancer. The patient successfully sued the large family practice where Merenstein was training, despite extensive documentation by Merenstein that the patient was fully informed of the tradeoffs when he made his initial choice not to get tested.

The outcome of such cases rests in part on the definition of *informed consent,* the legal standard for ensuring that patients understand what they are getting into when they agree to tests, such as the PSA, as well as elective surgery and other invasive procedures. Each state adheres to one of two definitions of informed consent, and both are an impediment to shared decision making. In a far-reaching article published in 2006 in the *American Journal of Law & Medicine,* Benjamin Moulton, who is the executive director of the American Society of Law, Medicine and Ethics, and Jaime Staples King, now a member of the faculty at Hastings School of Law, reviewed informed consent law in light of the unwarranted variation in preference-sensitive treatments.[4] They reached a startling conclusion: "... current legal concepts of informed consent are at odds with not only modern medical practice, but also individual autonomy rights .... Ironically, after placing autonomy at the center of informed consent, we have created a legal framework that fails to promote the personal values of individual patients" (see Box 14.1).

Both standards of informed consent assume that physicians understand what patients want and what they need to know in order to give consent. The reality, as I discuss in Chapters 3 through 5, is that physicians are not very good at diagnosing patient preferences or explaining the tradeoffs involved in medical decisions. Jaime and Ben recommended a substantial overhaul of the current informed consent system to balance patient autonomy with physician expertise and beneficence.

The King-Moulton article would soon contribute in a substantial way to the first legislative success story for shared decision making. In 2007, a Blue Ribbon Commission on Health Care Costs and Access, which included Washington state legislators and members of the community, issued a report on the state's health care system, relying in part on Dartmouth Atlas practice variations data. In November, I was invited by the Virginia Mason Medical Center, a large, multispecialty group practice in Seattle, Washington, to give a talk to which members of the state legislature were invited. State Senator Pflug and a senate staffer, Jonnel Anderson, heard my presentation on shared decision making and the article by Ben and Jaime. Senator Pflug then got in touch with them. Two months later, she introduced legislation to substantially revise the state's informed consent laws and promote shared decision making. Jaime, Ben, and I were subsequently invited to testify before the legislature in favor of the legislation.

Box 14.1.   *Informed Consent Laws Fail to Promote Personal Values of Individual Patients*

A central finding of the King-Moulton analysis is that informed consent laws fail to promote the personal values of individual patients. What explains this paradoxical outcome?

The laws of informed consent in the United States follow two lines of legal thinking: in about half of the states, the laws follow a physician-based standard, and in the other half, a patient-based standard is followed. The physician-based standard requires physicians to inform patients, as a "reasonably prudent practitioner" would do. The fundamental assumption is that physicians agree on the best treatment option and agree as well on what information patients need to achieve informed consent. In other words, the physician standard codifies the agency role of the physician (discussed in Chapter 2) and fails to promote the standard of informed patient choice for the many reasons outlined in this book.

The patient-based standard requires that physicians provide all information that a "reasonable patient" would want to know. The fundamental assumption behind this standard is that reasonable patients value information on risks and benefits similarly and that physicians know what reasonable patients need and they can diagnose their preferences. The flaws in this standard are evidenced by the practice variation phenomenon, particularly the randomized trials of shared decision making that show that patients who receive their care as part of "usual practice," even when conducted in practices governed by the patient-based standard for informed consent, are at risk for receiving surgery they do not want.

Both standards fail because neither provides physicians with a clear explanation of their legal disclosure obligations, nor patients with a valid understanding of what information they have a right to possess.

Again, it was the data on practice variations that seemed to gain the legislators' attention. They were fascinated, and I believe disturbed, by the great differences in the use of surgery among the communities they represent as elected officials. The male members of the legislature seemed particularly surprised by the striking differences in surgery for BPH surgery (Figure 14.1).

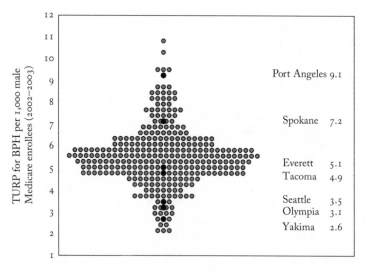

Figure 14.1. Rates of transurethral prostatectomy (TURP) for benign prostatic hyperplasia among hospital referral regions (*shaded circles*) and selected hospital service areas (*filled circles*) located in Washington State (2002 through 2003). (*Source*: Dartmouth Atlas Project database.)

A member of the legislature from Port Angeles could see that the rate for BPH surgery there was about nine procedures per 1,000 men, 3.5 times greater than that of Medicare men living in Yakima. Rates in Spokane were twice those of Seattle. By comparing the rates in Washington communities to the 306 regions across the United States, I was able to make the point that while practice variations were a national problem, it was one that needed a local solution—a change in the doctor-patient relationship to ensure that demand for preference-sensitive care is based on informed patient choice.

The bill, which was signed into law on May 2, 2007, represents the first time shared decision making and the normative importance of informed patient choice have been formally acknowledged by a state legislature[5] (Box 14.2). The benefit of using decision aids was also recognized in the law, as was the need for a process of certification to ensure their high quality. The bill provides superior legal protection from "failure to inform" malpractice suits against physicians who engage in shared decision making. The legislation also says that patients who agree to treatment as a result of shared decision making have given informed consent that can only be rebutted by "clear and convincing evidence," a higher standard of defense than that governing traditional informed consent, where rebuttal is based on "preponderance of evidence." (The latter standard requires a patient to demonstrate that it is more

Box 14.2.   *What Is in Washington State's Blue Ribbon Commission Health Bill (ESSB 5930)?*

An endorsement of shared decision making:

The legislature finds that there is growing evidence that, for preference-sensitive care involving elective surgery, patient-practitioner communication is improved through the use of high-quality decision aids that detail the benefits, harms, and uncertainty of available treatment options. Improved communication leads to more fully informed patient decisions. The legislature intends to increase the extent to which patients make genuinely informed, preference-based treatment decisions, by promoting public/private collaborative efforts to broaden the development, certification, use, and evaluation of effective decision aids and by recognition of shared decision making and patient decision aids in the state's laws on informed consent.

A definition of shared decision making:

... a process in which the physician or other health care practitioner discusses ... high quality, up-to-date information about the condition, including risks and benefits of available options and, if appropriate, the limits of scientific knowledge about outcomes; values clarification to help patients sort out their values and preferences; and guidance or coaching in deliberation, designed to improve the patient's involvement in the decision process.

A definition of patient decision aids (for purposes of this legislation):

... a written, audio-visual, or online tool that provides a balanced presentation of the condition and treatment options, benefits, and harms, including, if appropriate, a discussion of the limits of scientific knowledge about outcomes, and that is certified by one or more national certifying organizations.

A strong grant of immunity for physicians who use shared decision making and certified decision aids:

If a patient ... signs an acknowledgement of shared decision making [this] ... shall constitute prima facie evidence that the patient gave his or her informed consent to the treatment administered and the patient has the burden of rebutting this by clear and convincing evidence.

probable than not [i.e., a 50.1% chance] that the physician failed to provide all material information.)

In passing the bill, the legislature took an additional step to encourage Washington state physicians to adopt informed patient choice as the standard of practice. It called for the Washington State Health Care Authority—the agency overseeing all state agencies involved in health care, including state employee insurance plans and Medicaid—to conduct a "shared decision making demonstration project" at one or more group practice sites that provide health care purchased by the state. Since then, thanks in large part to an educational program run by the Milbank Foundation, a number of state legislators have attended seminars on the issue of shared decision making, and several have passed, or are contemplating, similar legislation.

The call of the Washington state legislators for demonstration projects appears to be paying off. At the time of this writing, four projects have been organized, including one undertaken by Group Health Cooperative, a large group practice that depends primarily on capitation as its payment model. Group Health is now developing clinical pathways to ensure the implementation of shared decision making for most common surgical procedures, and for care at the end of life, and integrating decision aids and decision quality reports into its electronic medical record system. Long-term follow-up of patients will soon be possible, just as was done in the original early 1990s collaboration between Group Health and the BPH and low back pain PORTs I reported on in previous chapters.

Over the years since then, I have kept in touch with the leaders of those early studies and shared their frustration that once the studies were finished, Group Health did not adopt (or champion) shared decision making as its model for managing preference-sensitive treatment decisions. It just seemed to make so much sense that it should do this, as Group Health physicians are primarily salaried and have no direct economic gain from doing surgery. Most Group Health members are capitated, so fee-for-service incentives do not drive physician practice patterns. Moreover, as Group Health providers had learned from the PORT studies, under shared decision making their patients were making more knowledgeable decisions, and decisions more in line with their preferences. And the use of shared decision making reduced the rate of surgery at Group Health, saving money without introducing fear among its members that they were being denied care they truly wanted.

So why did shared decision making not become the way medicine was practiced at Group Health? A considered answer would require extensive research and interviews with key personnel. However, the facts serve to illustrate just how difficult it is to change the culture of medicine when only a few seem to care. Employers, payers, and policy makers paid only passing attention to what was going on. At the time, information on practice variation was not generally available. The champions within Group Health remained a vocal minority without persuasive power.

By the mid-2000s, however, there was an awakening. The Governor's Blue Ribbon Commission on Health Care Costs and Access raised the question of shared decision making and presented data showing that medical practice varies substantially from place to place. Group Health leadership was part of that process and emerged as strong proponents of the legislative changes in support of informed patient choice. And once the bill was passed, the organization committed itself to change. According to Karen Merrikin, who serves as Group Health's executive director for public policy, practice variation data played an important role in gaining the attention of physicians throughout the Group Health organization and getting their commitment. Using its own claims data, Group Health analysts demonstrated variations among its own providers in terms of how Group Health members were treated, depending on the clinic they used.

Regulatory and Financial Incentives to Promote a Transition to Informed Patient Choice

Economic and regulatory incentives will be needed to push the transition from delegated decision making to shared decision making. Under the informed patient choice standard, *clinical appropriateness* would still be defined by medical experts (based to the fullest extent possible on evidence garnered from medical effectiveness research), and coverage decisions that establish the content of the benefit package would still be made by the payer. However, the necessity of care in the specific case would be determined by the patient, through participation in a high-quality shared decision-making process. Why the distinction between appropriateness and necessity? Because an individual patient can be an appropriate candidate for surgery based on clinical criteria, yet that patient may want an alternative (also appropriate) option. For this patient, surgery is unnecessary. As we found in our BPH work, and Canadian researcher Gillian Hawker and her colleagues found in the case of joint replacement, the number of patients who are appropriate candidates for surgery (as judged by evidence-based clinical criteria) far exceeds the number who actually want to have surgery.[6] Clinical trials of decision making also suggest that the number of patients who are appropriate candidates for many other surgeries and tests is larger than the number of patients who believe that the intervention is necessary, once they have undergone shared decision making.[7]

What are the regulatory and economic incentives that can promote shared decision making? In a recent paper in *Health Affairs*, my colleagues and I proposed a strategy for the Centers for Medicare & Medicaid Services (CMS) to address the economic barriers.[8] Our proposal initially targets eleven common conditions that account for about 40% of Medicare's spending for inpatient surgery. (See Table 14.1 for a list of these conditions and the primary treatment options.) If shared decision making can be implemented for these high-profile conditions, extending it to other conditions should be relatively easy. And there is all the more reason to implement shared decision making for other conditions for which the clinical evidence for efficacy is less clear, because patients deserve to know when the procedure being offered has not been shown to be effective.

The long-term goal of payers (not just Medicare) should be to ensure that all patients have access to shared decision making. Our *Health Affairs* proposal is a three-phase strategy intended to lead progressively over a decade to the point where delegated decision is replaced by high-quality shared decision making, and informed patient choice is established as the national standard of practice. Here is a brief summary. A pilot project phase of five or so years would give special attention to developing models that integrate shared decision making into everyday practice, including hospitals and the primary care medical home. During this phase, the federal government would support two key research and development tasks that are essential for the transition to informed patient choice. One is an analysis of the costs of supporting shared decision making in the various clinical settings, so that providers can be compensated fairly for providing shared decision making. The other is a process for certification. The reimbursement and legal reforms discussed in this chapter require the availability of patient decision aids that have been certified to meet certain quality standards. Although experts have reached consensus on what should be the standards for development and evaluation,[9] a formal certification process has not as yet been established. The Department of Health and Human Services should work with national accrediting organizations to develop this process. It should also develop a process for certifying that a given provider has put into place the key components for supporting high-quality shared decision making, including reporting on patient decision quality measures that would determine pay for performance incentive rewards.

Table 14.1. Treatment Options for Selected Conditions

Clinical Condition	Treatment Options
Chronic cholecystitis and silent gallstones	Watchful waiting
	Cholecystectomy (usually laparoscopic rather than open surgery)
Chronic stable angina (chest pain or other symptoms from coronary artery disease)	Medical treatment
	Angioplasty
	Bypass surgery
Hip and knee osteoarthritis	Medical treatment
	Hip replacement
Claudication (exertional leg pain from peripheral vascular disease)	Medical treatment, exercise
	Angioplasty
	Bypass surgery
Carotid stenosis (stroke risk from narrowing of carotid artery)	Aspirin
	Carotid endarterectomy
Herniated disc or spinal stenosis (causing back pain or other symptoms)	Medical treatment
	Chiropractic and other
	Back surgery
Early-stage prostate cancer	Watchful waiting
	Radiation (conventional or implant seeds)
	Radical prostatectomy
Early-stage breast cancer	Lumpectomy
	Mastectomy
Enlarged prostate (benign prostatic hyperplasia)	Surgical treatment (several methods)
	Drug treatment
	Watchful waiting

After four or five years, building on the accomplishments of the pilot projects, payers would undertake a national effort to change the standard for defining medical necessity. Group practices, hospitals, ambulatory surgery centers, and primary care physicians practicing in organized medical homes would be encouraged to implement certified shared decision-making processes and participate in a pay-for-performance program. Eventually (we suggest the target date be within ten years), payers would no longer reimburse providers for surgery if they fail to comply with the new standard for defining medical necessity. Compliance would be defined by the presence of a certified shared decision-making process and satisfactory scores on (audited) decision quality measures.

Primary Care as Professional Advocates for Informed Patient Choice

Experience shows that without strong professional advocacy, the transition to informed patient choice will take years, if it occurs at all. I am impressed by the fervor of the commitment to patient-centered care on the part of advocates for team-based primary care medicine. Patient-centeredness forms one of its central tenets: every American needs a long-term professional relationship with a personal physician who helps patients navigate the complexities of the heath care system and leads a team of health care workers, who collectively take responsibility for the patient's care. The job description calls for a comprehensive role of the personal physician to provide "all the patient's health care needs at all stages of life," including being responsible for arranging referrals to medical and surgical specialists.[10] How this assumption of responsibility unfolds could be key for the prospects of implementing informed patient choice. If the members of the medical home were to assume professional responsibility for shepherding patient preferences for treatment options, particularly those involving elective surgery and end of life care, a critical structural barrier to establishing informed patient choice would be overcome.

Traditionally, the referrals that primary care physicians make to surgical specialists have had two goals: one is to obtain an expert's diagnosis of the patient's condition, and the other to obtain a treatment recommendation. Not surprisingly, surgeons commonly diagnose a need for surgery, and recommend themselves to perform it. Progress in comparative effectiveness research, however, will change the primary care physician's dependency on specialist opinion. For a number of common procedures, including most of those listed in Table 14.1, evidence-based practice guidelines now make it possible for primary care physicians to diagnose conditions for which surgery is an option, and to determine which patients are clinically appropriate candidates. Implementing shared decision making would allow the primary care physician to determine if the patient also *wants* surgery. For example, our early work with BPH established the practice guidelines for diagnosing the condition and determining the patient's preferences. This could all be managed by the primary care physician. Indeed, most common surgical procedures can be similarly managed.

Structurally, primary care physicians and their team members seem the ideal professional advocates for informed patient choice and the appropriate guarantors of the integrity of the shared decision-making process. Unlike specialists who perform specific procedures or favor certain clinical options, primary care physicians, at least in theory, have no horse in the race, no financial interest in one treatment option over another. With the development of clinical effectiveness research along the lines of the PORT teams, primary care physicians can have access to up-to-date information on the outcomes of various treatment options. With the development of patient decision aids and other means of informing patients about treatment options, the primary care team has access to tools that facilitate the shared decision-making process. The physician's performance in achieving informed patient choice can be evaluated using patient decision quality instruments.

Thus, for a number of common conditions that involve elective surgery and tests, the medical home team can become accountable for managing the clinical problem, using practice guidelines to sort out which patients would qualify as clinically appropriate candidates and helping patients make the critical choices between the treatment options. At this juncture in the decision sequence, the primary care physician should be in a position to refer the patient who wants surgery to the specialist best qualified to perform the operation (Box 14.3). The process, ideally, would thus ensure that only patients who truly wanted a procedure would be referred to a surgeon, preferably one who scores well on technical competence. Naturally, not all conditions can be accurately diagnosed by the primary care physician, and in those cases the physician would need to refer the patient to the specialist before the patient has had access to a patient decision aid and undergone shared decision making. In such cases, the patient could share the treatment decision with the specialist, or return to his or her primary care physician before coming to a decision.

Payers should give special priority to a pilot project to test the medical home model for implementing shared decision making and estimating patient-driven demand for elective surgery. Using evidence-based guidelines, the primary care team can identify patients who meet up-to-date evidence-based guidelines for clinical appropriateness and then, through shared decision making, help patients decide if they want surgery or another treatment. Thus, primary care, because it serves a defined patient population, is well situated to help policy makers learn which rate is right: which utilization rates for preference-sensitive treatments approximate "true" demand.

Professional advocacy on the part of primary care physicians should also accelerate the establishment of informed patient choice as the standard of practice. It would increase the interest of other stakeholders in promoting shared decision making. Primary care advocacy in the state of Washington influenced legislators to take action, and primary care physicians could

Box 14.3. *Another Mission for the Science of Health Care Delivery*

Information on the outcomes of surgery according to the condition of the patient and the place where surgery is performed is essential in making a decision to undergo surgery and where to have it. Yet such information is rarely available in everyday practice; providing the infrastructure for achieving transparency should be a goal of comparative effectiveness research. Valid information depends on skill in accomplishing one of the most difficult tasks facing the epidemiologist—making inferences from observational data about the outcomes of care. In addition to skilled epidemiologists, it requires the data infrastructure to ensure the systematic follow-up of all patients treated at a given institution and the ability to analyze the data. For reasons of economy of scale, and for feedback and interpretation, the process is best organized with multiple institutions participating in a network designed around the principles of continuous quality improvement.

The Northern New England Cardiovascular Disease Study Group (NNECDSG) provides an example of how the science of health care delivery contributes to rationalizing surgical care for coronary artery disease. Organized in 1987 under the leadership of Dartmouth epidemiologist Gerald O'Connor, the NNECDSG maintains registries of all patients operated on in hospitals in Maine, New Hampshire, and Vermont who receive coronary artery bypass grafting, percutaneous coronary intervention, or heart valve replacement surgery. During the last seventeen years, information on 150,000 patients has been accumulated in the registries.

The database tracks clinical outcomes of all revascularization procedures, and outcome data for coronary artery bypass grafting are available on a center-specific basis on the website. Studies undertaken by the NNECDSG have resulted in more than eighty peer-reviewed articles in medical journals. Data feedback has fueled a number of interventions to improve quality. Using the registry data, O'Connor and his colleagues have developed risk-adjusted models of outcomes. Decision-making tools have been developed to help clinicians, patients, and families understand the likely outcomes of care according to the risk status of the individual patient. These tools are available on the NNECDSG website (http://www.nnecdsg.org).

also push CMS and private payers to provide the regulatory and economic incentives to make shared decision making part of everyday practice.

* * *

Replacing delegated decision making and informed consent with shared decision making and informed patient choice will not be easy. It requires a transformation in the culture of medicine. This chapter has suggested a strategy for achieving this transformation, based on changes in legal, economic, and regulatory incentives; improvements in clinical science; and a new role for primary care physicians as advocates and guarantors of the shared decision-making process. I believe these reforms hold promise for achieving a market for preference-sensitive care, a market in which the utilization of surgery and other costly preference-sensitive treatments is determined by patient demand. Available evidence suggests that this would lead to lower uptake of elective surgery and a reduction in Medicare spending. More important, patients would be less likely to undergo surgery that they do not want.

15

Five Ways to Control Costs and Accelerate Health Care Reform

So far, this book has concentrated on three of the four goals for health care reform: establishing informed patient choice, promoting organized systems of care, and improving the science of health care delivery. This chapter deals with the fourth goal—constraining undisciplined growth in capacity and spending. While the reforms discussed thus far should result in cost savings, counting on changes in the delivery system as the principal weapon for containing unwarranted growth in spending is extremely risky. How long it will take for delivery system reforms to take hold, and how effectively they will moderate rising health care costs, is far from clear. Left unchecked, the dynamics of growth that lead to overutilization and escalating costs will likely continue well into the future, becoming increasingly intolerable, and destroying our competitiveness in the world economy.

An understanding of practice variation, particularly the role that supply plays in influencing medical demand, suggests several concrete steps to check undisciplined growth and reduce unwarranted variation. The ideas discussed in this chapter could stabilize the health care economy and buy time, and even accelerate the transition from disorganized to organized care, and from delegated decision making to informed patient choice.

The first component of a cost-control plan is to put into place a "safety valve," a regulatory strategy to constrain spending for supply-sensitive care. The second is to impose obligatory copayments to address variation and growth in the use of discretionary surgery and other expensive preference-sensitive treatments. The third is to influence the size and specialty composition of the physician workforce as a means for reducing growth in spending and ensuring that tomorrow's physicians are skilled in coordinating care and supporting informed patient choice. The fourth step is to reduce transfer payments among regions by adjusting the cost of insurance premiums to reflect regional per capita spending, thus improving equity and creating awareness of the relationship between capacity and per capita costs. The fifth is to establish "real-time" feedback of information on performance of the delivery system, using routine claims data from private as well as public payers.

Constraining Spending for Supply-Sensitive Care

Our studies of practice variation have pinpointed the clinical conditions that are responsible for most of the variation in Medicare per capita payments among regions or states. It is not surgery—surgery rates and Medicare spending on surgery are about the same in regions with high and low overall Medicare spending per capita. It is the rate of the use of hospitals and post-acute care for managing acute and chronic illness that make up the bulk of the overuse problem in regions with high Medicare spending. This is the primary driver of variation in total Medicare spending among regions, and it is reimbursements for inpatient care that account for most of the spending. And, as discussed in Chapter 12, it is the high-spending regions that tend to grow fastest.

The Centers for Medicare & Medicaid Services (CMS) and other payers would find significant savings if they were to follow the money trail and limit reimbursement in regions and among providers that overuse care the most. One way to do that would be to impose an overuse penalty: setting an upper limit on the amount paid to hospitals and physicians for the inpatient care of patients with acute or chronic medical conditions—the causes of hospitalization that contribute most to overuse. Initially, the penalty could be quite modest. For example, payers could determine that hospitals with age-, sex-, race-, and illness-adjusted utilization rates that exceed the 98th percentile on the hospital care intensity (HCI) index should be reimbursed only at the level of the 98th percentile. The difference between the actual amount Medicare spent for managing chronic illness in these hospitals and the target budget set for the 98th percentile would be the amount an outlier hospital would forgo. Based on this benchmark for the volume of patient days and inpatient physician services, Medicare would have saved about $150 million—$127.7 million in reimbursements to hospitals (Part A) and $22.7 million for professional services (Part B)—in 2005.[1]

Reducing payments to the most highly inefficient providers by $150 million would not by itself achieve cost-containment goals, nor would it substantially reduce the regional transfer payments and disparities in patient copayments discussed in previous chapters. But it would be a powerful signal that the rules of game are changing. The effects on the health care economy would likely be profound, particularly if an overuse penalty were implemented in parallel with the shared savings programs discussed in Chapter 14, and if it were clear to providers that the Secretary of Health and Human Services (and private payers) reserved the option to use the target budget more aggressively if providers failed to limit growth and recover waste. It would signal a significant shift in Medicare policy away from fostering undisciplined growth and unwarranted variation, as it currently does, to a policy that rewards value and efficiency in managing acute and chronic illness.

One likely result of such a strategy would be that providers everywhere would become very interested in comparing their own performance to that of others, as measured by routine reports such as the Dartmouth Atlas reports discussed in Chapter 11. Physicians, boards of trustees of hospitals, and administrators would want to understand why overuse is such a problem and to consider options for their hospitals to avoid the penalty. The impact of imposing an overuse penalty and creating strong incentives to reduce excess acute care capacity would likely extend beyond the provider community. At the very least, such a move has the potential to disrupt the easy money traditionally afforded to hospitals by the bond and equity markets, putting a brake on further hospital expansion in high-use regions. For example, the frenzy of construction projects under way in Los Angeles is funded in large part by investors who assume that hospitals are low-risk borrowers. However, if uncertainty were to arise over the long-term commitment of Medicare to pay for utilization no matter how profligate, analysts rating hospital bonds or evaluating hospital stocks would be much more interested in looking at the Dartmouth Atlas utilization reports for the hospitals they are evaluating. It would also strengthen the hand of consumer organizations (such as the Consumers Union) that are seeking to draw the attention of their members to the dangers and financial costs of overuse.

Under this scenario, more aggressive use of the target budget option might not be needed. But if these efforts fail and costs continue to rise in an uncontrolled way, if Medicare spending grows to the point some now project and the consequences of inefficiency and waste become overwhelming, then a payment method that provides CMS with the means for limiting spending in a predictable way may become attractive, even inevitable. A simple way for CMS (and other payers) to obtain leverage over inpatient spending for supply-sensitive care would be to adjust the benchmark used to calculate the target budget to a percentile on the HCI index that meets policy objectives. Setting hospital-specific target budgets for supply-sensitive care, particularly if a similar policy were adopted by other payers, would force a reduction in overuse. It would also motivate providers to seek opportunities to gain control over their own budgets by taking advantage of shared savings programs, as discussed in Chapter 14.

Constraining Preference-Sensitive Surgery

Corralling health care cost growth can also be achieved by limiting spending for elective surgery. As discussed in Chapter 5, the pattern of regional variation in the use of surgery is remarkably consistent from year to year, without evidence of any significant regression to the mean, even though the per capita rate of surgery is growing rapidly for many operations. This consistency has been traced to the practice style of local physicians. Breaking the cycle of supplier influence on the utilization of surgery requires reform of the doctor-patient relationship, by replacing delegated decision making with shared decision making. Chapter 14 contained several suggestions of ways to achieve this goal, including changes in legal, economic, and regulatory incentives, improvements in clinical science, and a new role for primary care as advocates and guarantors of a shared decision-making process. I believe these reforms hold promise for creating a real market for preference-sensitive care, one in which the utilization of surgery and other expensive preference-sensitive treatments are determined by informed patient choice.

The transition to informed patient choice as the standard of practice is fully justified on ethical grounds alone. It is not a good idea to operate on patients who would not want surgery were they truly informed. However, evidence that the implementation of shared decision making often leads to lower uptake of surgery and substantial savings, at least in the short term, should certainly enhance the attractiveness to policy makers and payers of fostering the transition to informed patient choice. Our study of BPH surgery among patients enrolled in Group Health Cooperative and Kaiser Permanente (see Figure 6.1, pp. 87) registered a 40% drop in population-based rates of surgery following introduction of the shared decision-making decision aid. (This decline in utilization following the shift from supplier-influenced to patient-induced demand is all the more impressive for the fact that Group Health's rates were already in the bottom quartile of the rates for the country.) A recent Cochrane review of randomized clinical trials comparing shared decision making supported by decision aids to obtaining informed consent through usual care showed an average 24% decline in demand for a wide range of elective surgeries and tests.[2] There will be exceptions, of course, and shared decision making will lead to an increase in demand for at least a few procedures. But from a financial standpoint, an expected net reduction in utilization in the range of 25% would result in annual Medicare savings of $4 billion or more (in 2006 dollars) for the procedures listed in Table 14.1 (pp. 237). A more modest decline of 5% in demand would still result in substantial savings—about $800 million—and the amount would be $2.4 billion if the decline is 15%.

But changing the culture of medicine—and this is what shifting to shared decision making entails—will not happen overnight. In the meantime, Medicare could pursue a regulatory approach to signal its intention to work toward informed patient choice as the standard of care. Immediate savings would be available if CMS were to, in effect, set a quota and stop reimbursing providers in a region for certain procedures when the rates rise above a certain percentile rank in per capita incidence of surgery. But quotas—remember the hysterectomy story in Lewiston, Maine, from Chapter 5—fail to achieve the objective of informed patient choice and punish all surgeons in a region, not just those who fail to help their patients become fully informed.

Another approach would be to impose obligatory cost sharing for patients who choose expensive treatment options for selected conditions where the benefit of treatment is to increase the quality of life. Imposing differential cost sharing in situations where choice evolves around considerations of quality of life does not mean the abandonment of Medicare's commitment to pay for necessary care. As Victor Fuchs, the Stanford economist has argued, "When quality of life is the object of high-intensity care, the egalitarian imperative for collectively funding such care loses much of its force."[3] For example, Medicare could require that most patients with knee arthritis who elect the more expensive treatment option, joint replacement, are themselves responsible for at least part of the copayment for the operation, even when they have supplemental insurance. (Cost sharing for low-income patients could be waived.) Cost sharing would likely motivate patients to seek information on treatment options and thus accelerate the transition to informed patient choice. Although the evidence so far predicts that even in the absence of cost sharing, well-informed patients choose invasive, high-cost treatments less often, it is difficult to predict the *long-term* impact on utilization if informed patient choice were to become the standard of practice. In a market where demand for preference-sensitive care is based on informed patients, cost sharing for more expensive options would provide policy makers with a powerful means for keeping the overall utilization for preference-sensitive treatments within acceptable limits.

Influencing the Numbers, Specialty Composition, and Training of Physicians

In a health care economy prone to supplier-induced demand, the size and specialty composition of the physician workforce are key factors determining the level of utilization and thus health care spending. Having more physicians per capita means greater spending per capita. And the spending I am talking about is not just for the care the physicians themselves provide. It is all the other services they prescribe—the hospitalizations, stays in intensive care units, extended care, referrals to home health agencies, and drugs and medical devices—that account for the majority of physician-influenced health care spending. The Dartmouth Atlas provides an estimate of how much such costs increase along with an increase in physician inputs. For Medicare, increasing the full-time equivalent labor input of physicians by one physician per 1,000 enrollees is associated with about a $1,000 per enrollee increase in spending for the other services that physicians prescribe—and this amount does not include spending for drugs[4] (Figure 15.1).

The federal government plays a pivotal role in subsidizing postgraduate medical education for physicians, and thus a pivotal role in determining how many physicians there are in the United States. In 2007, Medicare paid teaching hospitals more than $8.6 billion to train some 89,000 residents, about $96,000 per physician.[5] But, so far, Medicare has not exercised its influence to ensure that these funds are used to construct a physician workforce whose numbers, specialty composition, and training experience are geared to the needs of the delivery system or the patients they serve.

Instead, it has relied on the suppliers of training programs—the teaching hospitals themselves—to decide what is needed. Relying on teaching hospitals to determine the need for physicians might not be such a bad policy if, in fact, there was a consensus among teaching hospitals on the number and specialty composition of physicians necessary to serve the nation. But, as discussed in Chapter 11, the teaching hospitals vary to an extraordinary degree in the way they use their physician workforces in providing care. New York University's teaching hospital, for example, allocated about fifty-one

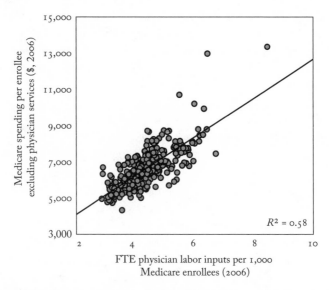

Figure 15.1.   The association between physician labor inputs and Medicare spending excluding physician services among hospital referral regions (2006). (Source: Dartmouth Atlas Project database.)

full-time equivalent physicians per capita in taking care of patients with serious chronic illnesses over the last two years of life, while the University of Wisconsin's hospital allocated only seventeen.[6]

A recent Internet posting by two noted workforce policy analysts, Fitzhugh Mullan and Elizabeth Wiley,[7] provides insight into an important dynamic that has shaped the nation's workforce. In the absence of consensus on the needs of tomorrow's delivery system, the daily staffing needs of the teaching hospitals have dominated the size and specialty composition of physicians-in-training:

> The complement of residents that hospitals need to staff their services is not the same complement that the nation needs to deliver health care to 300 million people—99% of whom are not in a hospital. The pattern of training in U. S. hospitals is heavily specialty oriented reflecting the intensivity [sic] of hospital care as well as the more lucrative payments associated with many specialty services.

In view of the variation in how teaching hospitals actually use physicians, their uniform opinion that the nation needs *more* residency positions seems ironic. Legislation has been introduced to increase the number of slots in teaching hospitals to produce 15,000 more physicians annually at a cost of over $1 billion per year. Mullan and Wiley issue a strong warning against this proposal:

> The 15,000 resident provision of these pieces of legislation, despite the rhetorical support for primary care, will bring us more of the same sub-specialty oriented training patterns well established in the past several decades.... [More residency positions are] unlikely to result in more primary care trainees and will ultimately play out as more subsidized specialty slots.

I believe the Dartmouth data speak loudly in support of not increasing the number of residency positions. As outlined in Chapter 12, care intensity for the Medicare population is increasing at an alarming rate, in concert with increasing physician labor input, particularly medical specialists. In light of the evidence that more is not better, it makes little sense to produce more physicians. Moreover, increasing the supply of physicians will not cure the symptoms of pseudo-scarcity that appear to be motivating the call for more physicians. *The difficulties most Americans experience in getting an appointment with their physician, or finding a physician who will accept them, should not be blamed on a lack of physicians.* Patients living in regions with more physicians experience more visits on a per-person basis, yet they have no less trouble finding a physician when they want one than do patients living in regions with fewer physicians. In fact, it is just the opposite.[8] Take the case of Massachusetts. In 2007, the state enacted legislation extending insurance to most of its citizens, but many of the newly insured were unable to find a physician who would accept them as a new patient. Others found themselves at the end of a long waiting list. These symptoms of scarcity have been widely reported in the press as evidence for a physician shortage and have led many to conclude that Massachusetts needs more physicians, particularly primary care physicians. Yet, according to data we obtained from the American Medical Association and the American Osteopathic Association, *Massachusetts has the highest number per capita of clinically active physicians of any state in the country.* This is so for primary care physicians as well as for medical specialists. Clearly, something other than a physician shortage (and lack of insurance) is responsible for the barriers to access recently experienced in the state. A likely explanation is that Massachusetts care is dominated by fee-for-service payment policies that discourage organized care. Payers there, like payers everywhere, have encouraged the "efficiency" of the ten-minute patient visit, thus creating incentives for physicians to schedule revisits by their established patients, with whom they are quite familiar, and to shun new patients, who may need extensive evaluation and careful, time-consuming care management.

I agree with Mullan's and Wiley's conclusion that it is time to rethink workforce policy:

> With the entire health system on the table for consideration, we have the opportunity to reassess and redirect federal support for physician training. We need a willingness to set aside interest-group-as-usual thinking if we are going to address the huge challenge of building a good, fair, and affordable health system. Rethinking our investments in the education and training of physicians is essential.[9]

In rethinking workforce policy, it is important to keep in mind that organized systems of care use many fewer physicians to provide high-quality care, and that based on benchmarks from prestigious practices such as the Mayo Clinic and Intermountain Healthcare, my colleague David Goodman has shown that we already have more than enough physicians to meet the needs of the aging Baby Boomer generation and any increase in need that may occur from insurance reforms that enfranchise the uninsured.[10] If facilitating the growth of organized care becomes a central goal of health care reform, we already have enough physicians to meet this need.

A rethinking of workforce policy should also consider the type of training required to produce the skills physicians will need in the future. When the goal of reform is to foster organized, coordinated systems, it makes little sense to continue training medical specialists in practice settings where their mentors' style of practice in managing chronic illness is marked by overuse and poorly coordinated care. It also seems foolish to train surgeons in hospitals that do not support shared decision making or fail to provide high-quality surgical outcomes. Finally, if the mission of primary care is to coordinate care and share decision making, it behooves us to stop training primary care physicians in care settings where these do not occur.

Adjusting Premiums to Regional Spending Levels

The amount of money the Medicare program spends varies substantially among regions (Figure 15.2). For example, Medicare spending per patient in 2005 varied by a factor of 2.7, from $5,280 per enrollee in Rapid City, South Dakota, to $14,360 in Miami, Florida. Variation in Medicare spending was

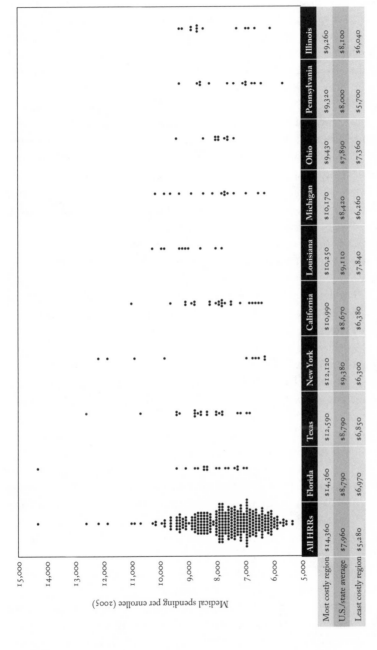

	All HRRs	Florida	Texas	New York	California	Louisiana	Michigan	Ohio	Pennsylvania	Illinois
Most costly region	$14,360	$14,360	$12,590	$12,120	$10,990	$10,250	$10,170	$9,430	$9,320	$9,260
U.S./state average	$7,960	$8,790	$8,790	$9,380	$8,670	$9,110	$8,420	$7,890	$8,000	$8,100
Least costly region	$5,280	$6,970	$6,850	$6,300	$6,380	$7,840	$6,260	$7,360	$5,700	$6,040

Figure 15.2. Medicare spending per enrollee among hospital referral regions: all regions and among regions in selected states (2005). (Source: Dartmouth Atlas Project database.)

substantial even among hospital referral regions located within the same state. In Sarasota, the lowest-spending region in Florida, Medicare spent $6,970 per enrollee, less than half the amount spent in Miami. In New York, spending in the highest-spending region, Manhattan ($12,120 per enrollee) was nearly twice as high as spending in the lowest region, Binghamton ($6,300). Among the nine states containing at least ten hospital referral regions, rates varied more than 60% from highest to lowest in six of the nine states.

As discussed in Chapter 12, the cost of health insurance is not adjusted to closely reflect regional variation in per capita spending and utilization. This lack of market-based pricing results in unjustified transfer payments from markets in which providers are more efficient to markets where they are less efficient. It is not that those living in high-cost areas are sicker or that they receive better care. They simply receive more care. This is so both for patients with private insurance plans and for Medicare patients, and judging from the experience of Medicare, we should expect at least a two-fold variation in private sector utilization and spending across regions.

The full impact of these differences in spending can be appreciated by looking at the estimated cumulative spending over the lifetime of a 65-year-old newly enrolled in Medicare—what economists call the "present value" of the Medicare benefit. For residents of Miami, the estimated present value in 2005 was $273,118; for Sarasota, it was $124,715; and the average for the nation as a whole was $138,700. Assuming that the residents of Miami are slightly above average with regard to their Medicare and income taxes, the net transfer of tax dollars from low-spending regions like Sarasota to Miami is more than $100,000 per resident of Miami (and much more per Miami physician).

It is not only because they are unfair that policy makers should pay attention to transfer payments. It is also because they distort market signals relating to the costs of care in a given region. For example, if the cost of health care insurance in Miami was directly determined by the rate of per capita spending in Miami, a decision to increase the capacity of the Miami delivery system would not be uniformly viewed as good for Miami. For years, I have argued for adjusting health insurance premiums and related taxation to reflect regional spending levels. This fairly simple change could set the stage for the emergence of public and private sector resolve to reduce unwarranted variation and growth in health care delivery. It would make transparent to patients, providers, employers, hospital boards, politicians, regulators, and others just how much the cost of care is in their own area and in other locations. It should create a broad incentive for payers, providers, and patients to pay attention to regional variation, in particular the overuse of acute care hospitals and the lack of community resources in caring for the chronically ill. It should also draw attention to the idiosyncratic and challenging patterns of surgical practice from one community to another.

While the response would likely differ from region to region and from state to state—with some locations and jurisdictions seeking competitive market solutions and others seeking regulation—the net effect should be increased awareness that today's health care market is not self-regulating and that steps need to be taken to move beyond the status quo. In order to set this dynamic into motion, the U.S. Congress should carefully consider the option to require the rating of health insurance premiums to reflect regional markets.

Establish Feedback of Information on Practice Variation

Another way to increase awareness about practice variation and foster reform is to make routine reports about practice variations available to payers, providers, regulators, and patients and their families on a continuing basis. This book provides a number of examples of how information feedback changed clinical practice in Vermont and Maine. Practice variation data played a major role in stimulating providers to reduce the overuse of tonsillectomies in Morrisville; to participate in our comparative effectiveness studies of prostate surgery in Maine; to organize the Maine Medical Assessment Foundation; and for the leadership of the American Urological Association to join in a national effort to reduce variation in urological practice. Practice variation data should play a similar role if this research agenda comes again into fashion. The Dartmouth Atlas Project provides examples of how such information can lead directly to health care reform, as illustrated by the role it played in stimulating the Washington State Legislature to change the law to favor informed patient choice. The decision on the part of Seattle-based Group Health Cooperative to undertake a large-scale project to implement shared decision making was motivated in part by the awareness of the variation that existed among its clinics in different parts of the state of Washington. More recently, Atlas data have become a vital and often quoted source of information in Washington, D. C., in the debate over health care reform.

Practice variation data can be used effectively by the press to write stories that challenge the conventional wisdom that health care is based on sound science and patient demand. The New York Times coverage of the epidemic of percutaneous coronary intervention surgery in Elyria, Ohio, is a case in point, as is *The New Yorker* article contrasting the patterns of care in McAllen and El Paso, Texas, and Grand Junction, Colorado. These articles, particularly *The New Yorker* report, coming as it did in the middle of the debate over health care reform, have widened the discussion over whether more care is better. I believe such a debate is essential to pave the way for the cultural changes that need to occur if we are to successfully reform health care.

Transparency about the relative efficiency of providers in managing chronic illness can open up new opportunities for real choice. Health care providers serving any individual region are not all alike. The consequences of choice in terms of cost will differ according to hospital, because Medicare spending and resource inputs per capita can vary widely from hospital to hospital, even within the same community. Dartmouth Atlas routine reports provide this information. It is not just that Medicare spending varies substantially among regions, even in the same state. It is that per capita spending varies about as much among the individual hospitals located in a given region (see Figure 15.3). For example, during the last two years of life, spending among the hospitals located in Miami (the most costly region on a per capita basis in Florida) varied 1.7-fold from the least to the most costly hospital; among Manhattan (the most costly region in New York) hospitals, spending varied 1.8-fold; and among Los Angeles hospitals, it varied 2.1-fold. The identities and locations of these hospitals, along with other information on resource inputs, utilization, and quality of care, are available on the Dartmouth Atlas Project website.

Knowledge of which hospital is which should be of great importance to insurers in contracting with hospitals to care for their patients and for employers trying to encourage their employees to seek an efficient provider. Information on capacity should be important to hospital administrators and trustees in making decisions to hire physicians or build beds (particularly if CMS were to impose an outlier penalty on high-rate hospitals, as I suggest they should).

State governments, particularly states that regulate the construction of hospitals or the purchase of capital equipment through Certificate of Need (CON) laws, should be vitally interested in population-based, hospital-specific information on resource inputs. In theory, CON laws should be a key strategy in stabilizing the health care economy because of the importance of the role that the supply of resources plays in influencing demand: a bed not built or a magnetic resonance imaging machine not purchased is a surefire way to constrain resource inputs and therefore reduce costs. But as we showed in Vermont, when regulators do not have the right information, they can mistakenly determine that the hospitals with the most beds per capita need still more beds, simply because the beds they have are fully occupied.[11] Dartmouth Atlas routine reports provide the intelligence required to avoid such regulatory errors. They profile resource inputs on a per capita basis among regions, as well as a hospital-specific basis. Population-based information based on claims data (or other large databases such as New York's and California's hospital discharge data sets) can support a rational approach to the administration of CON laws that, if effectively enforced, would reduce overuse and unwarranted variation.

Perhaps most important, provider-specific information helps patients and families and their physicians make an informed choice about where to seek care. Particularly for patients with chronic illness, the choice should involve finding a provider whose patterns of medical practice fits their preferences for care, including the intensity of acute care hospital use and end of life care. Here is a profile of the patient experience between two hospitals located in the San Gabriel-Arcadia section of Los Angeles, as reported in the 2008 Dartmouth Atlas.[12] Patients living there have a real choice. Alhambra

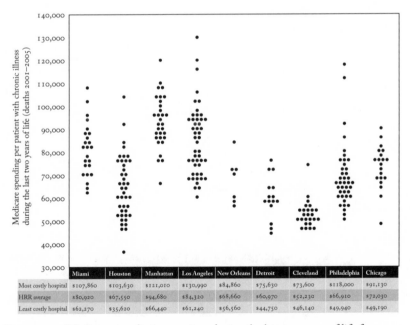

	Miami	Houston	Manhattan	Los Angeles	New Orleans	Detroit	Cleveland	Philadelphia	Chicago
Most costly hospital	$107,860	$103,630	$121,010	$130,990	$84,860	$75,630	$73,600	$118,000	$91,130
HRR average	$80,920	$67,550	$94,680	$84,320	$68,660	$60,970	$52,230	$66,910	$72,030
Least costly hospital	$62,270	$35,620	$66,440	$61,240	$56,560	$44,750	$46,140	$49,940	$49,190

Figure 15.3.   Medicare spending per patient during the last two years of life for patients with chronic illness receiving most of their care from a hospital located within selected regions. (Source: Dartmouth Atlas Project database.)

Hospital provides the more aggressive pattern of practice: during the last six months of life, patients using the Alhambra hospital can expect to spend an average of 30 days in hospital and incur 124 physician visits; 50% of patients using this hospital experienced a stay in a intensive care unit at the time of death; and only 11% of its patients were enrolled in hospice care. Methodist Hospital care is more conservative: its patients averaged 17 days in hospital and 59 physician visits; 31% of its patients experienced a intensive care unit stay at time of death; and 25% were enrolled in hospice.

Los Angeles is not unique. Figure 15.4 profiles the variation in the use of the intensive care unit at the time of death among hospitals located in selected urban regions. The percentage of deaths involving a stay in an intensive care unit varies by a factor of 2 or greater in every region except New Orleans and Chicago.

Finally, I suggest that routine feedback reports be based on merged data from all payers and be available in as close to "real time" as possible. The Dartmouth Atlas Project database has important limitations as an efficient

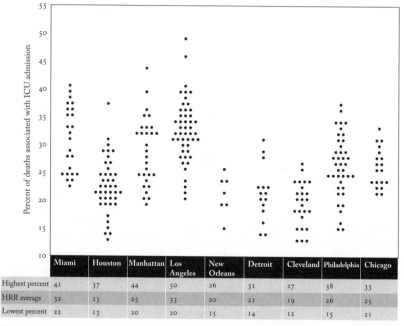

	Miami	Houston	Manhattan	Los Angeles	New Orleans	Detroit	Cleveland	Philadelphia	Chicago
Highest percent	41	37	44	50	26	31	27	38	33
HRR average	32	23	25	33	20	21	19	26	25
Lowest percent	22	13	20	20	15	14	12	15	21

Figure 15.4.   Percent of deaths associated with a stay in an ICU for hospitals in selected regions for death occurring 2001 through 2005. (Source: Dartmouth Atlas Project database.)

source of information for generating routine reports. First, it is available only after considerable delay because it is based on research files and cannot provide information on a "real-time" basis. To be maximally useful, feedback should be available as close as possible to the time of the actual event. This is particularly important if the data are to be used in shared savings programs, as advocated in Chapter 13. Second, it is limited to claims generated under traditional Medicare. Even though Medicare utilization rates appear to be highly correlated with the rates for populations under 65 years of age (see Figure 12.4, pp. 200), it can only tell part of the story and is silent about maternal and child health care and differences in prices negotiated with providers by commercial insurers. The missing information is hidden in the claims files of other payers, both public and private. The timely availability of an "all-payer" database, based on the merging of these disparate systems, would create an important tool for monitoring health care delivery, no matter where health care reform may lead.

Over the years, there have been a number of efforts to establish all-payer systems on a voluntary basis, but only recently have they met with some success, as in Maine, New Hampshire, and Minnesota. I believe that the U.S. Congress—or if not Congress, then the states—should take steps to ensure that these sources of data become available and are used to generate performance reports at the regional and individual provider levels of aggregation.

* * *

Reform of the health care delivery system requires major changes in the doctor-patient relationship, a transition from delegated decision making to shared decision making and informed patient choice. It also requires a transition from disorganized to organized care that can meet the needs of patients over the course of their illnesses. These changes will take time and experimentation before we get it right. In the meantime, the inexorable increases in health care costs must be held in check. This chapter suggests five strategies that federal and state governments could pursue to reduce the growth in spending, reduce variation, and set the stage for the necessary reforms. It remains to be seen how long it will take legislators and policy makers, providers, and payers to begin to move down the path of putting them into action.

16

The Challenge of Practice Variations

It is the thesis of this book that an understanding of unwarranted variation in health care delivery—variation that cannot be explained on the basis
of prevalence of illness, medical evidence, or patient preference—provides
a framework for interpreting the crisis in costs and the chaos that plagues
health care in the United States. The chaotic patterns of practice, first uncovered in Vermont and New England, and now documented by the Dartmouth
Atlas Project across the nation, are incompatible with the assumption that
clinical science and medical ethics govern the utilization of care. While policy makers recognize that delegating choice to the seller of services sets up
the possibility for abuse, most have assumed that undue influence on utilization by physicians was rare, the result of the action of an unscrupulous few
who transgressed the dictates of clinical science or the standards of medical
ethics. But supplier influence on utilization is not restricted to just a few
bad apples—a handful of greedy physicians. It is a ubiquitous phenomenon,
a central tendency of the market for health care services. It affects patients
everywhere, including those cared for by the nation's most famous academic
medical centers, and by the most caring and careful of physicians.

The mechanisms behind the influence that physicians exercise on utilization depend on the category of care. For preference-sensitive care, epito-
mized by elective surgery, the most important factor is the physician's opinion
about the outcomes of various treatment options and the physician's belief

about the patient's preference. When clinical science is weak, medical opinion is only loosely constrained by medical evidence, as we saw in the case of surgery for an enlarged prostate. There, an erroneous assumption about the life-extending power of surgery led to as many as 60% of men having their prostates removed in some areas of Maine. But even when the decision is "evidence-based," when outcomes are predictable and risks are well characterized, the treatment the physician recommends may not be the treatment an informed patient would prefer. Among Group Health Cooperative and Kaiser Permanente patients, only 22% of men who were severely symptomatic from their enlarged prostate gland chose surgery after being informed of the potential benefits and harms of their treatment options. In Ontario, only 15% of patients who met evidence-based appropriateness guidelines for knee and hip replacement actually wanted surgery when they were asked about their preference. Unless the decision process that leads to surgery is designed to untangle the patient's preference from the physician's opinion, the outcome of the decision process can all too often be the prescription for a treatment that the patient really does not want.

We now know enough to remedy unwarranted variation in preference-sensitive care—to complete the unprecedented and historic transition from a passive patient and a paternalistic physician to a doctor-patient relationship grounded in shared decision making and informed patient choice. When I began my studies in Vermont more than forty years ago, most patients played a passive role in the choice of their treatments, gladly delegating the decision to the physician under the assumption that only physicians know what patients truly need. Today the agency model is viewed with increasing skepticism, and the path forward has been blazed: the science of health care delivery can clarify what is at stake for patients depending upon their choice among treatment options; shared decision making, augmented by decision aids, results in better decisions that are more in keeping with patient values; and a health care delivery system based on informed patient choice that would establish patient-induced rather than supplier-induced demand as the most important determinant of utilization. If the United States can make this transition to a democratized doctor-patient relationship, it will be the first nation in the world to do so.

The influence of physicians on the utilization of what we call supply-sensitive care follows a different behavioral model. The primary issue is the frequency, or the intensity of use, of routine care—services like physician visits, referrals to specialists, imaging exams, hospitalizations, and stays in the intensive care unit. The frequency of these services varies remarkably from one clinical setting to another, and it is the primary reason for the more than

2.5-fold variation in Medicare spending among regions. Yet despite its importance in terms of overall costs, the question of appropriate use of supply-sensitive care runs below the radar screen of objective professional discourse. The medical literature is silent about how often and for which patients such care should be provided, in large measure because there is virtually no science to help physicians make such discretionary decisions. In the absence of scientific constraints on utilization, the assumption holds that more care is better care, and the agency role of the physician leads naturally to the use of available resources up to the point of their exhaustion.

Although the question of the appropriate frequency of the use of supply-sensitive care has been virtually untouched by clinical research, our studies have used the population-based methods of epidemiology to evaluate the "more is better" assumption. We find that patients with similar illnesses living in regions where the intensity of care is high have no better, and sometimes worse, outcomes than those living in regions where the intensity of care is low. Patients in high-intensity regions also are less satisfied with their care, and their providers tend to score worse on objective measures of the quality of care.

The good news is that the pattern of variation we see reflects overuse in high-cost regions, rather than the rationing of care in low-cost regions. We should not spend more to bring Minneapolis and Seattle up to the level of Miami and Los Angeles. Indeed, if the nation were able to bring care intensity down to the per capita benchmarks provided by such low-rate regions, savings of up to 40% in the costs of managing chronic illness would be realized, more than enough to offset any increases in public spending that might result from extending insurance coverage to the uninsured.

The bad news is that the remedies for unwarranted variation in supply-sensitive care will be difficult to implement. It will depend on simultaneously addressing the multiple problems that lie behind the variation: the virtual nonexistence of the clinical science on which to base guidelines concerning the frequency of use, the disequilibrium between resource capacity and utilization, and disorganized care systems that are presently incapable of coordinating care, controlling capacity, and learning from experience in ways that contribute to the advancement of clinical knowledge.

Chapter 13 presented some ideas on how to reform the delivery system to reduce unwarranted variation in supply-sensitive care. Supply-sensitive care goes mostly to patients with chronic illness, and the episode of illness for the chronically ill is indefinite, a trajectory that, for most patients, progresses until the end of life and involves many sectors of care and many different providers. This would suggest that we need to move beyond the emphasis on rescue medicine and the dominant role the acute care hospital now plays in managing care. This will entail care coordination and a strategy for transferring some of the capital now tied up in hospitals, skilled nursing facilities, and long-term care hospitals into community-based care. It remains to be seen, however, whether the economic incentives embedded in the shared savings concept outlined in Chapter 13 are strong enough to put high-quality, low-cost systems within the reach of every American.

Engaging Providers, the Federal Government and Payers

Practice variations pose a special challenge to medical science. The nation looks to academic medical centers and the National Institutes of Health (NIH) as the principal sources of medical innovation, and guarantors of the scientific basis of care. Yet the NIH and academic medicine have paid little attention to the science of health care delivery. The consequences of this neglect are evident in the inconsistent practice patterns of the academic medical centers themselves: the more than two-fold variation in the number of physicians and intensive care beds used in managing chronic illness, and the even greater variation in rates for preference-sensitive surgery.

Neglect of the sciences of health care delivery has other consequences. America's medical schools do not teach the skills required to understand patient preferences, evaluate medical practice, assess clinical evidence, design and test clinical pathways, improve quality, and understand the effect of systems of care on clinical practice. The mentorship of physicians-in-training takes place in the context of widely varying practice patterns, such that those trained in Los Angeles and Miami teaching hospitals encounter an entirely different strategy for managing chronic illness than those trained in teaching hospitals in Salt Lake City, Portland, Oregon or Minneapolis. Surgical training programs routinely take place in settings where informed patient choice is not yet the standard of practice for establishing the need for elective procedures.

This must change. Over the past 50 years, the NIH has been remarkably successful in promoting the growth of biomedical sciences. This success is a testimony to the responsiveness of the nation's medical schools and academic medical centers to the incentives embedded in an enlightened federal science policy. Now it is time for that science policy to provide similar incentives to establish the science of health care delivery. But it isn't just a stable source of research funds that is needed. The results of this research can change medical theories and practice patterns, and thus lead to economic gain or loss to clinicians, hospitals, device makers and pharmaceutical companies, to name just a few of the players in the health care market. Anything that threatens their revenue stream is vulnerable to attack, as I learned from experience (see Chapter 7). To avoid a fate similar to that of the Agency for Health Policy and Research and the patient outcomes research teams, it is essential that the federal agency responsible for managing the new medical research agenda—for setting priorities, conducting peer review and awarding grants and contracts to researchers—be strong enough to protect its agenda and the scientific teams that conduct the research.

The success of any reform effort to address unwarranted variation will also depend on the emergence of professional leadership. On this point, I am quite optimistic. When confronted with practice variation, practicing physicians, nurses and other health professionals have stood up and done the right thing. I have told some of their stories in this book: the actions of the physicians in Morrisville, Vermont, that led to a rapid drop in the misuse of tonsillectomy in their own hospital; the campaign of Dan Hanley to establish feedback on variation in practice patterns to providers in Maine, and create the Maine Medical Assessment Foundation; the engagement of Maine's urologists in a ten-year study of their own practice patterns, to name only a few.

The leaders of organized systems of care—private sector organizations such as the Mayo Clinic, Cleveland Clinic and Intermountain Healthcare, as well as the nation's largest public sector systems, the U.S. Military Health System and the Veterans Health Administration—bear a special responsibility for addressing unwarranted variation. First, because these systems are organized, they are uniquely situated to adopt the principles of informed patient choice as a standard of practice, coordinate care for their chronically ill patients across sectors of care and, because they serve a defined population, control capacity and growth through population-based planning of resource allocation. Second, because they have the necessary infrastructure, including electronic medical records, they are uniquely situated to conduct the science of health care delivery: to develop and validate clinical pathways to rationalize the use of supply-sensitive care and assure high quality shared decision making. From such research, they (and the nation) will learn the resources (the dollars, the per capita workforce and facilities) needed to provide cost effective care for those with chronic illness and understand the demand for discretionary surgery and other forms of preference-sensitive care. Finally, organized systems of care, particularly those in the private sector, should accept the responsibility to grow: to enter into new markets and help the nation convert disorganized systems of care. In Chapter 13, I discussed some ideas as to how shared savings programs could create the incentives to make this happen.

The challenge to payers emerges from the special requirements for meeting the financial needs of providers who implement shared decision making, reduce overuse, and coordinate care for patients with chronic illness over time and across sectors of care—in other words, who are committed to reducing unwarranted variation. To meet these needs, the financial incentives affecting a given provider need to be coherent across payers: for example, policies governing the sharing of savings and other "pay for performance" strategies must be similar for all chronically ill patients and incentives to provide shared decision making must apply to all candidates for surgery, not just those who are covered by a particular payer. The challenge is thus to move away from the traditional volume-driven model for reimbursement and competition among payers based on discounts on the price per unit of service, to new models that support, indeed promote, providers who struggle to implement the principles of health care reform.

The Challenge to Patients and Families

Ultimately, the success of any reform effort to make informed patient choice the standard of practice, to reduce overuse, and to promote organized care will require support from a broad constituency. The natural appeal of shared decision making to the patient, combined with the efforts on the part of state legislatures to promote it, bodes well for accelerating the transition to informed patient choice as the standard of practice. Strengthening the role of the primary care physician as professional advocate for shared decision making and the introduction of federal legislation to support its implementation give me hope that one day, perhaps in the not-too-distant future, patients will no longer receive elective services that they would not have chosen had they understood the tradeoffs.

Gaining support for addressing the problems associated with the overuse of acute care in managing chronic illness will be the greater challenge. Providers who are threatened with the prospect that limits might be placed on their high-intensity patterns of practice might resort to what Robert Evans, the Canadian economist, calls "shroud waving," raising the specter of health care rationing. Indeed, some already have. The epidemiologic evidence that greater care intensity is not producing longer life, higher quality of care, or greater patient satisfaction should help keep the debate focused; and Dartmouth Atlas data describing on a hospital-specific basis the patient's experience of care at the end of life could help patients and families avoid hospitals that deliver unnecessary care.

But statistics, it has been said, "are people with the tears wiped off." Getting beyond the "more is better" assumption will likely require a national debate on the limitations of medicine's power to heal and cure, and on the quality of care at the end of life. The decisive voice in such a debate may come from the experiences of the Baby Boomers, who are about to enter the period of life when chronic illness begins to take hold. Many are already gaining firsthand experience with the problem of overuse as they struggle to help their aging parents cope with chronic disease and care at the end of life.

Reforming our health care delivery system requires a transition from today's mostly disorganized care to organized, coordinated systems of care, and from delegated or "rational agent" decision making to shared decision making and informed patient choice. This will not be easy. After all, it requires transforming the culture of medicine and reengineering an industry that accounts for nearly 18% of the U.S. gross domestic product. But such is the eye of the needle through which we must pass to achieve significant reform.

Epilogue

The Patient Protection and Affordable Care Act, passed and signed into law in March 2010, is a landmark piece of legislation that not only covers the majority of the nation's uninsured but also begins to address the delivery system. While most of the public debate leading up to its passage centered on coverage, many members of the U.S. Congress also recognized the need to transform the way health care is delivered, and the law contains a number of provisions that specifically and deliberately promote three of the four goals for reform laid out in this book: building organized care, establishing informed patient choice, and building the science of health care delivery. A crucial mechanism for achieving these goals was built into the legislation in the form of a well-funded Innovation Center within the Centers for Medicare and Medicaid Services (CMS). This center is intended to stimulate and coordinate innovation in the way providers are paid and the measures used to reward them. The legislation also contains two policy levers for the fourth goal of reform, constraining undisciplined growth and spending, but it does not pursue this goal as directly as the other three.

The legislation attacks the task of building organized systems of care from several different angles. There are provisions for the creation of accountable care organizations (more or less along the line discussed in Chapter 13); the bundling of payments to ensure coordinated care for at least 30 days after discharge from hospitals; and the establishment of primary care "medical home" pilot projects. Each of these initiatives promotes greater continuity of care over time and provides for new payment models that free providers from the constraints of fee-for-service medicine. The bottom line here is that CMS now has authority to work with providers to modify Medicare's fee-for-service payment in support of organized systems of care that are capable of managing the illnesses of their patients over time. The savings gleaned when providers reduce their dependency on acute care hospital "rescue" medicine can be shared between CMS and the provider and reinvested in more efficient, community-based practices. Shared savings thus offer providers a "glide path," an incentive to improve efficiency coupled with a way of softening the blow of reduced volume of care (and thus reduced revenue). This should provide a mechanism for converting income that traditionally has been generated by providers through fee-for-service into budgets that will allow them to build organized care.

As outlined in Chapter 13, the shared savings programs could provide the incentives that group practices, academic medical centers, hospital systems, and primary care networks need to transform health care as fast as possible. But to do this, providers need to change the way they care for all patients, not just those covered by Medicare and Medicaid. What is missing is a public-private partnership that creates an integrated financial model for all insured patients who are cared for by any given organized provider system—a model that combines the Medicare and Medicaid payment reforms with new reimbursement methods from employers and private insurance companies. We hope the development of such a partnership becomes a major goal of public and private payers over the next few years.

The place to start such a partnership could be with the approximately 100 million Americans—more than half of workers—who are covered under self-insured plans, many of them through large private employers and state government. Federal regulations permit self-insured employers to contract directly with providers, opening the door for them to reward accountability and organization through shared savings in parallel with CMS projects. Robust experiments in the redesign of health care, ones that test an all-payer model for system transformation, may become possible. It would also help the process along if health services researchers and CMS had an all-payer database. Private insurers have thus far been reluctant to share claims data, and it would seem that legislation may be the only way to get meaningful access.

All-payer data will be particularly important for the states as they seek to implement the insurance exchanges called for in the legislation. Tracking unwarranted variation in utilization and the growth in per capita spending is not just a problem for Medicare. As suggested in Chapter 15, the gap in information can and should be filled by the pooling of claims data from various payers (and other relevant data) to provide population-based performance measures on a state, regional, and hospital-specific basis for all Americans. We hope the quality measure development provisions under Section 931 of the Act will stimulate the building of such databases.

Even before the bill passed, efforts to establish *informed patient choice* as a standard of practice seem to have reached a critical juncture. For example, the American Cancer Society, which has been an unwavering advocate of many cancer screening tests, published a new guideline in 2010, specifically promoting shared decision making and informed patient choice for middle-aged men facing the decision about whether to undergo a prostate specific antigen (PSA) test. The leadership of primary care physicians has also begun to embrace the task of promoting shared decision making. At the state level, several legislatures have passed, and others are contemplating, bills that would promote informed patient choice and the use of patient decision aids. The Patient Protection and Affordable Care Act takes further steps. It establishes a process for certification of patient decision aids that would ensure that they are up-to-date, accurate, and unbiased. It also provides funds for developing decision aids and calls for demonstration projects to establish payment models for integrating shared decision making into everyday practice. Once again, private payers should participate.

The legislation also takes important steps toward improving the knowledge base for clinical practice; by 2013, more than $500 million will be available annually for comparative effectiveness research, which will focus primarily on comparing the risks and benefits of drugs and devices. This will improve our understanding of the effectiveness of many treatment options. However, comparative effectiveness research as it is currently conceived is too narrowly focused. The priorities do not explicitly include research into ways to improve clinical decision making when choice should depend on patient preferences. This is essential to achieving the goal of reducing unwarranted variation in elective surgery and screening examinations such as the PSA test.

Nor does the legislation give priority to research that addresses the expensive differences in the way chronically ill patients are managed. This is crucial to bending the cost curve, because variation in care intensity—frequency in the use of physician visits, referrals, imaging examinations, and acute care hospitals—accounts for most of the variation in Medicare per capita spending among regions and academic medical centers. The legislation also does not provide the broad-based support necessary for securing a commitment to *the science of health care delivery* from the nation's medical schools and academic medical centers. This is unfortunate. Changing the culture of medicine depends on establishing the evaluative sciences as central to medical education, a core competency required for practicing medicine. A new federal initiative embracing the science of health care delivery, equivalent in scope to the founding of the National Institutes of Health or the National Science Foundation, remains to be made.

The fourth goal of health care reform listed in this book, *constraining undisciplined growth*, will be difficult to accomplish through comparative effectiveness research and the gradual promotion of greater organization in the delivery system, and we think it is risky to assume that these aspects of the legislation will control spending in a meaningful way in the near future. But the news is not all bad. The legislation contains two provisions that could stabilize the health care economy while buying time, and perhaps even accelerating the transition from disorganized to organized care and from delegated decision making to informed patient choice.

One of those provisions concerns the growth of the physician workforce. Given the importance of resource supply to utilization and costs, any decision that affects the size and specialty composition of residency slots will be among the most important choices that Congress will make in the next few years. To help legislators formulate a science-based workforce policy, the legislation establishes a Workforce Commission, whose responsibilities include an annual report to Congress that reviews the current workforce supply and distribution and makes projections on the demand for health care workers over the next 10 and 25 years. In view of the goal to promote organized care, we believe the Commission and Congress should pay special attention to the workforce requirements of organized delivery systems. As outlined in Chapter 15, the nation already has enough physicians to meet the employment needs of organized systems well into the future. Moreover, adding more physicians will not cure the symptoms of scarcity. Look at Massachusetts, the state with the most physicians per capita (including primary care). The difficulty the newly insured have finding physicians and getting care is the result of a disorganized system and financial disincentives to taking on new patients, not lack of supply. Adding more physicians will not cure the symptoms of pseudoscarcity in Massachusetts, or in other regions that already have a large supply of doctors, but it will raise costs. The opportunity to rethink the nation's workforce policies—particularly the needs of organized systems with advanced medical records—is also an opportunity to bend the cost curve.

The legislation's second policy lever for limiting growth and unwarranted variation lies in the establishment of the Independent Medicare Advisory Board. This new entity will have broad authority to develop proposals for new reimbursement strategies, which will be implemented if Medicare spending grows in excess of amounts specified in the legislation.[1] The Board must give priority to recommendations that "improve the health care delivery system," and it is instructed to target reductions in spending at the "sources of excess cost growth." Data about the rates of growth in utilization and spending, and the patterns of variation among regions and hospitals, could help the board carry out this task, and through its decisions, it could begin to limit spending according to the degree of overuse by specific providers in high-use regions. One strategy for identifying such outliers was outlined in Chapter 15. As argued there, we believe the mere existence of a clear policy to address overuse by outliers could have an immediate effect on market behavior: it should accelerate the growth of organized care, particularly in high-cost regions, where providers will be motivated to avoid penalties by participating in CMS's (much less onerous) shared savings programs. We also anticipate that CMS's newfound authority will make it increasingly difficult for hospitals that overuse care to obtain financing from the bond or equity markets,[2] thus further limiting the incentives for undisciplined growth.

Perhaps the most gratifying aspect of the legislation is that much of it reflects a growing recognition of the central role geographic variation plays in our health care markets. The critical first step to understanding practice variation and containing per capita spending is measurement—the tracking of providers' performance using routine, uniformly collected data. As the Dartmouth Atlas Project demonstrates, claims data can provide much of the information needed to document inefficiencies and overuse of care. Claims data permit the measurement of per capita spending and resource inputs such as physician labor and hospital beds, and key aspects of the patient experience such as care intensity at the end of life, use of screening examinations and surgical procedures, and copayments. Claims data can also provide information on the price of care as well as the volume of care in order to evaluate their relative contributions to overall per capita spending.

No one would argue that the legislation is perfect, or that the law as written has identified all the answers to our health care delivery system woes. It is a pastiche of programs, incentives, and experiments, some of which may wind up working against each other, and many of which will undoubtedly be abandoned if they fail to produce in short order the kinds of changes in the structure of health care delivery that are needed. It would be foolish of administrators and providers to give up too quickly if programs do not produce instant results. After all, we are talking about transforming a gargantuan industry whose growth has been driven in part by deeply held, but nonetheless faulty, beliefs about the nature of health care markets, the scientific underpinnings of medicine, and the power of more care to heal. By the same token, CMS and other payers should not cling to old remedies that are not working. Obviously there are many ways for health care reform to fail, but we are optimistic that this legislation, coupled with the growing understanding of geographic variation and the role of supply in influencing utilization, will lead to a better system.

John E. Wennberg and Shannon Brownlee

Appendix on Methods

Defining Hospital Service Areas

Hospital service areas (HSAs) represent local health care markets for community-based inpatient care. HSAs were originally defined in three steps using 1993 provider files and 1992 through 1993 utilization data. First, all acute care hospitals in the fifty states and the District of Columbia were identified from the American Hospital Association Annual Survey of Hospitals and the Medicare Provider of Services files and assigned to a location within a town or city. The list of towns or cities with at least one acute care hospital (N = 3,953) defined the maximum number of possible HSAs. Second, all 1992 and 1993 acute care hospitalizations of the Medicare population were analyzed according to ZIP Code to determine the proportion of residents' hospital stays that occurred in each of the 3,953 candidate HSAs. ZIP Codes were initially assigned to the HSA where the greatest proportion (plurality) of residents was hospitalized. Approximately 500 of the candidate HSAs did not qualify as independent HSAs because the plurality of patients resident in those HSAs was hospitalized in other HSAs.

The third step required visual examination of the ZIP Codes used to define each HSA. Maps of ZIP Code boundaries were made using files obtained from Geographic Data Technologies (GDT) and each HSA's component ZIP Codes were examined. To achieve contiguity of the component ZIP

Codes for each HSA, "island" ZIP Codes were reassigned to the enclosing HSA and/or HSAs were grouped into larger HSAs. (See the Appendix in the 1999 *Dartmouth Atlas of Health Care* for an illustration.) Certain ZIP Codes used in the Medicare files were restricted in their use to specific institutions (e.g., a nursing home) or a post office. These "point ZIPs" were assigned to their enclosing ZIP Code based on the ZIP Code boundary map.

This process resulted in the identification of 3,436 HSAs, ranging in total 1996 population from 604 (Turtle Lake, North Dakota) to 3,067,356 (Houston, Texas) in the 1999 edition of the Atlas. Thus, the HSA boundaries remained the same but the HSA populations might have changed between the two editions of the Atlas. In most HSAs, the majority of Medicare hospitalizations occurred in a hospital or hospitals located within the HSA. (See the Appendix in the 1999 *Dartmouth Atlas of Health Care* for further details.)

Defining Hospital Referral Regions

Hospital referral regions (HRRs) represent health care markets for tertiary medical care. Each HRR contained at least one HSA that had a hospital or hospitals that performed major cardiovascular procedures and neurosurgery in 1992 through 1993. Three steps were taken to define HRRs.

First, the candidate hospitals and HRRs were identified. A total of 862 hospitals performed at least ten major cardiovascular procedures (DRGs 103–107) on Medicare enrollees in both years. These hospitals were located within 458 HSAs, thereby defining the maximum number of possible HRRs. Further checks verified that all 458 HSAs included at least one hospital performing the specified major neurosurgical procedures (DRGs 1-3 and 484).

Second, we calculated in each of the 3,436 HSAs in the United States the proportion of major cardiovascular procedures performed in each of the 458 candidate HRRs in 1992 through 1993. Each HSA was then assigned provisionally to the candidate HRR where most patients went for these services.

Third, HSAs were reassigned or further grouped to achieve (a) geographic contiguity, unless major travel routes (e.g., interstate highways) justified separation (this occurred in only two cases—the New Haven, Connecticut, and Elmira, New York, HRRs), (b) a minimum population size of 120,000, and (c) a high localization index. Because of the large number of hospitals providing cardiovascular services in California, several candidate California HRRs met the above criteria but were found to perform small numbers of cardiovascular procedures. These HRRs were further aggregated according to county boundaries to achieve stability of cardiovascular surgery rates within the areas.

The process resulted in the definition of 306 hospital referral regions, which ranged in total 1996 population from 126,329 (Minot, North Dakota) to 9,288,694 (Los Angeles, California).

Measures of Association (R^2 and Regression Lines)

In this book, I am often interested in examining the degree to which one factor is related another—for example, how the number of beds that are available to serve the population of a region relates to the utilization of hospitals by those enrolled in the Medicare program. To capture the extent of the association between two factors or "variables" such as beds and hospitalization, we constructed a figure relating beds per 1,000 and Medicare hospitalizations per 1,000. Figure A.1 illustrates this relationship for Medicare enrollees who were hospitalized for medical (nonsurgical) conditions among the 306 hospital referral regions. If beds and hospitalization rates were negatively correlated, so that regions with higher acute care beds per 1,000 had lower hospitalization rates, the "dots" in the figure—each of which represents one of the 306 regions—would be tilted downward, running from northwest to southeast. Conversely, if positively correlated—which they in fact are—the dots would run from southwest to northeast.

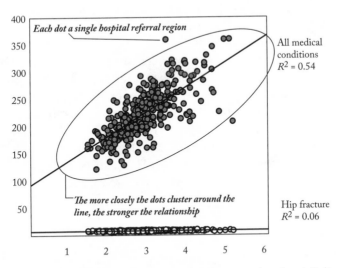

Figure A.1.   The association between hospital beds per 1,000 (1996) and discharges for medical conditions and for hip fracture (1995 through 1996) among hospital referral regions.

It is sometimes difficult to discern the relationship by inspection of the figure. A linear regression line provides the best fit of the data and summarizes the relationship between them. A measure of the "goodness of fit" or the extent to which hospital beds per 1,000 population predicts hospitalization per 1,000 Medicare enrollees is the coefficient of determination[1] or the "R^2 statistic," which measures the proportion of total variation in the Medicare hospitalization that is explained by variation in hospital beds. The R^2 statistic ranges from 0 to 1, where 1 is perfect correlation and 0 means the two variables are completely unrelated. In Figure A.1, the R^2 statistic is 0.56, which means the two are closely related—that 56% of the variation in medical hospitalization is related to bed supply.

Methods for Evaluating Care in the Last Two Years of Life

The methods were developed over the course of several years and have been described in detail in peer-reviewed publications.[2-4] This appendix provides a summary of these methods.

Databases used in the Analysis

The primary database is derived from seven Centers for Medicare & Medicaid Services (CMS) research files for traditional (fee-for-service) Medicare: the Denominator File (which provides information on all Medicare enrollees' demographic data, eligibility status, and date of death) and files that contain records of Medicare claims—the MedPAR file (acute care discharges and stays in skilled nursing, rehabilitation, psychiatric, and other long-stay facilities); the Inpatient File (used to classify intermediate- and high-intensity subtypes of intensive care unit stays); Physician/Supplier Part B (physician services for a 20% sample of Medicare enrollees); the Outpatient File (the facility [versus professional] component of outpatient services); and Home Health Agency, Hospice, and Durable Medical Equipment Files.

Study Populations

The follow-back from death studies are for two study populations, one based on assignment of decedents to the hospital they most frequently used in the last two years of life, and the other on the place of residence at time of death. To allow for two years of follow-back for all patients, the populations are restricted to those whose age on the date of death was 67 to 99 years, and to those having full Part A and Part B entitlement throughout the last two years of life. Persons enrolled in managed care organizations were excluded from the analysis.

Populations assigned to specific hospitals: We identified Medicare enrollees who died over the five-year period from January 1, 2001 through December 31, 2005 and who were hospitalized at least once during the last two years of life for a medical (nonsurgical) condition. Patients with surgical admissions only were excluded because the surgery may not have been offered by the hospital and medical staff that usually provide their care (e.g., patients with bypass surgery can only be assigned to hospitals that perform the surgery). Excluding these patients also reduces the likelihood that a surgical complication was the cause of death. We further restricted the analysis to patients who had one or more of nine chronic illnesses associated with a high probability of death.[3] Claims data were used to assign each patient to the hospital the patient was admitted to most often during the last two years of life. In the case of a tie, patients were assigned to the hospital associated with the discharge closest to the date of death. Because seriously ill patients are highly loyal to the hospital where they receive their care—as has been shown elsewhere[5]—hospital-specific utilization rates reflect the approach to chronic disease management of the physicians who practice in association with that hospital. In some instances there were too few deaths at that hospital to calculate reliable measures and the measure is listed as missing. The minimum population count for reporting measures based on the MedPAR, Inpatient, Home Health Agency, Hospice, and Durable Medical Equipment Files is 80 deaths; for the Part B and Outpatient Files it is 400 deaths.

Populations grouped by place of residence: The state and regional level analyses include patients who were residents of a given geographic area at the date of death. Data are a 20% sample of deaths occurring over the five-year period from 2001 through 2005 (i.e., those deaths that were included in the CMS Part B claims of a 20% enrollee sample). The state and regional analyses includes all hospitalizations (including the patients excluded in the hospital-specific studies who only had surgical hospitalizations) and all patients who had one or more of nine chronic illnesses, whether or not they were hospitalized. Nonhospitalized patients with chronic illness were identified as those with two or more physician encounters (on different days), with a diagnosis of one or more of the nine chronic conditions.

Table A.1 provides information on the number of decedents according to diagnosis for the *hospital-specific chronic illness cohort* and the *geographic chronic illness cohort*. Table A.2 describes the characteristics of decedents who were hospitalized, according to their cause of hospitalization (and thus whether they are included in the hospital-specific chronic illness cohort). Table A.3 describes the characteristics of decedents and chronic illness and hospitalization status.

Table A.1.   Number of Decedents according to Cohort and Primary Chronic Condition, 2001 through 2005

Primary Chronic Condition	2001 to 2005 Hospital-Specific Chronic Illness Cohort*	2001 to 2005 Geographic Chronic Illness Cohort[†]
	Number of Decedents	Number of Decedents
Malignant cancer/leukemia	815,409	207,807
Congestive heart failure	1,519,795	381,972
Chronic pulmonary disease	914,867	231,486
Dementia	614,170	166,396
Diabetes with end organ damage	56,906	18,196
Peripheral vascular disease	120,654	37,996
Chronic renal failure	277,821	59,240
Severe chronic liver disease	52,843	35,280
Coronary artery disease	359,983	109,568
Total number of decedents	**4,732,448**	**1,247,941**

*From a 100% sample of Medicare enrollees.
[†]From a 20% sample of Medicare enrollees.

Table A.2.   Hospital-Specific Chronic Illness Cohort and Excluded Hospitalized Decedents, 2001 through 2005

	2001 to 2005 Hospitalized Decedents	
	Number of Decedents	Percent of Decedents
Hospital-specific chronic illness cohort*	4,732,448	69.99
Hospitalized decedents excluded from cohort		
Chronic illness, surgery only	344,241	5.09
Other medical illness	487,331	7.21
Other surgery	99,568	1.47
Assigned to non-U.S. hospitals[†]	635	0.01
All hospitalized decedents	5,664,223	83.77

*Data are based on a 100% sample of Medicare enrollees.
[†]Non-U.S. hospitals include those in U.S. territories such as Puerto Rico, the U.S. Virgin Islands, Guam, American Samoa, and others.

Table A.3. Decedents 2001 through 2005, according to Cohort Membership Status

| | 2001 to 2005 *Geographic Database* | | |
| | *Number of Decedents* | *Percent of Decedents* | |
		Percent of Chronically Ill	*Percent of all Decedents*
Chronic illness cohort	1,247,941	100.00	92.36
Hospital-specific cohort*	946,458	75.84	70.05
Chronic illness, hospital surgery only	68,738	5.51	5.09
Hospital, other medical illness	65,361	524	4.84
Hospital, other surgery	13,656	1.09	1.01
Assigned to non-U.S. hospitals	179	0.01	0.01
Not hospitalized	153,549	12.30	11.36
Excluded decedents (without chronic illness)			
Hospitalized decedents	37,997		2.81
Not hospitalized	65,215		4.83
Total decedents	1,351,153		100.00

*The hospital-specific chronic illness cohort corresponds to the cohorts described in Tables A.1 and A.2, but is smaller due to the use of a 20% sample of enrollees.

Measures of Resource Inputs

Measures of resource inputs, including physician labor, hospital beds, intensive care beds, and Medicare program spending (reimbursements), are presented as summary measures over the last six months or two years of life. Bed input rates are calculated by summing patient days and dividing by 365. Physician labor inputs are measured by summing the work relative value units (RVUs) on a specialty-specific basis and dividing by the average annual number of work RVUs produced by that specialty. The measure is used to estimate the standardized full-time equivalent (FTE) physician clinical labor input. Both bed and FTE physician resources are expressed as inputs per 1,000 decedents. Inpatient reimbursements were calculated by summing Medicare reimbursements from the MedPAR record and reflect *total* reimbursements, including indirect costs for medical education, disproportionate share payments, and outlier payments. Part B payments are for all services included in the Part B Physician Supplier File; likewise, payments for Outpatient, Skilled Nursing Facilities, Hospice, Home Health, and Durable Medical Equipment services reflect all services included in their respective files. Inpatient reimbursements and payments from Part B and all other files are measured as spending per decedent. All resource input rates were calculated based on the total experience of the population over the given period of time, not only from the care received at the assigned hospital or physicians associated with that hospital. In the case of the geographic studies, it includes care given by providers located outside of the region as well as within the region.

Measures of Utilization

The measures of utilization are for inpatient care and physician services. We calculated hospital days, intensive care unit days (high-intensity and intermediate-intensity days, separately), and physician visits (overall and separately for primary care physicians and medical specialists) for each patient over the last six months and the last two years of life; additional measures included home health visits, and days spent in skilled nursing facilities, long-term and rehabilitation hospitals, and hospice. Physician visits were also calculated by the place of service. Utilization rates were calculated on the total experience of the cohort, not just the services provided by the hospital and the physicians associated with the hospital to which the decedent was assigned. The proportion of total hospital care provided by the assigned hospital (loyalty) is high, so the variations in utilization among hospital cohorts primarily reflect clinical choices made by the associated physicians. Similarly, in the geographic studies, most care is provided by hospitals and physicians located within the state or region. The measures of utilization—patient days in the hospital and other facilities, patient days in intensive care units, and physician visits—are traditional epidemiologic, population-based rates of events occurring over a designated period of time.

Quality of Care Indicators

Two claims-based quality-of-care measures were used. The percentage of patients seeing ten or more physicians is a measure of the propensity to refer patients. High scores on this measure may indicate lack of continuity of care. The percentage of deaths occurring during a hospitalization that involved one or more stays in an intensive care unit is an indicator of the aggressiveness with which terminal patients are treated. Similarly, the percentage of decedents receiving hospice benefits indicates less aggressive care at the end of life. In light of the evidence that more aggressive care in managing patient populations with chronic illness does not lead to longer length of life or improved quality of life, higher scores on this measure can be viewed as an indicator of lower quality of death.

We also report quality measures regarding the processes of care, specifically the underuse of effective care derived from the consensus measure set of the Hospital Quality Alliance (HQA), the first initiative to routinely report data on U.S. hospitals nationally. Data are posted on the CMS website.[6] We provide summary scores on five measures for managing acute myocardial infarction (AMI), two for congestive heart failure (CHF), and three for pneumonia, for all reporting hospitals located within each HRR. In addition, we report a composite score, which is the weighted average of the three condition-specific summary scores. For individual hospitals, summary scores are based on measures for which there are twenty-five or more eligible patients in calendar year 2005.[7]

Statistical Methods

We compared measures of resource inputs, utilization, and quality at fixed intervals prior to death among geographic regions and hospitals. All utilization and resource input measures are further adjusted for differences in age, sex, race, and the relative predominance of the nine chronic conditions, using ordinary least squares for Medicare spending variables[8] and overdispersed Poisson regression models for all other variables; 95th percentile confidence limits were calculated for all variables. The HQA technical process quality of care measures were not adjusted for differences in case mix among hospitals, as they are specifically restricted to those patients eligible for the specific treatment, and therefore do not need adjustment.

Caveats and Limitations

Certain limitations of our measures need to be mentioned.

Sample sizes and data issues. The data are for traditional Medicare (Part A and Part B) and do not include Medicare enrollees enrolled in managed care organizations under Medicare Part C. The measures of physician resource input and utilization are based on a 20% sample, reducing the precision of our estimates. For hospital-specific cohorts, we addressed this by limiting reporting for these services to 2949 hospitals with 400 decedents (expected 20% sample size for five years = 80 deaths). Data fields for measures based on Part B are left blank for hospitals with less than 400 decedents. Approximately 15% of hospitals failed to report on their use of intensive care beds, and for these hospitals, this measure is left blank. Our measure of the use of multiple physicians—the percentage of decedents seeing ten or more physicians—depends on the accuracy of the coding of individual physician encounters using the physician identification number; if a given patient is seen by multiple physicians but only one physician identification number is recorded, this would result in an underestimate of the number of individual physicians seen.

Denominator for hospital-specific cohorts. The hospital-specific studies are based on Medicare decedents with one or more medical hospitalizations during the last two years of life (as shown in Table A.2). Because we had no reliable method for assigning non-hospitalized patients with chronic illness to hospitals, decedents who were not hospitalized are not included in the denominator used in calculating population-based resource input and utilization rates for the hospital-specific cohort. This limitation does not exist at the regional level where patients are assigned to regions on the basis of their place of residence, making it possible to identify patients who were not hospitalized.

To estimate the impact of not including nonhospitalized patients with chronic illness in the denominator for calculating rates for the hospital-specific cohort, we compared rates for regions calculated without the inclusion of nonhospitalized chronically ill decedents in the denominator (Hospitalized Cohort Denominator Method) to rates calculated with the inclusion of nonhospitalized decedents (Full Cohort Denominator Method).

This analysis compared rates under each of these two methods, which were calculated for the 306 regions for deaths occurring in 2000 through 2003. The key findings were as follows:

- First, the proportion of Medicare decedents with severe chronic illness who were not hospitalized at least once for a medical (nonsurgical) admission varied substantially from region to region—from less than 15% to more than 35% among regions.
- Second, regions with *lower* percentages of decedents not hospitalized tended to have *higher* per capita utilization rates. The correlation among regions between the percentage of chronically ill decedents who were not hospitalized during the last two years of life and patient days per decedent calculated under the Hospitalized Cohort Denominator Method had an R^2 = 0.39 (negative association); the same correlation using the patient days calculated under the Full Cohort Denominator Method had an R^2 = 0.49 (negative association).

- Third, when we examined the estimates of patient days per decedent obtained by the two methods, it became apparent that (1) the correlation between the rates generated using the two methods was very high: R^2 = 0.97 (Figure C); and (2) variation was less (measured by the extremal range, interquartile ratio, and coefficient of variation) when the rates were calculated using the Hospitalized Cohort Denominator Method.

These studies show that the Hospitalized Cohort Denominator Method (which we use for our hospital-specific analyses) underestimates the "true" population-based rates to a greater extent in regions with lower utilization rates. A reasonable inference would be that our hospital-specific analyses underestimate the variation across hospitals and that those hospitals with lower patient day rates would actually be even more conservative (and have even lower rates) than we report if we were able to include all decedents cared for by the hospital and its associated physicians.

Exclusion of isolated surgical hospitalizations. The hospital-specific follow-back studies of chronic illness were designed to require at least one medical (non-surgical) hospitalization to qualify for inclusion. This was done to avoid confusing (1) a surgical referral as evidence that a given hospital was involved in the medical management of chronic illness and (2) a surgical death as a death from chronic illness. In the regional analysis, our interest in accounting for all Medicare spending and utilization in patients with chronic illness led us to include all Medicare hospitalizations (and Part B services) in the rates.

Glossary

CMS Centers for Medicare & Medicaid Services: United States federal agency that administers Medicare and Medicaid and the Children's Health Insurance Program

Clinically appropriate intervention A treatment or screening procedure to diagnose disease, whose use is sanctioned by clinical tradition or professional consensus and codified into clinical guidelines

Coefficient of variation (CV) A statistical measure of variation defined as the ratio of the standard deviation to the mean. The greater the ratio, the more the variation. The CV is used in this book to compare the dispersion of utilization rates among regions for different conditions or treatments.

Delegated decision making Traditional process of clinical decision making in which patients delegate decisions to physicians who act as their agents in defining medical need and prescribing treatments. Decisions are delegated by patients under the assumption that physicians know which treatment is best for a given patient. This process leads to informed consent.

Effective care Evidence-based interventions where the benefits are thought to exceed the harms and thus all patients in need are urged to be treated

Evidence-based intervention A treatment or screening procedure to diagnose a disease, whose use is supported by strong evidence concerning efficacy

Hospital service area (HSAs)   A geographic area in which most residents receive their care from local hospitals. Hospital service areas do not always fall within political boundaries, as patients may cross state lines to get to the nearest hospital. HSAs link populations with the hospitals that they use most and thus are useful for studying the influence of local providers on population-based rates of health care delivery (for details, see Appendix).

Hospital referral region (HRRs)   An aggregation of hospital service areas into larger regions based on use of cardiac surgery and neurosurgery (for details, see Appendix). HRRs are useful for studying regional systems.

Informed consent   The traditional normative standard for determining medical necessity based on patient consenting to the recommendation of the physician

Informed patient choice   A new normative standard for determining medical necessity based on patient understanding of the harms and benefits of treatment options and participation in a shared decision-making process to ensure that the treatment chosen is in keeping with the patient's own values and preferences

Population-based rate   A measure of utilization composed of a numerator (the number of events over a given period of time) and a denominator (the population eligible for the event over the same period of time)—for example, the number of hospitalizations experienced by residents of Maine in 2009 divided by the number of residents in Maine in 2009. Rates are typically expressed as events per 1,000 and are adjusted to remove the possible effects of age, sex, and race.

Preference-sensitive care   Procedures, tests, and surgeries for conditions for which there is more than one clinically appropriate treatment option. Under the informed patient choice normative standard, the choice of treatment should depend on the patient's preferences (e.g., the choice between lumpectomy and mastectomy for early-stage breast cancer).

R^2 statistic   A measure of the percentage of variation in one variable that is associated with variation in other variables. Called the coefficient of determination, it is frequently used in this book to measure association between two variables (see Appendix for further details).

Shared decision making   The best process for establishing need for a given preference-sensitive treatment option. In a shared decision, a health care provider communicates to the patient personalized information about the options, outcomes, probabilities, and scientific uncertainties of available treatment options, and the patient communicates his or her values and the relative importance he or she places on benefits and harms. The patient and physician work together to decide which treatment option best serves the patient's preferences. The aim of this process is to ensure informed patient choice.

Supply-sensitive care   Services such as physician visits, referrals, hospitalizations, and stays in intensive care units for patients with acute and chronic medical (non-surgical) conditions where the frequency of use (utilization) is closely association with the supply of available resources

Unwarranted variation   Variation in the utilization of health care services that cannot be explained by variation in patient illness or patient preferences

Notes and References

CHAPTER 1. IN HEALTH CARE, GEOGRAPHY IS DESTINY

1. Wennberg, John E., and Megan M. Cooper, eds., *The Quality of Medical Care in the United States: A Report on the Medicare Program. The Dartmouth Atlas of Health Care 1999* (Chicago, IL: American Hospital Association Press, 1999).

CHAPTER 2. THE VERMONT EXPERIENCE

1 James S. Coleman, *Introduction to Mathematical Sociology* (New York: Free Press of Glencoe, 1964).
2. These measures of resource input were corrected for boundary crossing such that hospitals or physician resources used in out-of-area locations were allocated back to the hospital area where the resident lived. The measures were thus estimates of the total resources allocated to the population living in each area.
3. Wennberg, John, and Alan Gittelsohn. 1973. Small Area Variations in Health Care Delivery: A Population-Based Health Information System Can Guide Planning and Regulatory Decision-Making. *Science* 182: 1102–1108.

4. Andersen, Ronald, and John F. Newman. Winter 1973. Societal and Individual Determinants of Medical Care Utilization in the United States. *The Milbank Memorial Fund Quarterly: Health and Society* 51(1): 95–124.

5. Wennberg, John E., and Floyd J. Fowler, Jr. 1977. A Test of Consumer Contributions to Small Area Variations in Health Care Delivery. *Journal of the Maine Medical Association* 68: 275–279.

6. The challenge of the Vermont studies to neoclassic economics is summarized in Wennberg, John E., Benjamin Barnes, and Michael Zubkoff. 1982. Professional Uncertainty and the Problem of Supplier-Induced Demand. *Social Science and Medicine* 16: 811–824.

7. Glover, Alison J. 1938. The incidence of tonsillectomy in school children. *Proceedings of the Royal Society of Medicine* 31:1219–1236 (Reprinted in the *International Journal of Epidemiology*, 2008; 37: 9–19).

8. Lembcke, Paul A. 1959. A Scientific Method for Medical Auditing. *Hospitals* 33: 65–71.

CHAPTER 3. TONSILLECTOMY AND MEDICAL OPINION

1. Chapter adapted with permission from the *International Journal of Epidemiology*, from Wennberg, John. 2008. Commentary: A debt of gratitude to J. Alison Glover. *International Journal of Epidemiology* 37: 26–29.

2. Glover, Alison J. 1938. The incidence of tonsillectomy in school children. *Proceedings of the Royal Society of Medicine* 31:1219–1236 (Reprinted in the *International Journal of Epidemiology*, 2008; 37: 9–19).

3. ibid.

4. American Child Health Association. "School Health Influence on Tonsillectomy," In: *Physical defects: The Pathway to Correction in Physical Defects* (New York: Lenz and Reicker, 1934), 80–96.

5. Bloor, Michael J., George A. Venters, and Michael L. Samphier. 1978. Geographical variation in the incidence of operations on the tonsils and adenoids. Part I. *Journal of Laryngology and Otology* 92: 791–801.

6. Bloor, Michael J., George A. Venters, and Michael L. Samphier. 1978. Geographical variation in the incidence of operations on the tonsils and adenoids. Part II. *Journal of Laryngology and Otology* 92: 883–895.

7. ibid.

8. ibid.

9. ibid.

10. ibid.

11. ibid.

12. Glover, Alison J. 1938. The incidence of tonsillectomy in school children. *Proceedings of the Royal Society of Medicine* 31:1219–1236 (Reprinted in the *International Journal of Epidemiology*, 2008; 37: 9–19).

13. ibid.

14. Wennberg, John E., Lewis Blowers, Robert Parker, and Alan M. Gittelsohn. 1977. Changes in Tonsillectomy Rates Associated with Feedback and Review. *Pediatrics* 59: 821–826.

15. Glover, Alison J. 1938. The incidence of tonsillectomy in school children. *Proceedings of the Royal Society of Medicine* 31:1219–1236 (Reprinted in the *International Journal of Epidemiology*, 2008; 37: 9–19).

CHAPTER 4. INTERPRETING THE PATTERN OF SURGICAL VARIATION

1. Wennberg, John E., John P. Bunker, and Benjamin Barnes. 1980. The Need for Assessing the Outcomes of Common Medical Practices. *Annual Review of Public Health* 1: 277–295.

2. Author's personal knowledge.

3. At the time of these early studies, laparoscopic removal of the gallbladder was not available. Since its inception, the rate of surgery for silent stones has increased substantially, yet the controversy concerning the risks and benefits of watchful waiting versus surgery remain. And even laparoscopic cholecystectomy carries a small risk of injury and death.

4. Duncan Neuhauser, "Elective inguinal hernia herniorrhaphy versus truss in the elderly," In: Bunker, John P., Benjamin A. Barnes, and Frederick Mosteller, eds., *Costs, Risks and Benefits of Surgery* (New York: Oxford University Press, 1977).

5. Root, Maurice T. 1979. Living with Benign Prostatic Hypertrophy (Letter to the Editor). *New England Journal of Medicine* 301(1): 52.

6. Barron H. Lerner, *The Breast Cancer Wars. Hope, Fear, and the Pursuit of a Cure in Twentieth-Century America* (New York: Oxford University Press, 2001).

7. Fisher, Bernard, Madeline Bauer, Richard Margolese, Roger Poisson, Yosef Pilch, Carol Redmond, et al. March 14, 1985. Five-Year Results of a Randomized Trial Comparing Total Mastectomy and Segmental Mastectomy with or without Radiation in the Treatment of Breast Cancer. *New England Journal of Medicine* 312(11): 665–673.

8. The picture has recently been further clouded by the rise in rates of ductal carcinoma in situ (DCIS), which is being detected with the use of increasingly sensitive screening technology. Some DCIS will develop into invasive cancer, but there is little agreement on how often this occurs or which women are most at risk. Because DCIS is often found scattered in multiple sites in the same breast, many women must undergo mastectomy if they choose to have all sites removed. The theory that aggressive treatment of DCIS reduces mortality or improves quality of life needs to be tested. [See also H. Gilbert Welch, *Should I Be Tested for Cancer? Maybe Not and Here's Why* (Berkeley and Los Angeles, CA: University of California Press, 2004, Chapter 4), 82–88.]

9. Wennberg JE, Cooper MM, eds, *The Dartmouth Atlas of Health Care in the United States* (Chicago, IL: American Hospital Publishing, Inc., 1996).

10. Green, Laura. November–December 1996. Geography is Destiny. *Mirabella* 154–158.

11. Fitzgibbons, Robert J., Jr., Anita Giobbie-Hurder, James O. Gibbs, Dorothy D. Dunlop, Domenic J. Reda, Martin McCarthy, Jr, et al. 2006. Watchful Waiting vs Repair of Inguinal Hernia in Minimally Symptomatic Men: A Randomized Clinical Trial. *Journal of the American Medical Association* 295: 285–292.

12. Flum, David R. 2006. The Asymptomatic Hernia: "If It's Not Broken, Don't Fix It," *Journal of the American Medical Association* 295: 328–329.

13. Boden, William E., Robert A. O'Rourke, Koon K. Teo, Pamela M. Hartigan, David J. Maron, William J. Kostuk, et al.; for the COURAGE Trial Research Group. 2007. Optimal Medical Therapy with or without PCI for Stable Coronary Disease. *New England Journal of Medicine* 356: 1503–1516.

14. In early 2009, preliminary results from two large, randomized trials conducted in Europe and the United States were published in the *New England Journal of Medicine*. The U.S. trial showed no mortality benefit from PSA screening [see Andriole, Gerald L., E. David Crawford, Robert L. Grubb, III, Saundra S. Buys, David Chia, Timothy R. Church, et al.; for the PLCO Project Team. 2009. Mortality Results from a Randomized Prostate-Cancer Screening Trial. *New England Journal of Medicine* 360(13): 1310–1319], whereas the European trial suggested that there might be some slight benefit, but the number needed to treat was fifty. In other words, fifty men had to undergo surgery or radiation, and suffer the side effects, in order for one man to avoid a premature death from prostate cancer [see Schröder, Fritz H., Jonas Hugosson, Monique J. Roobol, Teuvo L.J. Tammela, Stefano Ciatto, Vera Nelen, et al.; for the ERSPC Investigators. 2009. Screening and Prostate-Cancer Mortality in a Randomized European Study. *New England Journal of Medicine* 360(13): 1320–1328].

15. McPherson, Klim, John E. Wennberg, Ole B. Hovind, and Peter Clifford. 1982. Small-Area Variations in the Use of Common Surgical Procedures: An International Comparison of New England, England and Norway. *New England Journal of Medicine* 307: 1310–1314.

CHAPTER 5. UNDERSTANDING THE MARKET FOR
PREFERENCE-SENSITIVE SURGERY

1. Wennberg, John, and Alan Gittelsohn. 1975. Health Care Delivery in Maine, I: Patterns of Use of Common Surgical Procedures. *Journal of the Maine Medical Association* 66: 123–130, 149.

2. The population of the Lewiston was about 20,000 eligible women.

3. Wennberg, John E., Jean L. Freeman, and William J. Culp. 1987. Are Hospital Services Rationed in New Haven or Over-Utilized in Boston? *Lancet* 1(8543): 1185–1188.

4. Bunker, John P. 1970. Surgical Manpower: A Comparison of Operations and Surgeons in the United States and in England and Wales. *New England Journal of Medicine* 282: 135–144. Bunker's studies catalyzed a series of studies examining this relationship. Eugene Vayda and Gary Anderson found a strong correlation between the per-capita numbers of surgeons and the surgery rate among Canadian provinces. [See Vayda, Eugene, and Gary D. Anderson. 1975. Comparison of Provincial Surgical Rates in 1968. *Canadian Journal of Surgery* 18: 18–26.] Jan Mitchell and Jerry Cromwell demonstrated a positive correlation between surgeons per capita and surgery rates while holding demographic and economic factors constant. [See Cromwell, Jan, and Jerry B. Mitchell. 1986. Physician-induced Demand for Surgery. *Journal of Health Economics* 5(4): 293–313. See also Fuchs, Victor R. 1978. The Supply of Surgeons and the Demand for Operations. *The Journal of Human Resources*, Supplement: National Bureau of Economic Research Conference on the Economics of Physician and Patient Behavior 13: 35–56.] Leslie and Noralou Roos in Manitoba have also shown a positive correlation between surgeons and surgery, without evidence of differences in need on the part of patients. [See Roos, Nora P., and Leslie L. Roos. 1981. High & Low Surgical Rates: Risk Factors for Area Residents. *American Journal of Public Health* 71: 591–600; and Roos, Nora P., and Leslie L. Roos. 1982. Surgical Rate Variations: Do they Reflect the Health or Socioeconomic Characteristics of the Population? *Medical Care* 20: 945–958.] As reported in Chapter 1, we found that regions with more general practitioners who performed surgery experienced higher rates of less complicated surgeries such as tonsillectomies, while those served by more general surgeons had higher rates of more complicated surgeries such as gallbladder operations.
5. The coefficients of determination between supply of surgeons and procedure rates were as follows: supply of vascular surgeons and carotid artery surgery (R^2 = 0.00) and lower extremity arterial bypass procedures (R^2 = 0.02); general surgeons and mastectomy (R^2 = .00) and gallbladder surgery (R^2 = 0.00); and urologists and prostatectomy (R^2 = 0.03).
6. Hawker, Gillian A., James G. Wright, Peter C. Coyte, J. Ivan Williams, Bart Harvey, Richard Glazier, Annette Wilkins, and Elizabeth M. Badley. March 2001. Determining the Need for Hip and Knee Arthroplasty: The Role of Clinical Severity and Patients' Preferences. *Medical Care* 39: 206–216.

CHAPTER 6. LEARNING WHAT WORKS AND
WHAT PATIENTS WANT

1. Wennberg, John, and Alan Gittelsohn. 1975. Health Care Delivery in Maine I: Patterns of Use of Common Surgical Procedures. *Journal of the Maine Medical Association* 66: 123–130, 149.
2. Hanley, Daniel F. May 1975. A Tool for All Committees. Editorial. *Journal of the Maine Medical Association*: 149.

3. Keller, Robert B., David E. Wennberg, and David N. Soule. Summer 1997. Changing physician behavior: The Maine Medical Assessment Foundation. *Quality Management in Health Care* 5(4): 1–11.

4. Wennberg John E., and Robert Keller. Spring(I), 1994. Regional Professional Foundations. *Health Affairs* 13(1): 257–263.

5. Fowler, Floyd J., John E. Wennberg, Robert P. Timothy, et al. 1988. Symptom Status and Quality of Life Following Prostatectomy. *Journal of the American Medical Association* 259(20): 3018–3022.

6. Moses, Lincoln E., and Frederick Mosteller. 1968. Institutional Differences in Postoperative Death Rates: Commentary on Some of the Findings of the National Halothane Study. *Journal of the American Medical Association* 203: 492–494.

7. Bunker, John P., Benjamin A. Barnes, and Frederick Mosteller, eds., *Costs, Risks and Benefits of Surgery* (New York: Oxford University Press, 1977).

8. The Medicare database has other important uses. It serves as a registry of medical events that can be used to obtain information on outcomes that are not available directly in the claims. The Medicare claims data show the location of the patient's hospital records and these records can be reviewed to get additional information. Moreover, since the name and address of the patient can also be ascertained from the claims record, it is possible to obtain additional information directly from the patient through a structured interview. One can thus determine the incidence of problems associated with surgery and how they may affect the quality of life. In the course of our research, we have used each of these approaches for evaluating outcomes.

9. Grayhack, John T., and Ronald W. Sadlowski, "Results of surgical treatment of benign prostatic hyperplasia," In: Grayhack John T., J. D. Wilson, and M. J. Scherbenske, eds. *Benign Prostatic Hyperplasia* (Washington, D.C.: U.S. Government Printing Office, DHEW Pub. No. NIH 76–1113, 1976), 125–134.

10. We found two case series reports in the British medical literature. One study was done by a group of British general practitioners who decided to follow their patients (for a period of up to five years) to see how they fared. In that period of time, only about 10% progressed to the point where surgery was actually undertaken (and it was not clear for what reason surgery was done). (See Ball, A. J., R. C. L. Feneley, and P. H. Abrams. 1981. The Natural History of Untreated "Prostatism." *British Journal of Urology* 53: 613–616.) The second study was by a skeptical British urologist who conducted a similar study with more or less the same results. (See Muller, A. 1965. When is Prostatectomy Indicated? *British Journal of Surgery* 52: 744–745.) We also were able to use some information obtained from clinical trials—not from comparisons of surgery to watchful waiting (there were none) but from FDA-required clinical trials that compared patients with BPH treated with experimental drugs to those treated with a placebo.

11. Barry, Michael J., Albert G. Mulley, Floyd J. Fowler, and John E. Wennberg. 1988. Watchful Waiting vs Immediate Transurethral Resection for Symptomatic Prostatism. *Journal of the American Medical Association* 259(20): 3010–3017.

12. Fowler, Floyd J., John E. Wennberg, Robert P. Timothy, et al. 1988. Symptom Status and Quality of Life Following Prostatectomy. *Journal of the American Medical Association* 259(20): 3018–3022.

13. Barry, Michael J., Albert G. Mulley, Floyd J. Fowler, and John E. Wennberg. 1988. Watchful Waiting vs Immediate Transurethral Resection for Symptomatic Prostatism. *Journal of the American Medical Association* 259(20): 3010–3017.

14. Wennberg, John E., Albert G. Mulley, Daniel Hanley, et al. 1988. An Assessment of Prostatectomy for Benign Urinary Tract Obstruction. *Journal of the American Medical Association* 259(20): 3027–3030.

15. From our focus groups with patients, we learned that patients want to know what their chances were for a given outcome when they make up their minds about treatment for BPH. We had used various research strategies to come up with estimates for their probabilities. The array of probability estimates that are germane to decision making cannot be retained in memory. Based on their age, general health status, symptom level, and history of acute retention, we had classified patients into 64 major subgroups.

16. "Benign Prostatic Hyperplasia: Choosing Your Treatment," Shared Decision Making Program Video, The Foundation for Informed Medical Decision Making, 1998.

17. By the summer of 1992, over 1,000 patients with BPH had viewed the SDP. Most (87%) agreed that the information presented was the amount they needed to make their decisions, while 6% said they would like more and 7% said they learned more than they needed to know. Ninety-nine percent thought that everything or most things were clear. While those who had less than a high school education more often reported that they received more information than they wanted, only a small minority thought this way: 16% compared to less than 5% for high school graduates.

18. Barry, Michael J., Floyd J. Fowler, Albert G. Mulley, Joseph V. Henderson, and John E. Wennberg. 1995. Patient reactions to a program designed to facilitate patient participation in treatment decisions for benign prostatic hyperplasia. *Medical Care* 33(8): 771–782.

19. In answering this question, patients were asked to check one of seven categorical responses: delighted, pleased, mostly satisfied, mixed, mostly dissatisfied, unhappy, terrible. Based on these responses, patients were grouped into three classes: those who were positive (the first three responses), mixed, and negative (the last three categories). Data in Table 6.1 are from Fowler, Floyd Jackson, Jr. November 1994. "The Role of Patient Preferences in Medical Care," Paper presented at the Distinguished Lecture Series, 1994–1995, Office of Graduate Studies and Research, University of Massachusetts, Boston.

20. Wagner, Edward H., P. Barrett, Michael J. Barry, W. Barlow, Floyd J. Fowler, Jr. 1995. The Effect of a Shared Decision Making Program on Rates of Surgery for Benign Prostatic Hyperplasia. Pilot Results. *Medical Care* 33(8): 767–770.

21. Barry, Michael J., Abraham T. K. Cockett, H. Logan Holtgrewe, John D. McConnell, Stephen A. Sihelnik, and Howard N. Winfield. 1993. Relationship

of Symptoms of Prostatism to Commonly used Physiological and Anatomical Measures of the Severity of Benign Prostatic Hyperplasia. *Journal of Urology* 150: 351–358.

CHAPTER 7. THE BIRTH AND NEAR DEATH OF
COMPARATIVE EFFECTIVENESS RESEARCH

1. Gray, Bradford H. Winter 1992. The Legislative Battle over Health Services Research. *Health Affairs* (Millwood) (11)4: 38–66.
2. Agency for Health Care Policy and Research (AHCPR). July 1995. *Prostate Disease Patient Outcomes Research Team (PORT) Final Report.* Publication No. 95-N010 (Washington, D.C.: AHCPR) 1–59.
3. Wennberg, John, and Robert Keller. Spring(I), 1994. Regional Professional Foundations. *Health Affairs* 13(1): 257–263.
4. Gray, Bradford H., Michael K. Gusamo, and Sara R. Collins. January–June 2003. AHCPR and the Changing Politics of Health Services Research. *Health Affairs* (Millwood), Supplement, Web exclusives: W3–283–307.
5. Gormley, G. J., E. Stoner, R. C. Bruskewitz, J. Imperato-McGinley, P. C. Walsh, J. D. McConnell, G. L. Andriole, J. Geller, B. R. Bracken, J. S. Tenover, et al. 1992. The Effect of Finasteride in Men with Benign Prostatic Hyperplasia. *New England Journal of Medicine* 327: 1185–1191.
6. Lourenco, Tania, Robert Pickard, Luke Vale, Adrian Grant, Cynthia Fraser, Graeme MacLennan, James N. Dow, and the Benign Prostatic Enlargement Team. 2008. Minimally Invasive Treatments for Benign Prostatic Hyperplasia: Systematic Review of Randomized Controlled Trials. *British Medical Journal* 337: a1662.
7. Yang, Q., T. J. Peters, J. L. Donovan, T. J. Wilt, and P. Abrams. 2001. Transurethral Incision Compared with Transurethral Resection of the Prostate for Bladder Outlet Obstruction: A Systematic Review and Meta-analysis of Randomized Controlled Trials. *Journal of Urology* 165: 1526–1532.
8. Armitage, J. N., P. J. Cathcart, A. Rashidian, E. De Nigris, M. Emberton, and J. H. P. van der Meulen. May 2007. Epithelializing Stent for Benign Prostatic Hyperplasia: A Systematic Review of the Literature. *Journal of Urology* 177(5): 1619–1624.
9. Wasson, John H., Cynthia C. Cushman, Reginald C. Bruskewitz, Benjamin Littenberg, Albert G. Mulley, Jr., and John E. Wennberg. 1993. A Structured Literature Review of Treatment for Localized Prostate Cancer. *Archives of Family Medicine* 2: 487–493.
10. Barry, M. J., F. J. Fowler, Jr., M. P. O'Leary, R. C. Bruskewitz, H. L. Holtgrewe, W. K. Mebust, and A. T. Cockett. 1992. The American Urological Association symptom index for benign prostatic hyperplasia. *Journal of Urology* 148: 1549–1557.

11. Barry, Michael J., Floyd J. Fowler, Jr., Michael P. O'Leary, Reginald C. Bruskewitz, H. Logan Holtgrewe, Winston K. Mebust, and The Measurement Committee of The American Urological Association. Measuring Disease-specific Health Status in Men with Benign Prostatic Hyperplasia. 1995. *Medical Care* 4: AS145–AS155.

12. O'Leary, M. P., M. J. Barry, F. J. Fowler, Jr., and W. Lenderking. 1994. Measuring Sexual Function: The Sexual Function Symptom Index (Abstract). *Journal of Urology* 151: 322A.

13. Barry, Michael J., Albert G. Mulley, Floyd J. Fowler, and John E. Wennberg. 1988. Watchful Waiting vs Immediate Transurethral Resection for Symptomatic Prostatism. *Journal of the American Medical Association* 259(20): 3010–3017.

14. Wagner, Edward H., P. Barrett, Michael J. Barry, W. Barlow, and Floyd J. Fowler, Jr. 1995. The effect of a shared decision making program on rates of surgery for benign prostatic hyperplasia. Pilot results. *Medical Care* 33(8): 767–170.

15. Millenson, Michael. 1988. Managing Medicine. *Chicago Tribune*, November 27.

16. Roos, N. P., J. E. Wennberg, D. J. Malenka, E. S. Fisher, K. McPherson, T. F. Anderson, M. M. Cohen, and E. Ramsey. 1989. Mortality and Reoperation after Open and Transurethral Resection of the Prostate for Benign Prostatic Hyperplasia. *New England Journal of Medicine* 320: 1120–1124.

17. Andersen, Tavs Folmer, Henrik Bronnum-Hansen, Torben Sejr, and Christian Roepstorff. 1990. Elevated Mortality Following Transurethral Resection of the Prostate for Benign Hypertrophy! But Why? *Medical Care* 28: 870–879.

18. Sidney, Stephen, Charles P. Quesenberry, Marianne C. Sadler, Eugene V. Cattolica, Eva G. Lydick, and Harry A. Guess. 1992. Reoperation and Mortality after Surgical Treatment of Benign Prostatic Hypertrophy in a Large Prepaid Medical Care Program. *Medical Care* 30: 117–125.

19. Meyhoff, H., and J. Nordling. 1986. Long Term Results of Transurethral and Transvesical Prostatectomy: A Randomized Study. *Scandinavian Journal of Urology and Nephrology* 20: 27–33.

20. A subsequent study suggested that absorption of fluid at the time of surgery was responsible for higher mortality from heart disease following transurethral resection of the prostate See Hahn, R. G., and P. G. Perssen. 1996. Acute Myocardial Infarction after Prostatectomy. *Lancet* 347: 355; and Hahn, R. G., A. Nilsson, B. Farahmand, J. Ekengren, and P. G. Persson. 1996. Operative Factors and the Long-term Incidence of Acute Myocardial Infarction after transurethral Resection of the Prostate. *Epidemiology* 7(1): 93–95.

21. Malenka, D. J., N. Roos, E. S. Fisher, D. McLerran, F. S. Whaley, M. J. Barry, R. Bruskewitz, and J. E. Wennberg. August 1990. Further Study of the Increased Mortality Following Transurethral Prostatectomy: A Chart-Based Analysis. *Journal of Urology* 144: 224–228.

22. Fraser, Kenneth S. October 19, 1989. Letter to the Editor. *New England Journal of Medicine* 321(16): 1123.

23. "TU or not TU". Editorial. June 17, 1989. *Lancet* 333(8651): 1361–1362.

24. Barry, M. J., F. J. Fowler, Jr., M. P. O'Leary, R. C. Bruskewitz, H. L. Holtgrewe, W. K. Mebust, and A. T. Cockett. 1992. The American Urological Association Symptom Index for Benign Prostatic Hyperplasia. *Journal of Urology* 148: 1549–1557.

25. Bigos, Stanley J., O. Richard Bowyer, G. Richard Braen, Kathleen C. Brown, Richard A. Deyo, Scott Haldeman, John L. Hart, Ernest W. Johnson, Robert B. Keller, Daniel K. Kido, Matthew H. Liang, Roger M. Nelson, Margareta Nordin, Bernice D. Owen, Malcolm H. Pope, Richard K. Schwartz, Donald H. Stewart, Jr., Jeffrey L. Susman, John J. Triano, Lucius Tripp, Dennis Turk, Clark Watts, and James Weinstein. *Acute Low Back Problems in Adults: Assessment and Treatment.* Clinical Practice Guideline, Quick Reference Guide No. 14 (Rockville, MD: U.S. Department of Health and Human Services, Public Health Service, Agency for Health Care Policy and Research, AHCPR Pub. No. 95–0643, December 1994.) See also http://www.ncbi.nlm.nih.gov/books/bv.fcgi?rid=hstat6.chapter.34262.

26. Deyo, Richard A., Bruce M. Psaty, Gregory Simon, Edward H. Wagner, and Gilbert S. Omenn. 1997. The Messenger under Attack—Intimidation of Researchers by Special-Interest Groups. *New England Journal of Medicine* 336: 1176–1180.

27. U.S. Preventive Services Task Force. 1994. Screening for Prostate Cancer: Commentary on the Recommendations of the Canadian Task Force on the Periodic Health Examination. *American Journal of Preventive Medicine* 10: 187–193.

28. Mettlin, C., G. Jones, H. Averette, S. B. Gusberg, and G. P. Murphy. 1993. Defining and Updating the American Cancer Society Guidelines for the Cancer-Related Checkup: Prostate and Endometrial Cancers. *CA: A Cancer Journal for Clinicians* 43: 42–47.

29. In early 2009, preliminary results from two large, randomized trials conducted in Europe and the United States were published in the *New England Journal of Medicine.* The U.S. trial showed no mortality benefit from PSA screening [see Andriole, Gerald L., E. David Crawford, Robert L. Grubb, III, Saundra S. Buys, David Chia, Timothy R. Church, Mona N. Fouad, Edward P. Gelmann, Paul A. Kvale, Douglas J. Reding, Joel L. Weissfeld, Lance A. Yokochi, Barbara O'Brien, Jonathan D. Clapp, Joshua M. Rathmell, Thomas L. Riley, Richard B. Hayes, Barnett S. Kramer, Grant Izmirlian, Anthony B. Miller, Paul F. Pinsky, Philip C. Prorok, John K. Gohagan, and Christine D. Berg; for the PLCO Project Team. 2009. Mortality Results from a Randomized Prostate-Cancer Screening Trial. *New England Journal of Medicine* 360(13): 1310–1319], whereas the European trial suggested that there might be some slight benefit, but the number needed to treat was fifty. In other words, fifty men had to undergo surgery

or radiation, and suffer the side effects, for one man to avoid a premature death from prostate cancer. [See Schröder, Fritz H., Jonas Hugosson, Monique J. Roobol, Teuvo L. J. Tammela, Stefano Ciatto, Vera Nelen, Maciej Kwiatkowski, Marcos Lujan, Hans Lilja, Marco Zappa, Louis J. Denis, Franz Recker, Antonio Berenguer, Liisa Määttänen, Chris H. Bangma, Gunnar Aus, Arnauld Villers, Xavier Rebillard, Theodorus van der Kwast, Bert G. Blijenberg, Sue M. Moss, Harry J. de Koning, and Anssi Auvinen; for the ERSPC Investigators. 2009. Screening and Prostate-Cancer Mortality in a Randomized European Study. *New England Journal of Medicine* 360(13): 1320–1328.]

30. Flood, Ann Barry, John E. Wennberg, Robert F. Nease, Jr., Floyd J. Fowler, Jr., Jiao Ding, Lynda M. Hynes, and Members of the Prostate Patient Outcomes Research Team. 1996. The Importance of Patient Preference in the Decision to Screen for Prostate Cancer. *Journal of General Internal Medicine* 11: 342–349.

31. Volk, Robert J., Alvah R. Cass, and Stephen J. Spann. 1999. A Randomized Controlled Trial of Shared Decision Making for prostate Cancer Screening. *Archives of Family Medicine* 8(4): 333–340.

32. Wolf, Andrew M. D., Jonathan F. Nasser, Anne M. Wolf, and John B. Schorling. 1996. The Impact of Informed Consent on Patient Interest in Prostate-Specific Antigen Screening. *Archives of Internal Medicine* 156(12): 1333–1336.

33. Gattellari, M., and J. E. Ward. 2003. Does Evidence-based Information about Screening for Prostate Cancer Enhance Consumer Decision-Making? A Randomised Controlled Trial. *Journal of Medical Screening* 10(1): 27–39.

34. Sakr, W. A., D. J. Grignon, G. P. Haas, L. K. Heilbrun, J. E. Pontes, and J. D. Crissman. 1996. Age and Racial Distribution of Prostatic Intraepithelial Neoplasia. *European Urology* 30(2): 138–144.

35. Ries, L. A. G., D. Melbert, M. Krapcho, D. G. Stinchcomb, N. Howlader, M. J. Horner, A. Mariotto, B. A. Miller, E. J. Feuer, S. F. Altekruse, D. R. Lewis, L. Clegg, M. P. Eisner, M. Reichman, and B. K. Edwards, eds., *SEER Cancer Statistics Review,* 1975–2005, National Cancer Institute. Bethesda, MD, http://seer.cancer.gov/csr/1975_2005/, based on November 2007 SEER data submission, posted to the SEER Web site 2008.

36. Raffle, Angela E., and J. A. Muir Gray, *Screening: Evidence and Practice* (Oxford, UK: Oxford University Press, 2007), 68.

37. Morgan, Matthew W., Raisa B. Deber, Hilary A. Llewellyn-Thomas, Peter Gladstone, R. J. Cusimano, Keith O'Rourke, George Tomlinson, and Allan S. Detsky. 2000. Randomized, Controlled Trial of an Interactive Videodisc Decision Aid for Patients with Ischemic Heart Disease. *Journal of General Internal Medicine* 15(10): 685–693.

38. Deyo, Richard, Daniel C. Cherkin, James Weinstein, John Howe, Marcia Ciol, and Albert G. Mulley, Jr. 2000. Involving Patients in Clinical Decisions: Impact of an Interactive Video Program on Use of Back Surgery. *Medical Care* 38(9): 959–969.

39. McPherson, K. 1994. The Cochrane Lecture. The Best and the Enemy of the Good: Randomized Controlled Trials, Uncertainty, and Assessing the Role of Patient Choice in Medical Decision Making. *Journal of Epidemiology and Community Health* 48: 6–15.

40. Birkmeyer, Nancy J. O., James N. Weinstein, Anna N. A. Tosteson, Tor D. Tosteson, Jonathan S. Skinner, Jon D. Lurie, Richard Deyo, and John E. Wennberg. 2002. Design of the Spine Patient outcomes Research Trial (SPORT). *Spine* 27: 1361–1372; and Weinstein, James N., Jon D. Lurie, Tor D. Tosteson, Brett Hanscom, Anna N.A. Tosteson, Emily A. Blood, Nancy J.O. Birkmeyer, Alan S. Hilibrand, Harry Herkowitz, Frank P. Cammisa, Todd J. Albert, Sanford E. Emery, Lawrence G. Lenke, William A. Abdu, Michael Longley, Thomas J. Errico, and Serena S. Hu. 2007. Surgical versus Nonsurgical Treatment for Lumbar Degenerative Spondylolisthesis. *New England Journal of Medicine* 356: 2257–2270; and Weinstein, James N., Tor D. Tosteson, Jon D. Lurie, Anna N.A. Tosteson, Emily Blood, Brett Hanscom, Harry Herkowitz, Frank Cammisa, Todd Albert, Scott D. Boden, Alan Hilibrand, Harley Goldberg, Sigurd Berven, and Howard An, for the SPORT Investigators. 2008. Surgical versus Nonsurgical Therapy for Lumbar Spinal Stenosis. *New England Journal of Medicine* 358: 794–810.

CHAPTER 8.   UNDERSTANDING SUPPLY-SENSITIVE CARE

1. Wennberg, J. E., K. McPherson, and P. Caper. 1984. Will Payment Based Upon Diagnosis-Related Groups Control Hospital Costs? *New England Journal of Medicine* 311: 295–300.

2. Wennberg, John E. 1984. Dealing with Medical Practice Variations: A Proposal for Action. *Health Affairs* 3(2): 6–32.

3. Wennberg, John E., Jean L. Freeman, and William J. Culp. 1987. Are Hospital Services Rationed in New Haven or Over-Utilized in Boston? *Lancet* 1(8543): 1185–1188.

4. Wennberg, J. E., J. L. Freeman, R. M. Shelton, and T. A. Bubolz. 1989. Hospital Use and Mortality among Medicare Beneficiaries in Boston and New Haven. *New England Journal of Medicine* 321: 1168–1173.

5. Hospital case-fatality rates are calculated by dividing the number of patients who die while in hospital by the number of patients admitted to hospital. Patients in Boston hospitals had significantly lower chances of dying while in the hospital: 18.4% of hospitalizations ended in death, compared to 23% for New Haven patients.

6. Fisher, Elliott S., John E. Wennberg, Thérèse A. Stukel, and Sandra M. Sharp. 1994. Hospital Readmission Rates for Cohorts of Medicare Beneficiaries in Boston and New Haven. *New England Journal of Medicine* 331(15): 989–995.

7. Roemer, M. I. November 1961. Bed Supply and Hospital Utilization: A Natural Experiment. *Hospitals* 1(35): 36–42.

8. Wennberg, J. E., K. McPherson, and P. Caper. 1984. Will Payment Based Upon Diagnosis-Related Groups Control Hospital Costs? *New England Journal of Medicine* 311: 295–300.

9. Because hysterectomy is relatively infrequent in post-menopausal women and performed for different indications, we selected knee replacement as the boundary between moderate and high variation conditions.

10. In 2005, 29% of patients with primary diagnosis of heart attack patients were classified by CMS as surgical patients. We analyzed rates separately for surgical and non-surgical heart attack patients as well as for a combined group. Variation exceeded knee replacement in each case.

CHAPTER 9. CHRONIC ILLNESS AND PRACTICE VARIATION

1. Andersen, Ronald, and John F. Newman. Winter 1973. Societal and Individual Determinants of Medical Care Utilization in the United States. *The Milbank Memorial Fund Quarterly: Health and Society* 51(1): 95–124.

2. Wennberg, John E., and Floyd J. Fowler, Jr. 1977. A Test of Consumer Contributions to Small Area Variations in Health Care Delivery. *Journal of the Maine Medical Association* 68: 275–279.

3. The nine chronic diseases are cancers, congestive heart failure, peripheral vascular disease, dementia, diabetes with end-organ failure, chronic pulmonary disease, chronic renal failure, severe chronic liver disease, and coronary artery disease.

4. The nonblack category includes all other race-ethnicity Medicare codes, made necessary largely because Hispanics are sometimes classified as white.

5. Bach, Peter B., Deborah Schrag, and Colin B. Begg. December 8, 2004. Resurrecting Treatment Histories of Dead Patients: A Study Design that Should Be Laid to Rest. *Journal of the American Medical Association* 292: 2765–2770.

6. Fisher, Elliott S., David E. Wennberg, Thérèse A. Stukel, Daniel J. Gottlieb, F. L. Lucas, and Etoile Pinder. 2003. The implications of regional variations in Medicare spending: Part 1. Utilization of services and the quality of care. *Annals of Internal Medicine* 138: 273–287.

7. Wennberg, John E., and Megan M. Cooper, eds., *The Quality of Medical Care in the United States: A Report on the Medicare Program. The Dartmouth Atlas of Health Care 1999* (Chicago, IL: American Hospital Association Press, 1999).

8. We estimated the number of beds needed for a given level of illness based on the average utilization rates.

9. Wennberg, John E., Elliott S. Fisher, David C. Goodman, and Jonathan S. Skinner. *Tracking the Care of Patients with Severe Chronic Illness: The Dartmouth Atlas of*

Health Care 2008 (Lebanon, NH: The Dartmouth Institute for Health Policy and Clinical Practice, Dartmouth Atlas Project, online and print editions).

10. The SUPPORT Principal Investigators. 1995. A controlled trial to improve care for seriously ill hospitalized patients. The Study to Understand Prognoses and Preferences for Outcomes and Risks of Treatments (SUPPORT). *Journal of the American Medical Association* 274: 1591–1598.

11. Physicians in the intervention group received estimates for their patients of the likelihood of six-month survival as well as periodic reports on functional disabili-ty—to make them aware of their poor prognosis and raise the need for advanced planning. Specially trained nurses were part of the intervention. Their job was to make "multiple contacts with the patient, family, physician and hospital staff to elicit preference, improve understanding of the outcomes, encourage pain control and facilitate advance care planning and patient-physician communication."

12. The sample included 479 SUPPORT patients—56% died in the hospital, 25% died at home, 9% died in a nursing home, 9% died in a hospice, and 1% died on the way to the hospital.

13. Pritchard, R. S., E. S. Fisher, J. M. Teno, S. M. Sharp, D. J. Reding, W. A. Knaus, J. E. Wennberg, and J. Lynn, for the SUPPORT Investigators. 1998. Influence of patient preferences and local health system characteristics on place of death. *Journal of the American Geriatric Society* 46: 1242–1250.

CHAPTER 10. IS MORE BETTER?

1. Enthoven, A. C. 1978. Shattuck Lecture—Cutting Cost without Cutting the Quality of Care. *New England Journal of Medicine* 298(22): 1229–1238; and Alain C. Enthoven. *Health Plan: The Only Practical Solution to the Soaring Cost of Medical Care* (Reading, MA, and Menlo Park, CA: Addison Wesley, 1980).

2. Skinner, Jonathan S., Douglas O. Staiger, and Elliott S. Fisher. 2006. Is tech-nological change in medicine always worth it? The case of acute myocardial infarction. *Health Affairs* (Millwood) 25: w34–w47.

3. Wennberg, John, and Alan Gittelsohn. 1973. Small Area Variations in Health Care Delivery: A Population-Based Health Information System Can Guide Planning and Regulatory Decision-Making. *Science* 182: 1102–1108.

4. Wennberg, J. E., J. L. Freeman, R. M. Shelton, and T. A. Bubolz. 1989. Hospital Use and Mortality among Medicare Beneficiaries in Boston and New Haven. *New England Journal of Medicine* 321: 1168–1173.

5. Skinner, Jonathan S., Elliott S. Fisher, and John E. Wennberg, "The Efficiency of Medicare," In: D. A. Wise, ed., *Analyses in the Economics of Aging* (Chicago: University of Chicago Press, 2005), 129–157.

6. Fisher, Elliott S., David E. Wennberg, Thérèse A. Stukel, Daniel J. Gottlieb, F. L. Lucas, and Etoile Pinder. 2003. The Implications of Regional Variations

in Medicare Spending: Part 1. Utilization of Services and the Quality of Care. *Annals of Internal Medicine* 138: 273–287; and Fisher, Elliott S., David E. Wennberg, Thérèse A. Stukel, Daniel J. Gottlieb, F. L. Lucas, and Etoile Pinder. 2003. The implications of regional variations in Medicare spending: Part 2. Health outcomes and satisfaction with care. *Annals of Internal Medicine* 138: 288–298.

7. For every 10% increase in spending, the relative risk of death was 0.3% greater for patients with hip fracture, 1.2% for patients with colon cancer, and 0.7% for patients with acute myocardial infarction. The 95% confidence limits on the estimates for two of the three cohorts showed "statistical significance": for colon cancer, the lower bound estimate for the increase in mortality was 0.5% and the upper bound was 1.9%; for acute myocardial infarction, these bounds were 0.1% and 1.4%, respectively. The 95% confidence limit overlapped 1.0 for hip fracture: the lower bound suggested a 0.1% reduction in mortality, and the upper bound suggested a 0.6% increase.

8. In the typical RCT, patients are assigned by the toss of a coin to a "control" group (the group who receives usual care or no active treatment) and a "treatment" group (the group who receives the experimental intervention). The assumption is that randomization results in two groups of patients who are alike in all essential features affecting health care outcomes, save one—the treatment they receive.

9. Skinner, Jonathan S., Elliott S. Fisher, and John E. Wennberg. "The Efficiency of Medicare," In: D. A. Wise, ed., *Analyses in the Economics of Aging* (Chicago: University of Chicago Press, 2005), 129–157.

10. Baicker, Katherine, Amitabh Chandra, Jonathan S. Skinner, and John E. Wennberg. 2004. Who You Are and Where You Live: How Race and Geography Affect the Treatment of Medicare Beneficiaries. *Health Affairs* (Millwood) (Supplement, Web Exclusives): VAR33–VAR44; and Baicker, Katherine, and Amitabh Chandra. 2004. Medicare Spending, the Physician Workforce, and Beneficiaries' Quality of Care. *Health Affairs* 23: w184–w197 (published online April 7, 2004).

11. Yasaitis, Laura, Elliott S. Fisher, Jonathan S. Skinner, and Amitabh Chandra. 2009. Hospital Quality and Intensity of Spending: Is There an Association? *Health Affairs* (published online May 21, 2009).

12. Fowler, Floyd J., Jr., Patricia M. Gallagher, Denise L. Anthony, Kirk Larsen, and Jonathan S. Skinner. 2008. Relationship between Regional Per Capita Medicare Expenditures and Patient Perceptions of Quality of Care. *Journal of the American Medical Association* 299(20): 2406–2412.

13. Wennberg, John E., Kristen Bronner, Jonathan S. Skinner, Elliott S. Fisher, and David C. Goodman. January/February 2009. Inpatient Care Intensity and Patients' Ratings of Their Hospital Experiences. *Health Affairs* 28(1): 103–112.

14. http://www.hcahpsonline.org/home.aspx.

CHAPTER 11. ARE "AMERICA'S BEST HOSPITALS" REALLY THE BEST?

1. http://health.usnews.com/articles/health/best-hospitals/2008/07/10/a-look-inside-the-hospital-rankings.html.
2. Even so, there are some differences in average reimbursements per day in hospital. What explains these differences? It does not appear to be due solely to differences in labor costs. While Medicare does adjust its DRG payments to account for local differences in cost of labor, the average hourly wages for these hospitals are essentially unrelated to their differences in reimbursements per day in hospital. For example, the wage index for Johns Hopkins was 1% below the national average, while the wage index of the Mayo Clinic's St. Mary's Hospital was 11% above. Yet the average reimbursement per day was 40% higher for Johns Hopkins than for the Mayo Clinic. Nor is the difference between the two adequately explained by differences in supplemental payments tied to the formulas for hospital reimbursement that subsidize medical education or help pay for care of the uninsured. For example, per capita reimbursements for inpatient care net of disproportionate share and indirect medical education were 70% greater for UCLA's patients than for the Mayo Clinic's during the last two years of life.
3. Stobo, John and Tom Rosenthal. Health Costs—No Quick Fix. *Los Angeles Times*, July 27, 2009, Opinion.
4. Baicker, Katherine, Elliott S. Fisher, and Amitabh Chandra. May/June 2007. Malpractice Liability Costs and the Practice of Medicine in the Medicare Program. *Health Affairs* 26(3): 841–852.

CHAPTER 12. THE TOP TEN REASONS WHY WE NEED TO REFORM THE WAY WE MANAGE CHRONIC ILLNESS

1. About 21% is spent on community-based care. Ambulatory care—primarily physician services—garners about 16% of spending, while home health care and hospice care account for about 5% each.
2. There are a number of reasons why inpatient care prices may vary among regions. One is cost of living, which Medicare takes into account by adjusting DRG prices. Another is the differences in average length of stay. Yet another is that under traditional Medicare, average per diem spending includes supplements for graduate medical education and so called DSH payments to offset costs of providing uncompensated care. These supplements vary from hospital to hospital and region to region. Average reimbursement per day can also reflect differences in DRG coding practices and a hospital's propensity for use of the outlier payment provision.

3. Wennberg, John E., and David E. Wennberg, eds., *The Dartmouth Atlas of Health Care in Michigan* (Hanover, NH: The Center for the Evaluative Clinical Sciences, Dartmouth Medical School, 2000).

4. http://www.lhcqf.org/links/51-health-care-quality-reports.html.

5. Baker, Laurence C., Elliott S. Fisher, and John E. Wennberg. 2008. Variations in Hospital Resource Use for Medicare and Privately Insured Populations in California. *Health Affairs* 27(2): w123–w134 (published online February 12, 2008).

6. Stiefel, Matt, Paul Feigenbaum, and Elliott S. Fisher. Winter 2008. The Dartmouth Atlas Applied to Kaiser Permanente: Analysis of Variation in Care at the End of Life. *The Permanente Journal* 12(1): 4–9.

7. This compares the present value of Medicare spending, that is, where future spending, starting at 2006 per-capita measures of $10,810 in Los Angeles and $6,705 in Minnesota, is assumed to grow at the average per capita real (inflation-adjusted) rate of growth from 1992–2006 (3.5% annual rate). This future spending is further discounted both by a 4% real interest rate and by the risk of dying, taken from United States life tables: http://www.cdc.gov/nchs/data/nvsr/nvsr54/nvsr54_14.pdf.

8. Wennberg, John E., Elliott S. Fisher, and Jonathan S. Skinner. 2002. Geography and the debate over Medicare reform. *Health Affairs* (Web Exclusive, published online February 13, 2002).

9. Feenberg, Daniel R., and Jonathan S. Skinner. September 2000. Federal Medicare Transfers across States: Winners and Losers. *National Tax Journal* 53(3): 713–732.

CHAPTER 13. PROMOTING ORGANIZED CARE AND REDUCING OVERUSE

1. Kronick, Richard, David C. Goodman, John Wennberg, and Edward Wagner. 1993. The Marketplace in Health Care Reform: The Demographic Limitations of Managed Competition. *New England Journal of Medicine* 328: 148–152.

2. Wennberg, John E., John H. Wasson, and James Heimarck. March 14, 1997. "A Plan for Implementing Managed Care among Medicare Populations living in Regions where Medical Care Economies of Scale Result in Natural Monopolies" (unpublished grant proposal narrative) (Hanover, NH: The Randolph Project, The Center for the Evaluative Clinical Sciences).

3. Harrington, Paul. 2004. Quality as a System Property: Section 646 of the Medicare Modernization Act. *Health Affairs* (Millwood), Supplement (Web Exclusive, published online October 7, 2004): VAR136–9. Available at http://content.healthaffairs.org/cgi/content/abstract/hlthaff.var.136.

4. Fisher, Elliott S., Mark B. McClellan, John Bertko, Steven M. Lieberman, Julie J. Lee, Julie L. Lewis, and Jonathan S. Skinner. March-April 2009.

Fostering accountable health care: moving forward in Medicare. *Health Affairs* (Millwood) 28(2) (published online January 27, 2009): w219–w231.

5. The estimate of savings is based on the use of Medicare claims to identify medical causes of hospitalization and calculate hospital-specific inpatient reimbursements under Part A and Part B Medicare. Compensatory increases in medical admissions in the other two hospitals have not been taken into account but would be limited unless bed capacity at these institutions was increased.

6. McCullough, Dennis. 2008. *My Mother, Your Mother: Embracing "Slow Medicine," the Compassionate Approach to Caring for Your Aging Loved Ones* (New York; HarperCollins).

CHAPTER 14. ESTABLISHING SHARED DECISION MAKING
AND INFORMED PATIENT CHOICE

1. O'Connor, Annette M., John E. Wennberg, France Légaré, Hilary A. Llewellyn-Thomas, Benjamin W. Moulton, Karen R. Sepucha, Andrea G. Sodano, and Jaime S. King. 2007. Toward the Tipping Point: Decision Aids and Informed Patient Choice. *Health Affairs* 26(3): 716–725.

2. The Cochrane Collaboration is a group of over 15,000 volunteers in more than ninety countries who review the effects of health care interventions tested in biomedical randomized controlled trials and cohort studies.

3. O'Connor, A. M., C. L. Bennett, D. Stacey, M. Barry, N. F. Col, K. B. Eden, V. A. Entwistle, V. Fiset, M. Holmes-Rovner, S. Khangura, H. Llewellyn-Thomas, and D. Rovner. "Decision aids for people facing health treatment or screening decisions (Cochrane Review)," In: The Cochrane Library, Issue 2, 2009, The Cochrane Collaboration. Published by John Wiley & Sons, Ltd. (http://www.thecochranelibrary.com).

4. King, Jaime Staples, and Benjamin W. Moulton. 2006. Rethinking Informed Consent: The Case for Shared Medical Decision-Making. *American Journal of Law & Medicine* 32(4): 429–501.

5. For more information on Engrossed Second Substitute Senate Bill (E2SSB) 5930, Chap. 259, Laws of 2007, see *Red Orbit News*, "Washington Becomes First State to Endorse Shared Medical Decision Making," Press Release, May 2, 2007, http://www.redorbit.com/news/display/?id=922404 (accessed June 10, 2009); and Washington State Legislature, "SB 5930–2007–08," http://apps.leg.wa.gov/billinfo/summary.aspx?year=2007&bill=5930 (accessed June 10, 2009).

6. Hawker, Gillian A., James G. Wright, Peter C. Coyte, J. Ivan Williams, Bart Harvey, Richard Glazier, Annette Wilkins, and Elizabeth M. Badley. March 2001. Determining the Need for Hip and Knee Arthroplasty: The Role of Clinical Severity and Patients' Preferences. *Medical Care* 39: 206–216.

7. O'Connor, A. M., C. L. Bennett, D. Stacey, M. Barry, N. F. Col, K. B. Eden, V. A. Entwistle, V. Fiset, M. Holmes-Rovner, S. Khangura, H. Llewellyn-Thomas, and D. Rovner. "Decision aids for people facing health treatment or screening decisions (Cochrane Review)," In The Cochrane Library, Issue 2, 2009, The Cochrane Collaboration. Published by John Wiley & Sons, Ltd. (http://www.thecochranelibrary.com).

8. Wennberg, John E., Annette M. O'Connor, E. Dale Collins, and James N. Weinstein. 2007. Extending the P4P Agenda, Part 1: How Medicare Can Improve Patient Decision Making and Reduce Unnecessary Care. *Health Affairs* 26(6): 1564–1574.

9. The group is the International Patient Decision Aids (IPDAS) Collaboration, a consortium of over 100 researchers, practitioners, patients and policy makers from fourteen countries. They have rated quality criteria in the following domains: information, risk communication, values clarification, balanced guidance in deliberation, systematic development, evidence base, disclosure of sources of support and conflicts of interest, and evidence of positive effects on decision quality. This work provides the basis for developing certification process called for in this chapter. For more information, go to this URL: http://ipdas.ohri.ca/.

10. American College of Physicians policy statement, March 2007. A copy of the policy statement can be downloaded at http://www.acponline.org/advocacy/where_we_stand/medical_home/approve_jp.pdf.

CHAPTER 15. FIVE WAYS TO CONTROL COSTS AND ACCELERATE HEALTH CARE REFORM

1. The simulation is based on a sample containing 2,891 hospitals that together accounted for 94.3% of Medicare inpatient reimbursements in that year. Altogether, the penalty would have affected about 3.4% of hospitals (0.8% of hospitals exceed the 98th percentile for both volume of patient days and physician visits; 1.3% for inpatient days only and 1.0% for physician visits only).

2. O'Connor, A. M., C. L. Bennett, D. Stacey, M. Barry, N. F. Col, K. B. Eden, V. A. Entwistle, V. Fiset, M. Holmes-Rovner, S. Khangura, H. Llewellyn-Thomas, and D. Rovner. "Decision aids for people facing health treatment or screening decisions (Cochrane Review)," In: The Cochrane Library, Issue 2, 2009, The Cochrane Collaboration. Published by John Wiley & Sons, Ltd. (http://www.thecochranelibrary.com).

3. Fuchs, Victor R. 2004. Perspective: More Variation in Use of Care, More Flat-of-the-Curve Medicine. *Health Affairs* (Web Exclusive, published online October 7, 2004): VAR.104.

4. The Dartmouth Atlas Project database does not include Medicare's costs for drugs, which are paid for under a different entitlement program.

5. http://www.cms.hhs.gov/CostReports/02_HospitalCostReport.asp.

6. Wennberg, John E., Elliott S. Fisher, David C. Goodman, and Jonathan S. Skinner. *Tracking the Care of Patients with Severe Chronic Illness: The Dartmouth Atlas of Health Care 2008* (Lebanon, NH: The Dartmouth Institute for Health Policy and Clinical Practice, Dartmouth Atlas Project, online and print editions).

7. Mullan, Fitzhugh, and Elizabeth Wiley. Beware the Siren Song of New GME: Graduate Medical Education and Health Reform. *Health Affairs* (blog), June 15, 2009. http://healthaffairs.org/blog/. Copyright ©2006 Health Affairs by Project HOPE—The People-to-People Health Foundation, Inc.

8. In Vermont, we found that patients who lived in the regions with the most physicians, particularly medical specialists, had the greatest difficulty in getting an appointment (Chapter 1). In the Fowler study (Chapter 10), patients living in Atlas regions with the greatest numbers of physicians per capita had the greatest difficulty in getting an appointment, even though the Medicare patients living there had the highest rates for visiting their physicians.

9. Mullan, Fitzhugh, and Elizabeth Wiley. Beware the Siren Song of New GME: Graduate Medical Education and Health Reform. *Health Affairs* (blog), June 15, 2009. http://healthaffairs.org/blog/. Copyright ©2006 Health Affairs by Project HOPE—The People-to-People Health Foundation, Inc.

10. Goodman, David C., Elliott S. Fisher, Thomas A. Bubolz, Jack E. Mohr, James F. Poage, and John E. Wennberg. 1996. Benchmarking the US Physician Workforce. An Alternative to Needs-Based or Demand-Based Planning. *Journal of the American Medical Association* 276(22): 1811–1817; Goodman, David C. 2004. Trends: Twenty-year Trends in Regional Variations in the US Physician Workforce. *Health Affairs (Millwood)* Supplement, Web Exclusives): VAR90-7; Goodman, David C. 2005. The Physician Workforce Crisis: Where is the Evidence? *Health Affairs (Millwood)* Web Exclusive: W5-108-W5-110; and Goodman, David C., Thérèse A. Stukel, Chiang-hua Chang, and John E. Wennberg. 2006. End-of-life Care at Academic Medical Centers: Implications for Future Workforce Requirements. *Health Affairs (Millwood)* 25: 521–531. See also Weiner, Jonathan P. January/February 2002. A Shortage of Physicians or a Surplus of Assumptions? *Health Affairs* 21: 160–162; and Weiner, Jonathan P. 2004. Prepaid Group Practice Staffing and U.S. Physician Supply: Lessons for Workforce Policy. *Health Affairs* (published online February 4, 2004). Available at http://content.healthaffairs.org/cgi/content/abstract/hlthaff.w4.43.

11. Wennberg, John, and Alan Gittelsohn. 1973. Small Area Variations in Health Care Delivery: A Population-Based Health Information System Can Guide Planning and Regulatory Decision-Making. *Science* 182: 1102–1108.

12. The 2008 edition of the Dartmouth Atlas compares the patient experience in several Los Angeles medical communities, providing maps and information

on variation among local hospitals, all within close proximity. The interested reader can access this report on the Dartmouth Atlas website.

EPILOGUE

1. For example, by 2018, the target growth rate in Medicare spending is the average 5-year increase in GDP plus 1 percentage point. So if GDP has been growing at 2 percent, the target is 3 percent. If Medicare's growth is faster than that, then the Independent Medicare Advisory Board is charged with saving the lesser of (1) the difference between the target growth rate and the real growth rate or (2) 1.5 percentage points off the projected growth rate. Its authority to contain costs is unique: if Congress fails to vote to accept or reject the Board's proposal, it goes into effect anyway. If Congress votes against the recommendation and the president vetoes it, it will still go into effect unless Congress finds the two-thirds votes needed to overcome the veto. The Board's recommendations are turned down only if Congress votes against them and the president agrees.
2. Moody's Investor Service recently announced that health care reform legislation might lead the service to downgrade the bond ratings of the most costly hospitals. With limited access to the bond market, these providers will find it difficult to expand capacity.

APPENDIX ON METHODS

1. For a description of the coefficient of determination, see http://en.wikipedia.org/wiki/Coefficient_of_determination.
2. Wennberg, John E., Elliott S. Fisher, Thérèse A. Stukel, Jonathan S. Skinner, Sandra M. Sharp, and Kristen K Bronner. 2004. Use of Hospitals, Physician Visits, and Hospice Care during Last Six Months of Life among Cohorts Loyal to Highly Respected Hospitals in the United States. *British Medical Journal* 328: 607–610.
3. Wennberg, John E., Elliott S. Fisher, Laurence Baker, Sandra M. Sharp, and Kristen K. Bronner. 2005. Evaluating the Efficiency of California Providers in Caring for Patients with Chronic Illness. *Health Affairs* (Web exclusive, published online November 16, 2005).
4. See Iezzoni, Lisa I., Timothy Heeren, Susan M. Foley, Jennifer Daley, John Hughes, and Gerald A. Coffman. 1994. Chronic Conditions and Risk of In-Hospital Death. *Health Services Research* 29: 435–460. Over the five-year period, 6,762,021 deaths occurred among Medicare enrollees who were enrolled in Medicare Parts A and B (and not enrolled in managed care organizations). The vast majority (92.4%) had serious chronic illnesses, defined as the presence

of one or more of nine conditions specified by Iezzoni et al. Almost 90% of these were hospitalized at least once (87.7%). Our study population for the hospital-specific analyses was comprised of 4,732,448 enrollees who had one or more nonsurgical admissions for chronic illness during the five-year period.

5. Wennberg, John E., Elliott S. Fisher, Thérèse A. Stukel, and Sandra M. Sharp. 2004. Use of Medicare Claims Data to Monitor Provider-Specific Performance among Patients with Severe Chronic Illness. *Health Affairs* Supplement (Web exclusive): VAR5-18.

6. http://new.cms.hhs.gov/HospitalQualityInits/25_HospitalCompare.asp.

7. The five performance measures for acute myocardial infarction are the percentage of eligible patients receiving (1) aspirin at time of admission, (2) aspirin at time of discharge, (3) ACE inhibitor for left ventricular dysfunction, (4) beta blocker at admission, and (5) beta blocker at discharge. The two congestive heart failure measures are percentage of patients with (1) assessment of left ventricular function and (2) ACE inhibitor for left ventricular dysfunction. For pneumonia, the three measures are percentage of patients with (1) oxygenation assessment, (2) pneumococcal vaccination, and (3) timing of initial antibiotic therapy. The summary scores are equally weighted averages for the items in each category. Hospital-specific summary scores are given only for those hospitals for which four of the five acute myocardial infarction measures and all of the congestive heart failure and pneumonia measures were based on twenty-five or more patients. See Jha, Ashish K., Zhonghe Li, E. John Orav, and Arnold M. Epstein. July 21, 2005. Care in U.S. Hospitals—the Hospital Quality Alliance program. *New England Journal of Medicine* 353(3): 265–274. (Regional scores in this study are based on the average for each measure, obtained by summing numerator and denominator information across all reporting hospitals.)

8. Where hospital spending is reported by sectors (e.g., Part B spending by place of service), a "partitioning approach" has been used: each hospital's (fully modeled) total Part B payments were partitioned into components based on the proportional distribution of its *crude* component spending rates. Similarly, MedPAR payments for inpatient, long-term and SNF stays and hospice, home health, and DME payments were partitioned from the hospital's (fully modeled) total reimbursement rate based on the sum of payments from all these 100%-type files.

Index

Note: Page numbers followed by "*f*" and "*t*" denote figures and tables, respectively.